The

Savvy Woman's Guide

to

PCOS

The Many Faces of a 21st Century Epidemic...
And What You Can Do About It

by Elizabeth Lee Vliet, M.D.

The Savvy Woman's Guide to PCOS
by Elizabeth Lee Vliet, M.D.
Copyright © 2006 Elizabeth Lee Vliet, M.D.

Published by:
HER Place Press
PO Box 64507
Tucson AZ 85728-4507
www.herplace.com

Disclaimer:
The ideas and suggestions in this book are based on the clinical experience and medical training of the author and scientific articles available. All of the patient vignettes described in the book are actual patients from the author's medical practice and have not been created just for this book. Names and some identifying details have been changed to preserve patient confidentiality but this did not alter basic clinical information, lab results, patient comments, or treatment presented. Patient quotes are used with permission as given to the author.

Every attempt has been made to present current and accurate information as of the time of publication. Peer-reviewed references from the medical literature are included in the Appendix. Suggestions in this book are not meant to be a substitute for careful medical evaluation and treatment by a qualified, licensed health professional. Each woman's health needs, risks, and goals are different and should be developed with medical supervision for personalized advice, answers to specific medical questions, and individual recommendations. The author and publisher specifically do not recommend starting any new treatment, changing any medication you may be taking, or using over-the-counter hormone or other preparations without consulting your personal physician.

This book is intended for educational purposes only, and the use of the information is entirely at the reader's discretion. The author and publisher cannot be responsible for any adverse reactions arising directly or indirectly from the suggestions in this material, and specifically disclaim any liability from the use of this book.

Cover Design: Kitty Werner, RSBPress and New West Agency
Book Design: Kitty Werner, RSBPress
Production and Prepress: Kitty Werner, RSBPress

Printed by Central Plains Book Manufacturing, Winfield KS
        Printed on New Life Opaque 100% recycled paper

ISBN 1-933213-01-9
Printed and bound in the United States of America
0 9 8 7 6 5 4 3 2 1

From Readers, From Patients

Dear Dr. Vliet,

Thank you for the gift and privilege of reading your new book *The Savvy Woman's Guide to PCOS*. Your new book offers much needed hope to many as it is written in such a clear, concise manner that delves into the multi-faceted mystery of PCOS. Each chapter takes the reader through a step-by-step process of looking at PCOS from its earliest onset, implications, and possible causes. In particular, Chapter 5 provides the most comprehensive list and explanations of possible PCOS causes that I have ever come across in one book.

Thank you for your dedication to providing the public with quality medical information about PCOS. I will be honored to recommend this book to any woman who is searching for direction on how to best address PCOS.

Sincerely,
Tracy S

"...we read your book and found it to be very informative on PCOS. It is well written and systematically educates lay people on the symptoms and treatment."

—John M, father of a PCOS patient

I made an appointment with an internist who discovered my blood pressure had sky-rocketed from normal to 160/120. At this time I was referred to an endocrinologist to rule out Cushing's Syndrome. I thought for sure the endocrinologist would comment on the unusually high cholesterol and triglycerides in addition to the LH/FSH ratio from my previous blood tests, but he did not.

I was still not seriously being considered for PCOS. I can't believe doctors do not take the big picture into consideration. Each symptom was being treated individually.

—Laura H, PCOS patient

The Savvy Woman's Mantra

"Nothing is obvious
to the uninformed."
—Salada tea bag tag

Dedication

To my patients…and readers…whose stories and struggles inspire me to be inquisitive, keep an open mind, and learn more…

To the women who have been told, "just eat less and exercise more," for your courage in persisting to find answers

To Gordon, Kitty, Tom, Kathy, Polly, Claudia, and Berit —who made it possible for me to meet the challenges and deadlines of writing *another* book while still seeing patients.

To God who guides it all.

Author's Note

Polycystic Ovarian Syndrome is seriously under-recognized and under-diagnosed. You may have it and not know it.

Polycystic Ovarian Syndrome is the most common endocrine cause of infertility and serious weight gain in young women. It affects millions—experts estimate 6–10% of reproductive-age women struggle with this devastating metabolic imbalance. That translates to perhaps a staggering 5 to 7 million women in the United States alone.

Look around schools and malls in this country and you see the impact of this burgeoning epidemic: obese young women are everywhere. Not all obese girls have budding PCOS. Nor are all PCOS patients overweight. But about 50–65% of PCOS patients *are* obese. PCOS is a frequently overlooked *cause* of significant obesity. Childhood and adolescent obesity are clues that something is wrong.

Many overweight teenaged girls, for whom strict diet and exercise are not working, have a form of PCOS, and don't even know it. Why is this? One reason is that many doctors think of PCOS as mainly a problem affecting fertility. If a woman is not trying to get pregnant, doctors don't often think to do an evaluation for PCOS as a cause of "just" weight gain. Besides, weight gain in teenagers is often viewed by doctors as more of an appearance issue than a serious medical problem.

Doctors haven't taken PCOS as seriously as it deserves; they often minimize symptoms such as excess body hair, weight gain, acne or thinning scalp hair, thinking they are just "cosmetic" problems of over-anxious young women. Gynecologists focus on helping women get pregnant rather than treating acne or weight gain. Endocrinologists typically consider ovarian problems as the "turf" of gynecologists. Mood swings in PCOS can be severe, but psychiatrists typically don't check hormones, so they don't identify PCOS either. Who's looking at the problem? What's a woman to do?

That's why I felt this book was needed. I want to go beyond the fertility problems in PCOS and help those of you—whatever your age—who are struggling with weight gain, excess body hair, irregular periods, or severe acne, but are not necessarily trying to get pregnant.

I hear from women every day who see these types of changes happening and want to know what is wrong. That's why I wrote this book. You need to know what PCOS is, how to get properly tested, and what treatment options are available today.

PCOS is not something to ignore. Aside from the effects on your appearance that can rob you of your confidence and self-esteem, its other health risks are enormous—from increased risk of teenaged diabetes to young mothers with heart attacks or strokes, to early onset of uterine cancer.

Early treatment is key to preventing serious health risks. But if you are among the sufferers who don't even know they have PCOS, then it's hard to take proactive steps to prevent damage.

It's not enough for doctors to tell you to just "eat less and exercise more." You need a practical guide to help you understand the disorder, what tests to ask for, what the tests mean, what treatments are available, and how to take a step-wise approach to healthy hormone balance, sound meal plans, exercise and stress management. I want to share with you my clinical experience and insights, as well as the latest research findings from international PCOS specialists and researchers.

It isn't about a "quick fix." I will teach you about learning to manage PCOS with an integrated approach using a variety of strategies so you can be as healthy as possible. I will talk briefly about approaches to helping fertility, but this book isn't about getting pregnant as much as it is about helping you become—and stay—healthier for life.

I hope you find that my book provides a practical, user-friendly guide for your journey to find answers and help. I want you to be successful in getting help for this devastating disorder before it ruins your life and your health.

Elizabeth Lee Vliet, M.D.

Edinburgh, Scotland

May 10, 2005

Acknowledgments

My deepest thanks and appreciation to all who have made this book possible—especially the dedicated researchers and clinicians world-wide who have led the way in providing the science to show how serious a problem PCOS is.

Kudos to Kitty Werner, designer and typesetter par excellence, whose boundless enthusiasm for this book and always positive, "can-do" at-titude helped to get this project off the ground. I am grateful for her wisdom, expertise, and guidance! She's a *real* savvy woman!

Thanks also to Tom Wadkins, business and financial overseer, com-puter whiz, and operations manager who has made my job easier. Thanks for always willingly being available to solve my technical challenges and glitches to keep the projects moving ahead.

Much appreciation again to Kathy Kresnik, who helped with the research, writing, reading and re-reading tasks to bring this book into being.

Special thanks to Berit Jones, Claudia Sawyer, and Polly Leigh. Your positive attitude, dedication, and commitment to support my work, and to be a caring presence for our patients, have been invaluable. Thank you for your support and encouragement while I take the time and energy to focus on researching and writing.

My deepest gratitude to my husband, Gordon Vliet, the "the wind beneath my wings," who once again has gone through all the pres-sures and joys of working with me on another book, as well as helping to run the office and care for our patients. You are, and have always been, the best support and encouragement I could have.

I am grateful for the trust placed in me by my patients, many of whom have had long struggles trying to find answers and help for puzzling PCOS-related problems. You have honored me by sharing your experi-ences and had the confidence to allow me to guide you on the journey to better health. Your observations have taught me much that goes beyond the textbooks of medicine. This book becomes part of your legacy too, as I pass on your experiences so that they can help other women know the truth of their own body experiences.

I also appreciate those of you who are not patients, but have read my books, found them helpful and enabled you to use the information to work with your own physicians. Thank you for letting me know that my books have made a difference and served to extend my reach beyond the four walls of my patient office.

Thanks to Becky Simpson of New West Agency, who was invaluable with her design input for the cover. And thanks to Lynne O'Hara and her team at Chelsea Green Publishing, and Melody Morris and the team at Central Plains Manufacturing, for all their work in production, printing, distribution and sales to help get this important message out to more women. My appreciation to my business advisors, David Cohen, C.P.A., and Tony Rickert—who guide me through the complexities of accounting and legal aspects of running the medical practices.

Thanks to the friends, colleagues, and patients who reviewed the early stages of the manuscript and gave me important guidance to make this book even better. All of my reader-editor "team" know firsthand the trial and tribulations of the "hormonal challenges" woman face, and how important this information is to women of all ages.

I thank the many health professionals—physicians, nurse practitioners, registered nurses, psychologists, physical therapists and others—have read my books, thought they made sense and were scientifically "sound" to the point that they have sent patients, or have come themselves, for hormone evaluations. I thank you for the validation that your comments have given me.

Together, we all make a difference. Together we continue to make positive changes toward a healthcare model for the future that will incorporate our unique hormone makeup as women into all our health assessments and treatment planning.

Elizabeth Lee Vliet, M.D.

Contents

Introduction

"I had always been a happy, carefree person and nothing seemed to faze me. Now it feels like an alien has taken over my body and I don't recognize myself anymore."

—16-year-old patient

"The only people who understand how profoundly devastating PCOS has been to me are my parents. I have suffered profoundly over the past 13 years, and this suffering defies description. In the past five months alone, I have had to quit my summer legal clerkship, withdraw from law school because of the exhaustion and problems concentrating. I feel like the acne, my appetite and weight are out of control. At times, I feel so depressed I just want to die. I must find a way to live a more normal life."

—25-year-old patient

"I experienced puberty much earlier than my friends, then I started getting horrible acne. I started getting fat when I was in middle school, and just keep gaining every year, no matter what I do. I also remember I was in middle school when I started getting a lot of hair on my face, chin, and stomach. I was so embarrassed I hardly wanted to go out of the house. It's been a long struggle and I feel miserable most of the time. No one seems to be able to tell me what's really wrong with me."

—31-year-old patient

"I'm tired of not feeling well and being on so many medicines from so many different doctors. And no one has addressed the connections with my menstrual cycles. No one will check my hormone levels. I feel these hormone imbalances are a major ignored part of what's wrong with me."

—38-year-old patient

"I have been on a lifelong quest to solve the mystery of why I can't eat a normal amount of food without menstrual irregularities, blood sugar problems, facial hair, and severe weight gain. I have been to many doctors and spent many thousands of dollars…the doctors suspect me of lying or just pass me off to the next referral, without regard for the physical and emotional damage they are causing me."

—*47-year-old patient*

Polycystic Ovarian Syndrome

PCOS for short, lurks as the culprit for all these women. It is a disease that is still relatively unknown and frequently unrecognized

All these women share common problems: the body getting fatter and fatter and acne bursting out on the face, neck, back and chest… hair seeming to come out of nowhere, dark and coarse and thick, on arms, legs, inner thighs, abdomen, face, and even around the breasts. Menstrual periods come, and then disappear for months. "What is this?" they ask. "What's happening to my body?"

Mothers gnash their teeth and stay awake at night, worrying about what is happening to their daughters. They seek medical help, and doctors just say, "It couldn't be hormonal. Your daughter just needs to eat less and exercise more." What's really going on here?

You ask, "What is PCOS? Why doesn't my doctor recognize it? Why haven't I heard more about it?"

PCOS is an endocrine-metabolic disorder that results in over-production of male hormones in women, called **androgens**, which lead to many of the unwanted body changes. The havoc PCOS causes is made worse by over-production of another hormone, **insulin,** that regulates sugar and fat metabolism in our bodies.

PCOS is the most common endocrine disorder affecting reproductive-age women. It is also the most common hormonal imbalance causing infertility and serious weight gain in young women. It affects millions—experts estimate about 6–10% of reproductive age women struggle with this devastating metabolic imbalance.

Look around schools and malls in this country and you see young women with the body build that suggests the beginnings of PCOS. It is on the rise today, for a variety of reasons we will explore further later on.

Here are some mind-boggling statistics to help you see the enormity of this problem:

- 90 to 120 million women worldwide suffer from some type of androgen excess disorder.
- In the United States alone, experts estimate that between 5 and 8 million women have an androgen excess disorder.
- 80–90% of women with androgen excess have a form of PCOS
- PCOS causes loss of ovulation (and infertility) in more than 50% of patients
- Excess body hair (hirsutism) in a male pattern (face, arms, chest, back, abdomen, thighs) occurs in about 80 to 90% of women with PCOS. Hirsutism is one of the most common signs of excess androgens in women.

Even though statistics show that millions of women are affected with this hormonal disorder, traditional medical approaches rarely include checking hormone levels. Basic hormone testing could quickly reveal developing PCOS and related problems.

If PCOS is left undiagnosed, it insidiously robs women of energy, vitality, fertility and often, self esteem. The heartbreak of infertility for young women can be profound, particularly if no one checks for PCOS.

As women get older, PCOS, and the metabolic Syndrome X that typically goes with it, are deadly diseases. They cause heart attacks and premature death in women in their 30s and 40s, 20 years earlier than we see in women without PCOS. They increase risk of serious depression. They increase risk of uterine cancer. They increase risk of early stroke.

As you see from the patient comments at the beginning, women suffer enormously when doctors fail to recognize its symptoms and offer appropriate treatments.

I am shocked at the number of calls from mothers of girls as young as 9 and 10, asking for a hormone evaluation because of their daughter's ominous body changes even before menses have started.

I am convinced the rise in PCOS, diabetes and obesity represent an overlooked part of the spectrum of the damage to our endocrine system from environmental pollutants, high sugar diet, and chemical additives in foods that affect us from the womb onward.

There are other causes as well. PCOS also can be inherited. Important genetic connections have been identified in recent years, and research is ongoing to identify the genes responsible for this serious problem.

Early *detection* is a prelude to getting the right treatment, and getting treated early, before more serious problems hit you. Blood tests are widely available and reliable. Pelvic ultrasounds can help identify cysts on the ovaries, or abnormal thickening of the lining of the uterus.

Early *treatment* is key to preventing serious health risks, but most sufferers don't even know they have PCOS.

It's time for that bleak picture to change. It's time for you to become more savvy about your health, and about the hidden saboteurs that make you feel sick, depleted, and depressed, and sagging in energy and vitality.

Some years ago, I wrote the following Self Test to use in my medical practice to help us identify new patients who were at risk for PCOS but may not have known it. It has turned out to be a valuable tool, for me, to assist our new patients in getting the right tests done. There are no "right answers" or agreed-upon set scoring "cut offs" for this test. I have provided the scoring ranges I find useful, based on my clinical experience with patients and what the medical studies have shown to be important components of the PCOS picture.

If you suspect you have PCOS, take the self-test. Use this Self Test to identify pieces of your health puzzle.

DR. VLIET'S SELF TEST:
AM I AT RISK FOR PCOS?

YES NO   1. I gain weight easily, even if I am careful about my diet.

YES NO   2. I have gained more than 25 pounds since high school.

YES NO   3. I have difficulty losing weight with diet and exercise.

YES NO   4. I crave sweets and carbohydrate foods.

YES NO   5. My waistline is greater than 35 inches.

YES NO   6. I have now, or in the past, problems with severe acne.

YES NO   7. My acne is worse a week or so before I have a period.

YES NO   8. I have noticed changes in my skin color or dark patches on my neck or groin or under arm areas.

YES NO   9. I have excess facial hair.

YES NO 10. I have balding or thinning hair in the front of my scalp.

YES NO 11. I have hair around the nipples on my breasts.

YES NO 12. I have excess hair on my upper or inner thighs.

YES NO 13. I have pubic hair that grows in a line up my stomach to my navel.

YES NO 14. My menstrual cycles are frequently longer than 35 days between periods.

YES NO 15. I have fewer than 6 menstrual periods a year.

YES NO 16. I have erratic, unpredictable menstrual bleeding.

YES NO 17. My menstrual bleeding sometimes lasts longer than a week.

YES NO 18. I have had problems getting pregnant.

YES NO 19. I have needed fertility treatment to get pregnant.

YES NO 20. I have high blood pressure.

YES NO 21. I have diabetes, or a history of gestational diabetes.

YES NO 22. I feel extremely hungry, irritable, moody, sleepy, fatigued, or "fuzzy-brained" within two-three hours of eating sweets or simple carbohydrates.

YES NO 23. I have a family history of obesity and/or diabetes.

YES NO 24. I have a family history of heart disease or stroke.

YES NO 25. I have a family history of uterine cancer.

SCORING GUIDELINES:

I. Score TWO points for each YES answer to the following questions: 5, 8, 15, 19, 21.

Add up this total:_____

II. Score ONE point for each YES answer to the remaining questions.

Add up this total:_____

TOTAL score (I + II): _____

If you have two or more YES answers in I and more than 4 YES answers in II, I encourage you to get properly tested for PCOS as outlined in later chapters.

The more YES answers you have, the more likely it is that you have PCOS. The earlier you start an integrated treatment plan, the better you can feel now, and the better your chances of reducing your risks of serious diseases later on.

©Elizabeth Lee Vliet, MD 2001-2005

Once you know your risk score, you'll know whether this book is for you to help you learn more about PCOS. Read about your options to get tested, or options for treatment to help you feel better and decrease long-term health risks. Then, use the self-test as a guide for you to discuss these issues with your own physician.

You can't afford to ignore the early warnings of PCOS.

Be a savvy woman, and take charge of your health!

Chapter 1
PCOS
The Overlooked Epidemic

One Woman's Saga

Laura was 29 years old, and had been experiencing severe unexplained weight gain, fatigue, excess body hair, and cystic acne. She had done a great deal of her own reading and suspected she had PCOS. After a long frustrating journey trying to get help, she came across one of my books and scheduled a consult with me. She had kept a diary of her experiences, and shared this with me to include in this book. These are her emails to friends and family in her words:

She said, "I hope by sharing my story, I can help other women keep from having to go through what happened to me."

"This is my story from the start when I first told my doctor that I was inexplicably gaining weight in addition to headaches and fatigue… If I won't take the doctor's crazy pills, then the doctors will make me crazy :)

My OB/GYN: Although your LH/FSH ratio is indicative of PCOS your insulin is fine. I don't think you have PCOS.

Me: The insulin test may not be accurate. Because no one explained to me the purpose of the post prandial insulin/glucose test, I had only eaten an egg between blood draws. The only way to control my weight recently is to eliminate carbs.

*OB/GYN: (in an agitated, accusing voice) So what is it you want, **DRUGS** to lose weight? I won't give you drugs if your insulin is fine, it isn't good for you.*

Me: I don't want drugs, I just want to know what is

wrong with me and I think that the tests may not have been done properly since I didn't eat a normal meal. I think the 5-hour IGTT (insulin response to glucose tolerance test) would give a better result.

OB/GYN: (hurried) The post prandial test was fine, concentrate on diet and exercise if you want to lose weight. If you are still concerned you should speak with an internist. I have to go to surgery. Bye.

Well, soon after that appointment I had gone off the pill for an unrelated reason. Shortly thereafter I made an appointment with an internist who discovered my blood pressure had sky-rocketed from normal to 160/120. She began sending me for every test under the sun to find out why (rightfully so), but refused to do the IGTT because she did not believe my suspicion about PCOS. To further prove that going off the pill was also contributing to my blood pressure, I even collected my blood pressure data from all my doctors of the past five years and graphed it in order to illustrate the sudden change. The internist felt this may be something to explore later after performing the more involved tests including an MRA of the renal artery and a chest X-ray. I still don't see why my doctors were so reluctant to do a IGTT. I have insurance and it has got to be a much cheaper test than an MRA/X-ray. It wasn't like I was asking for drugs or invasive medical treatment.

At this time I was also referred to an endocrinologist to rule out Cushing's Syndrome (even though my cortisol had tested fine) and to a nephrologist with a specialty in hypertension. I thought for sure the endocrinologist would comment on the unusually high cholesterol and triglycerides in addition to the LH/FSH ratio from my previous blood tests, but he did not.

I was still not seriously being considered for PCOS. I also can't believe the doctors did not take the big picture into consideration: acute onset of hyperlipidemia, hypertension, weight gain, acne, fatigue, and headaches. Each symptom was being treated individually. At that time both my OB/GYN and internist were also recommending medication and dietary changes to lower my cholesterol.

Following that appointment I accidentally came across Dr. Vliet's book It's my Ovaries, Stupid. *After reading the book I was more certain than ever PCOS was the culprit. Since my blood pressure chart did not convince my internist, I decided to make an appointment to plead my case again to my OB/GYN. It went something like this…*

Me: I'm not looking for drugs, I just want my hormone levels tested because my research leads me to believe the pill I was on may not have had sufficient estradiol. This could have contributed to the headaches and fatigue. Also, my research indicates my blood pressure could have spiked due to the loss of estradiol when I went off the pill.

OB/GYN: The pill you were on was fine. I have prescribed it for thousands of women. You just need to lose weight and your blood pressure will come down. As for the brain fog, headaches and fatigue, stop eating carbs. Besides hormone tests are not representative due to normal fluctuations.

Me: (frustration and desperation present in my voice) I really limit carbs so I do not think that is the problem. And weight does not cause a significant blood pressure increase virtually overnight.

She did acknowledge at this point that I would benefit from oral contraceptives based on my recent acne out-break. Oddly enough, she also admitted that hormone levels could contribute to my headaches and fatigue, and possibly blood pressure, but she made it perfectly clear that because my blood pressure was so high, there was no way in hell she was going to prescribe them. Talk about a catch 22…

OB/GYN: You sound upset. How about I give you an anti-depressant?

Me: No thanks. I am upset because, between my fatigue and headaches, I can barely make it through a day of work and spend my weekends on the couch, I am very upset because I am gaining weight at an unbeliev-able rate, and I'm upset because no one will listen to me So anyway how often do hormone levels fluctuate throughout the day?

OB/GYN: (literally yelling as she walks out the door) I really think the anti-depressants will help you, but FINE!!! WHAT WILL MAKE YOU HAPPY? THE BLOOD TEST? THEN, FINE! YOU CAN HAVE THE BLOOD TEST BUT IT WON'T TELL YOU ANYTHING ANYWAY!

Well the hormone tests did show very low levels of estradiol but she did not feel the result was abnormal since it was "in range." Of course the range was very large and I was at the lower limit. My next step was to go see a reproductive endocrinologist. A short time later I had another appointment with my OB/GYN for what I thought was my bi-annual physical. It went something like this...

OB/GYN: So how are things?

Me: I recently saw a reproductive endocrinologist who gave me the 5-hour IGTT, which of course I failed. It was abnormal, as I had thought all along.

OB/GYN: Have you started metformin?

Me: No. The doctor prescribed it, but I didn't want to start since I will no longer be seeing her. She would not acknowledge that PCOS could cause high blood pressure and when I questioned her response based on my research, she told me my research was wrong. Additionally she did not schedule a follow-up appointment with me. I don't feel comfortable being treated by a doctor like this.

OB/GYN: (in an excited voice) How about I prescribe the drugs!?! I'll schedule a follow-up with you. I really think this will help you lose weight and correct your other symptoms.

Me: (in my mind) What!!??!! 6 months ago you would not give me the 5-hour IGTT and you accused me of trying to manipulate you for these very drugs. Now you want to be the hero and prescribe them!!!! Now you believe they will make me better!!!! You are just excited because you get to write a prescription. Writing prescriptions is what doctors like you do best, certainly not listening and problem solving.

Me: (what I really said) Actually I have an appointment with a specialist next week.

OB/GYN: *Who?*

Me: *A nationally-recognized doctor in Arizona.*

OB/GYN: *Arizona!?! You don't need to go there, I will give you the metformin. That is all she is going to prescribe anyway.*

Me: *The appointment is a done deal and I think there may be more to it than just the metformin.*

OB/GYN: *OK you did your research. Why are you here then?*

Me: *I thought I was here for my bi-annual physical.*

OB/GYN: *No. Since you are no longer on birth control I only need to see you once a year. This is a follow-up to the last time we talked.*

Me: *(in my mind) What!!??!! Last time we talked you ran out the door screaming at me that nothing was wrong with me after trying to shove anti-depressants down my throat because I was obviously a hysterical female. What in the world is there to follow-up on????*

Me: *I'm sorry, that wasn't explained to me when the appointment was made.*

OB/GYN: *OK. At least we had time to chat. See you in March :)*

Well after going to Arizona and finally getting the appropriate oral contraceptives, I feel much better. So this past Monday I go back to my OB/GYN for the annual physical. I tell her that I am on OCs and I am feeling much better. She then asks if I would talk with my Arizona doctor about taking me off the pill since she still isn't comfortable with the OCs being prescribed to someone with a history of high blood pressure. She didn't pay attention to what I said about my blood pressure now has been under control for quite some time now back on the birth control pill. I re-explain that my blood pressure was not a problem until I had discontinued the birth control pills the first time. Since starting the OCs my blood pressure has been fine, as I have verified every week by a nurse at Health Services. I told her, "No way I'm stopping!!!" She pleads with me one more time to go off the pill, and I again decline. Out of nowhere she then writes a prescription for the OCs Dr.

Important Advice:
I would strongly encourage any woman to take control of her own healthcare. You are your best, and maybe only, advocate. Do your research and continue to look until you find a doctor who will listen.
—*Laura*

Vliet had prescribed for me and gives me a bunch of free samples before leaving the room. Bizarre!!! :)

So you wonder why I still go to this OB/GYN? Well, in my journey I have found worse doctors than her. Besides, before I challenged her with my "mystery illness," I thought she was pretty good. In addition there is no good way to properly screen new doctors so it could take me a lot of time to find one better.

I'm also still convinced some doctors do not feel doctor-like unless they write a prescription for something. So in the game of Doctor, if you fail to get a diagnosis for which they can give an appropriate drug, they write a script for anti-depressants (also known as parting gifts—thanks for playing the game).

Think I'm kidding? This is what they gave my aunt because they refused to look past her loss of appetite as anything other than depression considering her husband had passed away 5 years ago. Stage IV kidney cancer wasn't a possibility until they just happened to notice an enlarged lymph node when she pushed them to look further. She died 3 months later. When my golden retriever became lethargic and stopped eating, the vet did a full medical work-up and diagnosed cancer immediately. There was no prescription for doggy Prozac. He was also allowed to die with a lot more compassion and dignity.

I would strongly encourage any woman to take control of her own healthcare. You are your best, and maybe only, advocate. Do your research and continue to look until you find a doctor who will listen.

What really amazed me through all of this is that my opinion was not respected by most of the doctors. As a chemical engineer specializing in pharmaceutical manufacturing, I had considered myself rather intelligent. Yet because I did not have a degree in medicine, most of my doctors treated me as if I was incapable of contributing to my own healthcare.

Please do not let doctors intimidate you or convince you that your beliefs about your body are illogical or without merit.

Laura H.

Polycystic Ovary Syndrome (PCOS): Hormonal Havoc Wrecking Your Health

Polycystic ovary syndrome (PCOS) has finally come out of the dark and has begun to get attention in women's magazines and physician offices, even though it was first described in 1935. PCOS was initially called Stein-Leventhal Syndrome, named for the doctors who first described the characteristic body changes and tiny cysts covering the ovaries.

Finally
Now, it is known that it isn't just the ovaries that are affected.

At that time, doctors thought it was a disorder that just affected the ovaries, causing excess body hair, irregular menses, infrequent ovulation, and follicles that become multiple tiny cysts instead of developing properly to become an egg.

We now know the name "polycystic ovarian syndrome," is seriously misleading. It is a multi-system, complex endocrine disorder. It has many faces. It presents in a variety of different ways. It is a dynamic, changing disorder, not static. Even in the same person, features don't stay the same over time.

Attention!
The hormonal imbalance of PCOS leads to a metabolic syndrome with widespread effects that can wreak havoc throughout the brain and body.

Ominously, it is on the rise in young women today. In fact, PCOS is the most common endocrine disorder of women in their childbearing years, affecting between 6–10% of women, with symptoms often beginning in pre-pubescent girls or young teenagers. And that statistic doesn't include girls who have budding PCOS no one has yet recognized.

In the past, it was "an infertility problem," meaning it is only a concern if a woman is trying to get pregnant. That label is also woefully inadequate: PCOS is far more dangerous, and potentially deadly.

PCOS: Alarming Statistics

PCOS dramatically increases your risk of many serious health problems, beginning in your early teens. Consider these alarming trends:

Vicious Cycle

The fatter you get, the more insulin resistant you become, and the more abnormal your hormone ratios become. This makes you gain even more middle body fat, which pushes you into more severe insulin resistance. It becomes a terrible vicious cycle, spiraling out of control unless you get the right combination of treatment.

> By age 30, 50% of women with PCOS have either impaired glucose tolerance, significant insulin resistance, or full-blown diabetes.

> Women with PCOS have an *eleven*-fold increased risk of cardiovascular disease that can appear as early as the 20s and 30s.

> Women from 39 to 49 years old with PCOS have a heart attack risk that is *four times* that of women without PCOS in this age group, based on newer studies.

> Women with PCOS also have a higher risk of uterine cancer that occurs at younger ages than seen in women without PCOS.

> Studies on breast cancer in PCOS are conflicting: some studies show a higher risk of breast cancer at a younger age in women with PCOS, while other studies show no increased risk.

Hormone Imbalances in PCOS

Today, we know these diverse complications of PCOS are caused primarily by several critical hormone imbalances:

> elevated levels of androgens (testosterone, DHEA, DHEA-s, DHT, and androstenedione)

> higher-than-normal free testosterone

> high estrone-to-estradiol ratio

> elevated insulin levels, insulin resistance

> elevated cortisol

> elevated prolactin, in about half the patients with PCOS

The combination of elevated androgens and excess insulin, especially if free cortisol is also too high, causes rapid waistline and upper body fat deposits. It also causes what often feels like uncontrollable overall weight gain. This abdominal male fat pattern, unlike the typical female pattern of fat around the hips and thighs, is what contributes to such a marked increase in heart disease risk and diabetes.

How Do I Recognize the Symptoms of PCOS?

The most obvious ones are changes in your body. Rapid weight gain is one of the most noticeable ones, but not all patients with PCOS are overweight, some are quite thin. Acne, excess face and body hair, and thinning scalp hair are also tell-tale symptoms. Many women with PCOS experience irregular periods, have difficulty getting pregnant, or frequent miscarriages. Less noticeable changes include energy, sleep, mood stability, sex drive and mental clarity. I will describe these problems in more detail in upcoming chapters.

Warning: Undetected PCOS leads to far greater risks for the future.

Why Is PCOS Often Missed?

Why is PCOS so often missed? Why are women told these problems are "all in your head" or just due to depression? If diagnostic tests are widely available, why isn't it diagnosed more often, and earlier, than it is?

Why do so many young women go years and spend thousands of dollars trying to get the answer to what is causing the dramatic body changes I have described?

I think there are a variety of reasons that contribute to PCOS being under-recognized or not diagnosed:

Tip: Too many doctors treating different aspects of your health care don't always connect the symptoms.

- ❧ factors related to the organization of medical practice, with different specialists treating different parts of the body.
- ❧ the fact that it isn't the usual "standard of care" to check women's hormone levels unless they are trying to get pregnant.
- ❧ problems agreeing on a specific set of diagnostic criteria for PCOS
- ❧ disagreement among specialists about how many of the abnormal findings have to be present to "qualify" for the diagnosis of PCOS
- ❧ the many different presentations of PCOS, and its variability over time
- ❧ lack of awareness that brain symptoms (mood, sleep, memory, etc.) can be *caused by* hormone imbalance

These are some of the major obstacles I think contribute to women with PCOS having such difficulty getting a timely and accurate diagnosis. Let's take a closer look at them.

The Body Divided: The Problem of Multiple Specialists

PCOS produces a spectrum, of symptoms that cross the borders of many medical specialties. To illustrate how confusing this can be for both patients and doctors, let me list some of the areas of dysfunction in PCOS and the medical specialties that would normally treat each area:

Family Practitioners ("GPs") and Internists are usually a woman's first stop, especially for problems that don't easily fit into another specialty—heart palpitations, low energy, insomnia. These doctors don't usually check ovarian hormone levels; they assume the gynecologist will do that. They will offer extensive information about the dangers off being overweight, but unless they understand PCOS, their advice on losing weight will tend to be of the "exercise more / eat less" type. (And if that worked, you wouldn't be in the doctor's office in the first place!)

Gynecologists are traditionally trained as surgeons to handle matters related to the uterus and ovaries. Their focus is pregnancy, birth, and surgery for anatomical problems like fibroids and endometriosis. They

Sympton/Problem:	Physician Specialist:
ovarian function:	gynecologist
pancreas/insulin problems:	endocrinologist
thyroid:	endocrinologist
infertility:	reproductive endocrinologist
acne:	dermatologist
depression/mood swings/anxiety:	psychiatrist or psychologist
weight gain:	few physicians have any training in this area; they will usually refer a patient to a dietician, whose knowledge of PCOS weight problems is usually just as sparse
excess body hair/thinning scalp hair:	dermatologist
heart palpitations:	cardiologist
low sex drive.	psychologist, gynecologist

don't routinely check hormones, and—in my experience—when they do check hormones, they often underestimate what is needed to feel well, under-prescribe appropriate hormone therapy and over prescribe anti-depressants.

Many women don't realize, moreover, that OB/Gyn is a surgical specialty. The emphasis during residency and fellowship training is on performing hysterectomies, Caesarean sections, laparoscopies, and surgery for reproductive cancers. The problems caused by PCOS just don't seem as serious in a busy surgical practice.

Endocrinologists are medical specialists who focus primarily on diabetes and thyroid problems. Like internists and GPs, they stay out of gynecologists' "turf" and don't usually check ovarian hormone levels. Although more endocrinologists these days are looking at the "pre-diabetes" conditions (known as metabolic syndrome or Syndrome X) most of them still don't realize that PCOS goes hand in hand with these metabolic issues.

Psychiatrists in this country are not taught much about the brain effects of ovarian hormones. Rarely do they do blood or hormone tests at all, except in cases when the patient is on a psychiatric medication that needs careful monitoring, such as lithium. Ironically, psychiatrists usually don't know that some of the mood-stabilizer medicines like Depakote and others can actually aggravate hormone imbalances of PCOS. Because so many symptoms of PCOS (depression, anxiety, mental fogginess) are emotional in nature, psychiatrists naturally look for psychiatric explanations, diagnosing things like Bipolar Disorder, Dysthymia, or Depression.

The patients I see have often wasted years on medication trials for different antidepressants and tranquilizers with only partial relief (if any) of their symptoms.

Psychologists cannot order lab tests or do physical exams because they are not medical doctors (MDs) but have Ph.D. or M.S. degrees. Like other therapists (counselors, social workers, and so on), their orienta-

> **Frustrating:** Individual specialists are not likely to look at the whole symptom picture. Not only are few of them trained to recognize (or treat) PCOS, but each doctor's specialty brings with it unique blind spots.

Tip:
If you think you have PCOS, don't take a quick "No, couldn't be" for an answer without proper testing of your hormones.

Dangerous
This "split" of a woman's endocrine system means different doctors address different body parts, which obviously makes it hard for a woman with PCOS to get properly diagnosed.

tion will be toward "talk therapy," stress management, and similar areas.

Dermatologists are often consulted for excess hair, hair loss, or acne. Again, though, they don't often check hormone levels. They will help you to treat the problem., but they probably will have little idea of how to test to find the source of the problem.

What happens when all these specialty groups overlook the underlying metabolic changes in PCOS? Women are simply told to "not worry, everybody misses periods sometimes," or "just go exercise and lose weight and your periods will come back. You'll be fine," or, "just take this antidepressant or mood-stabilizer and you'll feel better."

This was exactly what happened to a 35-year-old patient who then went on to have 3 heart attacks by the time she was 38, occurring with the onset of her menstrual periods. She had almost died during the third one before she had the consult with me and we found the markedly abnormal hormone levels.

She had PCOS that had not been previously recognized, and the high androgens and low estradiol caused constrictions of her coronary arteries triggering the heart attacks that happened with the beginning of her periods. Fortunately, we found a way to keep her hormone levels steady with a constant dose birth control pill, and she did well when that was added to her other medications.

Misguided Views of *Women's Problems*

Tragically, many physicians see PCOS as a "cosmetic" problem when young women complain of excess face or body hair, and weight gain, and don't realize the far-reaching consequences of PCOS.

There appears to be an underlying attitude conveyed to patients that medicine has more serious matters to take care of than whether a woman is gaining weight, has acne, facial hair, or feels too tired.

There also seems to be a underlying belief among physicians that simply being a woman means not feeling well a lot of the time, and that's just the way it is. This underlying attitude has roots in the Biblical story of Eve being punished for giving in to temptation and eating of the forbidden fruit. There isn't much to do about "woman's lot" except "grin and bear it." This is nonsense!

Gynecologists have traditionally been taught that a hallmark characteristic of PCOS is a lack of menstruation, called *amenorrhea*. If a woman is still having periods, she could not have PCOS. We now know this is not correct. Many women with PCOS still have periods.

Sometimes women with PCOS can even have regular menstrual cycles for a while, and may even become pregnant without having to undergo fertility treatment. Most of the time, however, the periods are irregular and don't produce optimal levels or the normal balance of ovarian hormones, or reliable ovulations.

Infertility is a common reason women with undiagnosed PCOS see a physician. Women may go to a reproductive endocrinologist, who typically does check for PCOS as part of a thorough evaluation.

But what if you are *not* trying to become pregnant? Especially if you still have menstrual periods, based on our traditional teaching, it isn't likely that most physicians would be thinking about the possibility of PCOS.

And with women's health care so fragmented among various specialities, PCOS is likely to be overlooked, even though you may have all the *other* metabolic changes of PCOS.

Lack of Recognition That Brain Symptoms Can Be Caused by Hormone Imbalances

There is another misguided belief in medicine that "fatigue" or sleep disturbance, depression, anxiety and other mood changes in women are due to the *psychiatric* disorder of depression, not due to hormone problems.

Myth
Fatigue, low mood and anxiety are always a psychiatric problem in women.
Not so!

Myth
Simply being a woman means not feeling well a lot of the time, and that's just the way it is.
Not so!

Many brain symptoms, such as insomnia, palpitations, anxiety, depression, memory loss and others, can be triggered by hormone levels that are too low OR too high.

Tip:
Excess weight isn't the only symptom of PCOS

Psychiatrists, internists, gynecologists, and family doctors rarely check ovarian hormone levels, saying that they vary too much. But if they don't check hormone levels, they miss the possible hormonal connection with the symptoms!

That's why so many women are given antidepressants without having any hormone treatment first, even though the psychiatric diagnostic manuals all clearly state that endocrine (i.e. hormonal) disorders *must be ruled out before a diagnosis of depression is given.*

Do it!:
Don't give up! If your doctor isn't listening, *find one who does.*

Remember, cholesterol and glucose also vary constantly, but doctors check those measures to help decide if a person needs treatment, and to monitor treatment once it is started. Ovarian hormone levels are measured regularly by fertility specialists; other doctors need to learn how to use these tests too.

How Do I Find Out Whether I Have PCOS?

If you feel that you may have PCOS, read Chapter 8 about the tests I think you need. Then be assertive about asking your doctor to help you get them done. Your health is too important for you to go quietly away, and not have the proper tests done.

Chapter 2

What is PCOS?

The Spectrum of PCOS Presentations

PCOS is a master of disguise. Not all women have all of the classic symptoms. Not all women have all the known laboratory abnormalities. Not all women with PCOS are obese; some are quite thin. Not all women with PCOS will have irregular menstrual periods or difficulty getting pregnant.

This is different from diabetes, for example, where we have national standards for glucose levels that clearly alert doctors to the presence of diabetes. The diagnostic confusion in PCOS is also different from hypertension, hypothyroidism, or high cholesterol, where we also have nationally-accepted guidelines that tell us when the disease is present.

In a number of studies, women with abnormal ovaries on ultrasound overlapped with those who had abnormal hormone levels. Whether cysts are present on ultrasound does not, however, have much predictive value in determining who has the abnormal hormone levels characteristic of PCOS. Some women may have cysts on ultrasound and yet have normal hormone levels. Other women with the characteristic elevated androgens may not have any cysts seen on ultrasound of the ovaries.

Likewise, body size or hair patterns alone don't always predict who will have elevated androgens and insulin resistance. Some women, particularly if from an Asian ethic group, may have severe insulin resistance and rela-

Warning: The variability in how the syndrome presents itself makes it difficult to create a specific set of criteria that every woman has to have for the diagnosis.

tively little excess body hair. Other women, such as those of Mediterranean background, may have excessive body hair and not have significant elevations of insulin.

Important
The key point is to look at the entire picture, and not focus on whether one particular finding is present or not.

Problems agreeing on a specific set of diagnostic criteria

Doctors who specialize in researching and treating PCOS are the first to tell you there is disagreement both about the tests to do, and how many criteria must be met to confirm the diagnosis. In 1990, the National Institutes of Health (NIH) in the United States developed diagnostic criteria for PCOS in hopes of creating a more uniform way of identifying patients.

The NIH criteria in 1990 required the presence of both (1) chronic anovulation, and (2) clinical and/or biochemical hyperandrogenism. It did not specify the presence of polycystic ovaries.

Interesting
The NIH criteria were not universally accepted.

Doctors in different countries focused on different aspects in deciding whether a woman had PCOS or not. Some centers required cystic ovaries to be seen on ultrasound, other centers focused on the presence of elevated androgens and infertility. This made it hard for doctors and researchers to compare studies from different centers and areas of the world.

2003 Rotterdam Consensus Conference Diagnostic Criteria

In 2003, the Rotterdam Conference, composed of leading PCOS specialists from around the world, recommended modifying the diagnostic criteria so that *any two of the following three features were required for a diagnosis of PCOS:*

1) Reduced frequency of ovulatory cycles (oligo-ovulation), OR lack of ovulation (anovulation),

2) clinical and/or biochemical hyperandrogenism, and

3) polycystic ovaries.

Confusion persists, however. An Australian survey published in 2005 showed major differences between gynecologists and endocrinologist in diagnosing PCOS: 70% of endocrinologists felt that the diagnosis of PCOS required menstrual irregularity with evidence of elevated androgens on body changes or laboratory measures. Less than half of the gynecologists thought that menstrual irregularity was essential for the diagnosis of PCOS.

No wonder! Perhaps this helps you understand why it may be hard for patients to get properly diagnosed!

Gynecologists, on the other hand, were more likely than endocrinologists to require presence of polycystic ovaries for the diagnosis, by 61% to 14%. In this study, only 9% of gynecologists and only 38% of endocrinologists were in line with the 1990 NIH criteria, and only 16% of gynecologists and only 41% of endocrinologists used the more current Rotterdam criteria. The situation in the United States doesn't appear to be much better, based on our national statistics, what my patients tell me about difficulties getting diagnosed, and what you read of Laura's experiences at the beginning of this chapter.

A 2004 study by Dr. Souter and colleagues illustrates another reason it can be hard to pin down a rigid set of diagnostic criteria for PCOS. Dr. Souter's group studied 228 women and found that 65% of the women who had menstrual irregularities had an androgen excess disorder, but 22% of the women with normal menses and no hirsutism *also had an underlying androgen excess disorder*. This study was surprising in showing a fairly high percentage of women with normal menses who were discovered to have excess androgens.

Caution If we limit the diagnosis of PCOS to just those women with irregular menstrual cycles and excess body hair, we could miss almost one-quarter of women who may have it and not have those particular features!

But even if doctors can't agree on "diagnostic criteria," for the full-blown disorder, some of the abnormal findings can still wreak havoc on your hormone balance and health. **Even mild forms of PCOS can cause a lot of damage.** Treatments that improve symptoms and help you feel better are similar, regardless of whether you have many or only a few of the features of PCOS. Early treatment is your best chance to cut your risks of future diabetes and heart disease.

Medicine has also become overly focused on "evidence-based medicine," which emphasizes results from randomized clinical trials (RCT) to guide clinical decision-making and treatment.

The sad part of this focus on "evidence-based medicine" today is that the "evidence" from the individual patient often gets overlooked or discounted as not the same degree of importance as randomized clinical trials, as you saw with Laura's description of her experiences.

What Are Some of the Symptoms of PCOS?

The most obvious ones are changes in your body, but there are other, more subtle, symptoms affecting the brain that also are common due to the hormone imbalances.

But first, let's hear from a young woman, age 18, who struggled with many of these changes, and had been diagnosed as having a psychiatric disorder and started on multiple psychotropic medications before I saw her for her evaluation. Here is her story, in her words.

"PCOS? What is that? Well, it was something that I had no idea about when I was in high school. In general, it is not something doctors usually consider a fourteen-year-old to have. The first evident signs of my PCOS cropped up when I was in 9th grade.

Looking back, I realize that my symptoms then were too abnormal to be considered part of growing up, but that's what the doctors kept telling me. I was growing heavy, dark, thick hair all over my body, even though that was unusual in my family. I had severe acne that made me feel awful about myself when it hit. I felt like my moods were wild and out of control, like some force took me over. I would have periods that seemed to go on forever, sometimes lasting for three weeks. After one period's end, there would only be a one week break and

Alert!
If you have the symptoms and body changes, you need thorough testing and appropriate treatment

So true
I think that sometimes in medicine we get so hung up on "proof" of a diagnosis that we forget to focus on the person who is suffering and what we can do to help alleviate the suffering.

then the next would begin. Then other times, there were be a couple of months between cycles.

I went to multiple appointments with my family practitioner, I saw a gynecologist in town, and I even went to a specialist gynecologist at UCLA Medical Center. They all said the same thing; that these symptoms were normal and would eventually go away. I went on birth control, and I even took Depoprovera shots. But they only provided temporary relief from the frustrations of having to deal with a seemingly never-ending periods.

Having a 'syndrome' at the age of 14 seemed too far out there for me to even think of and apparently, it was too 'out there' for my doctors to consider as well, since they never diagnosed it properly. My friends would ask why I was going to the doctor and for what reasons. This would prompt me to lie or dismiss it as a "regular" checkup; although, it was far from it.

Coping with having some unknown problem as a teenager was extremely difficult. Not only did I have to learn to deal with feeling strange compared to my girlfriends, but I also had all the other parts of growing up. I used to feel embarrassed by my situation. I was teased a lot. I felt awful that I couldn't be normal like my sister and all my friends. It seemed incredibly unfair that I had to deal with all these problems while no one else I knew had anything like this.

At home, my mother was always worrying about me and why my body was "behaving in such a manner." That in itself was a hassle; the typical nagging mom. At first, both of us believed that everything would even out in the end; sometimes the irregular periods would stop and return to normal. It was not until I struggled with all these changes during high school that I finally found after I graduated a possible answer for what was wrong with me.

After four years of having to deal with irregular periods, excessive hair growth, and acne (mostly on my back,

"Time and time again, I was given the same explanation: that all my irregularities were just a part of growing up."

"It would only be later on, that we would find out that we had been kidding ourselves about the "normalness" of a never-ending period."

now called "backne" by magazines), I was introduced to that fact that I might have PCOS, not from a gynecologist, but from a doctor I was seeing for laser hair removal treatments.

During the appointment, this doctor asked if I had irregular periods. I was slightly startled by this question, because it seemed like an odd one to ask when getting laser hair removal. He told me that my hair growth was a lot thicker compared to most women, especially Asian-Indian women, and suggested I get my testosterone levels checked. My blood tests revealed a very high testosterone level, way out of the normal range for a teenager.

I then scheduled an appointment with an endocrinologist who confirmed that I had PCOS. Sitting there as he explained this was a relief because finally after so many years everything seemed to tie together. At the same time though, it was mildly depressing to hear that I had this serious 'problem' because doctors had always told me that I was just going through a 'phase' and it would go away on its own.

My story didn't end there though.

My mother thought it was strange that the endocrinologist just wanted to prescribe a high dose of Glucophage, a medicine we thought was for people with diabetes. My mother felt I was too young and too thin to be taking such a high dose. Since I was going off to college, she was also worried that if I had drops in my blood sugar, there would be no one to help. At the time, like most kids, I thought she was overreacting; but, in retrospect, she was right.

Because my mood swings were so bad, and I was having trouble sleeping, they sent me to a psychiatrist, who put me on Seroquel for sleep, and thought I was bipolar and needed to be on Lamictal for that. But my mother didn't want me to start Lamictal yet. She had read Dr. Vliet's book, It's My Ovaries, Stupid and had begun to think that maybe my mood swings were caused by the hormone imbalance. My mother wanted me to see Dr.

"Now, here I was being told I had this major disorder that could even keep me from having children. It was a big blow. It meant I had to get serious about taking care of myself; something no young person wants to hear, especially since I could imagine myself living off pizza while in college!"

Vliet to get a better idea of the whole picture and what types of treatment I might need.

After seeing Dr. Vliet, now I finally know that while I do have PCOS, it is manageable. Before, it seemed like PCOS was something that was going to destroy any attempts of normalcy. As it turned out after further tests, I really didn't need Glucophage or Lamictal or Seroquel at this point in my life. Instead, Dr. Vliet thought I should go back on a birth control pill called Yasmin to help decrease the hair growth and the acne. She also suggested I take the pills without a break so that I wouldn't have those awful, heavy, long periods anymore. Now that's an idea that appealed to me!

It's been several months since my first consult and I am amazed at how much better I feel now. I sleep well without the Seroquel, I don't have irregular and heavy periods anymore, and my acne has cleared up... which is a great relief! My body hair is getting less and less the longer I am on the Yasmin.

And it has turned out that what I do to manage my PCOS is much less complicated than what I thought I would have to do. It is such a relief to know that I don't have to spend the majority of my day trying to remember what medicine to take next.

I do have to maintain a healthy diet and get a lot of exercise, which in the long run is beneficial to anybody. The exercise has helped not only in managing my PCOS, but is a great stress reliever and is tons of fun, especially taking dance-aerobics with an instructor who tells you to move like a dancer!

I finally am out of all that frustration that I went through in high school trying to deal with a body that was doing all these weird things I didn't understand. I feel like I know what's wrong and what I have to do about it now. I now know that PCOS can happen to girls even younger than I was at fourteen. And I now know that being thin does not eliminate the chance of having PCOS.

"In the short period of time that my PCOS has been managed properly, I have noticed an incredible difference in my overall well-being. I don't have the horrible mood swings I used to go through."

I can be healthy and have my normal energy and feel good if I take care of myself and follow the treatment I need. I've learned that having PCOS isn't the end of the world... and it's manageable!

—Suki

PCOS: Characteristic Symptoms and Signs

PCOS can be devastating. The effects of high androgens hit women in many serious ways. Let's look at some of these problems.

Marked weight gain

Obesity is a common finding in PCOS, present in at least 50–60% of patients with this syndrome. The pattern of weight gain holds clues to the presence of PCOS:

1. The weight gain is usually rapid, often without change in food intake. Many of my patients say the weight seems to come from nowhere, and feels like the cookie monster running amuck inside their body. They describe feeling like the pounds pack on faster than they can shop for new clothes. They are puzzled and frightened. They diet, they exercise, and nothing seems to halt this inexorable growth in girth.

2. The excess fat is typically deposited around the waist, upper body, shoulders and arms, rather than hips and thighs. Women tell me they feel like a fire-plug or a barrel. Breasts get larger, fat sticks like glue under and around the arms and upper chest. The waistline? It disappears. The hormone imbalance creates the damaging male pattern apple-shaped body. Weight gain that happens when women overeat is usually more symmetrical and distributes in a woman's usual pear shape.

3. The weight gain of PCOS is commonly accompanied by acne and excess face and body hair, and thinning scalp hair. Weight gain from simply over

eating and under exercising isn't usually associated with these other problems.

4. The weight gain with PCOS typically doesn't respond normally to the usual dieting. The metabolic abnormalities of PCOS make it almost impossible for a woman to lose weight by simply eating less. The endocrine imbalances must be treated first. Effective help for this weight gain usually requires a combined approach with medication(s), the right type of meal plans, and aerobic exercise.

The caveat
PCOS can occur in thin women. Studies have found that some thin PCOS women have a more severe form of insulin resistance than obese PCOS women.

A 16-year-old young woman I saw for a consult had the severe hormonal imbalance typical of PCOS, with a very high level of free testosterone, high DHEA and DHEA-s, and a very low estradiol. She had gained 50 pounds over six months in spite of a healthy diet and exercise regimen.

She had PCOS, but her gynecologist had not recognized it. He saw her as simply a teenager obsessed with weight gain and complaining of PMS. His advice to her and her mother was for her to "eat less, and exercise more, and you'll lose weight." She had already been diligently doing just that, but her weight continued to balloon up. Weight loss is not that simple if you have PCOS.

Excess facial and body hair

About 60–70% of women with PCOS have excessive body hair, called *hirsutism*. The excess hair growth in PCOS can be profoundly distressing and embarrassing to women. It tends to occur in a male pattern, with coarse, dark hair on the chin, cheeks, upper lip, chest, around the nipples, on the stomach and inner thigh, back and buttocks.

Fact:
Hirsutism itself is not a disease; it is a symptom of an underlying hormonal imbalance.

In PCOS, high levels of the male hormones, androgens, are the primary culprits causing excess facial and body hair. There are several androgens made by the ovaries and adrenal glands in women: testosterone, DHEA, DHEA-s, dihydrotestosterone (DHT), androstenedione). There is also over-activity of an enzyme called

5-alpha reductase that converts testosterone to a more potent form called dihydrotestosterone (DHT) in the hair follicle, causing increased male-type hair growth.

Thinning scalp hair, or hair loss

Fact:

Scalp hair loss occurs in about 10–20% of women with PCOS.

Excess androgens also cause male-pattern balding or thinning of the scalp hair, called *androgenic alopecia*. Hair is thinner overall with loss of hair on the top of the head and around the forehead. Excess androgens may also cause changes in body hair texture, making it coarser and thicker.

These same types of changes can also occur in women with PCOS who have low estradiol, or menopausal women who have lost estradiol. The drop in estrogen unmasks the androgen effects.

Severe acne

Fact:

In PCOS the acne doesn't always confine itself to your face. You can have cystic acne outbreaks on your neck, upper chest, back, arms, and legs.

The acne in PCOS is typically far worse than just simple adolescent "zits" the week before your period and happens in 30–40% of women with PCOS. The acne can be large, painful, inflamed cysts that look and feel like boils. If you have acne that is this severe, or is not responding to the usual treatments, it is very important to have tests for excess androgens.

One young woman had become severely disfigured from the cystic acne, but had never been checked for possible PCOS despite the telltale signs. It took six months of aggressive management with the right birth control pill and spironolactone for her acne to resolve.

Skin Abnormalities

Skin tags, called *acrochordons*, occur often in women with PCOS, commonly found on the eyelids, neck, armpits and back. They are usually painless and don't grow or change, except to become irritated or inflamed due to friction from clothing. If bothersome, they can easily be removed in the doctor's office under simple local anesthesia.

Darkening of the skin, called *acanthosis nigricans* (AN), occurs in PCOS as a result of excess insulin production. The darker, thickened skin tends to occur on the inner thighs, vulva, neck, underarms, under the breasts and other areas where there are skin folds. Lowering excess insulin with combined approaches of diet, exercise and medication can result in lightening of the skin or even resolution of the AN.

Fact: *Acanthosis nigricans* (AN) is a definitive indication of excess insulin, so if you have noticed such pigment changes, you should be evaluated for insulin resistance.

Irregular menstrual cycles

About 70–80% of women with PCOS have menstrual irregularities of various types. Sometimes women with PCOS go months without a period, other times periods may still be relatively regular.

Amenorrhea means lack of menstrual periods and can occur in 30–40% of women with PCOS who began menstruation at puberty and then later stopped having periods.

Oligomenorrhea means "fewer than normal" periods. This type of irregular menses is even more common than complete lack of periods, and happens in 85–90% of women with PCOS.

Polymenorrhea refers to periods that come more frequently than once a month and may also be quite heavy.

Some PCOS sufferers have very heavy bleeding; others have periods that are barely there. Excessive bleeding occurs in PCOS for the same reasons that periods come less often in other women—the ovaries aren't functioning normally and there is no ovulation that leads to a regular menstrual period.

Loss of ovulation is common in PCOS, and one of the major causes of infertility. Some women with PCOS do still ovulate occasionally, even if not every cycle. If they become pregnant without major difficulty, they may not find out they have PCOS until later in life when other manifestations appear.

Difficulty getting pregnant, or frequent miscarriages

PCOS is the leading cause of infertility in young women, accounting for about 75% of anovulatory infertility. The excess levels of male hormones combined with excess body fat lead to increased conversion of androstenedione (an androgen found in high concentration in body fat), to the estrone form of estrogen. Excess production of estrone feeds back to the brain and alters the pituitary secretion of FSH and LH, which in turn means that development of follicles in the ovary can be abnormal.

Follicles in the ovary become stalled as multiple, tiny cysts, and the usual progression from follicle to ovulation and release of an egg doesn't occur. Then, if there is no ovulation, there is no corpus luteum to produce progesterone. Without the normal rise and fall in progesterone in the second half of the menstrual cycle, bleeding becomes unpredictable.

High prolactin, whatever the cause, suppresses the normal menstrual cycle production of estradiol and progesterone.

These several factors combine to increase the problem of infertility: decreased ovulation, lower levels of both estradiol and progesterone, high levels of estrone and prolactin, excess androgens, and excess insulin and cortisol, to name a few.

Miscarriages are more likely because the estradiol and progesterone levels are lower than needed for ovulation and for normal development of the uterine lining to receive a fertilized embryo and sustain the early pregnancy until the placenta can take over hormone production. High androgens can also impair normal follicle development. There may be many other causes of miscarriages as well.

Treatment of PCOS-induced infertility may itself cause health problems later in life. International specialists in the field of climacteric (menopause) medicine have

Key point 1

PCOS can affect your menstrual cycle in many different ways, from no periods to infrequent periods to heavy or prolonged bleeding.

Key point 2

Lack of menses, or extremely irregular menses, should always be checked out carefully and PCOS considered as a potential cause.

studies showing that drug treatments such as clomiphene citrate (Clomid) to stimulate ovulation, as well as laparoscopic ovarian treatments to remove cysts, can cause premature menopause and a higher risk of ovarian cancer later.

Invisible Brain and Body Changes

The changes inside the body that you don't see can be even more ominous, and rob you of energy, sleep, mood stability, sex drive, and clarity of thinking while increasing the later risks of heart disease and diabetes:

High androgen levels (testosterone—both free and total, DHEA-s, DHEA, androstenedione)

This is the most consistent hormone abnormality in PCOS, seen in more than 70–80% of sufferers. In addition to the hair, skin and weight changes I just described, high levels of androgens can cause muscle pain, irritability, anxiety, insomnia, and angry-agitated or depressed moods.

High estrone (E1) to estradiol (E2) ratio

Even if the ovarian levels of estradiol are lower than optimal, estrone can be high because it is also produced in body fat. PCOS is often described as a syndrome of both elevated androgens and elevated estrogen. But don't be misled. The terms "elevated estrogen" or "excess estrogen" or "estrogen dominance" or "hyperestrogenic and hyperandrogenic" that some health writers use to describe PCOS is not very definitive, and may not be accurate.

In my clinical experience of measuring hormone levels in thousands of women over the last 20-plus years, I find that it is not estradiol that is elevated but estrone, the estrogen made in body fat, which is too high. I have consistently found that estradiol is actually lower than expected in my patients with PCOS, which may occur as a result of abnormal follicle development.

Fact:
High levels of a pituitary hormone, prolactin, occur in about 60% of women with PCOS.

Fact:
Women with PCOS may have a double whammy— they often need specialized treatment to get pregnant, and some of those treatments can lead to later health problems.

High concentrations of Luteinizing Hormone, LH

Current studies have found that serum LH concentrations are significantly elevated in 40–60% of PCOS patients, and that women with PCOS also have more frequent "pulses" of LH release than do other women.

Doctors have said in the past that the diagnosis of PCOS required the presence of a reversed ratio of LH to FSH. Newer studies have shown, however, that this is not a reliable marker to use. It is present in some, but not all, women with PCOS. The LH to FSH ratio is no longer considered needed or useful for the diagnosis of PCOS.

Lower than normal sex hormone binding globulin (SHBG)

SHBG is a carrier for the sex hormones in the bloodstream. Low levels of SHBG means more androgens are "free" and more available to bind at receptors. More "free" androgens, especially if estradiol is too low, means more of the adverse body changes I have described.

Glucose intolerance

Glucose intolerance, leading to "blood sugar swings" from too high to too low that disrupt memory, concentration, mood, and sleep, as well as cause weight gain. This is one factor that causes women with PCOS to have "sugar cravings" or feel the need to eat more carbs, which perpetuates the problems with glucose regulation.

Insulin resistance

The majority of women with PCOS tend to produce excessive amounts of insulin. High levels of insulin stimulate the ovaries to make more of the androgens, and also make you store more fat, instead of burning fat for fuel. Insulin resistance makes you get fatter and fatter, even if you are eating less and exercising more. Then the fatter you get, the more insulin resistant you become.

High cholesterol and triglycerides with low HDL ("good") and high LDL ("bad") cholesterol

Women with PCOS often have abnormal cholesterol profiles at much younger ages than seen in women who don't have PCOS. High triglycerides are a separate, independent risk factor for heart disease in women, even if cholesterol isn't overly high.

Elevated prolactin, with or without nipple discharge (galactorrhea)

High prolactin can occur in 40–50% of women with PCOS, and may contribute to ovarian dysfunction, lack of ovulation, and weight gain. If prolactin remains high even with appropriate treatment of PCOS, it may be necessary to check for a possible pituitary adenoma as a cause, and to use medication to lower prolactin.

Excess production of the adrenal stress hormone, cortisol

High morning cortisol is common in PCOS, even in women who do not have primary Cushing's Disease. High cortisol contributes upper body and abdominal weight gain, insulin resistance, and diabetes.

High blood pressure, even in very young women

High blood pressure in younger women with PCOS can have a number of causes, such as low estradiol and high androgens, weight gain, and high cortisol. Effective treatment of PCOS usually helps lower blood pressure, but sometimes antihypertensive medication may be needed in addition to the usual treatment approaches for PCOS.

Recurrent ovarian cysts

The classic PCOS cysts on the ovary appear on ultrasound like a "string of pearls." Some doctors still mistakenly think that if a pelvic ultrasound shows no cysts, a woman can't have PCOS. This is not the case, for several reasons.

Alert: Abnormal LH release contributes to poor follicle development, anovulatory cycles, decreased chance of becoming pregnant, as well as increased risk of miscarriage.

Not every woman with PCOS has visible cysts. Many times the cysts are so tiny they can't be seen on ultrasound and are only found during surgery that is done for other reasons.

Other problems
↑ TG
↑ Chol
↑ cortisol
↑ prolactin
↑ BP

Another reason you may not see the cysts on ultrasound is that they are not present all the time. Cysts may not be there the day the ultrasound is done, so they elude detection.

Recent studies have also shown that there is a high degree of variation among people who interpret pelvic ultrasounds, making the predictive value of this test much more subjective than we used to think.

Summary

All of these hormonal and metabolic changes wreak havoc with your moods, energy level, fertility, and also cause young women with PCOS to have an especially high risk for diabetes. Diabetes then causes more damaging changes in the heart and blood vessels throughout the body and increases the risk of early angina, heart attacks, or even stroke.

Warning:
Not every PCOS sufferer has visible cysts. Some cysts can't even be seen. And, they come and go!

It's not a pretty picture. But there is hope, and help, available to turn this around and stop the vicious cycle of progressive damage.

So read on. In the next chapters, I will help you better understand PCOS, how to get diagnosed and what treatments are available.

Chapter 3

Your Menstrual Cycle and What Goes Awry in PCOS

Introduction

Our ovarian hormones play many roles in our overall health and well-being: maintaining bone and muscle strength, keeping our brain sharp, maintaining sleep, overseeing immune function, regulating blood pressure and heart function, and of course, our sexuality—not only its reproductive function, but our sexual thoughts, feelings and actions.

Here is one patient's story, from her mother, to show how complicated this situation can be.

Fact: Our ovaries and brain are delicately balanced, exquisitely sensitive, and closely intertwined.

When my daughter Brooke got her first pubic hair at the age of six, I knew something was wrong. Our pediatrician told me not to worry. Two years later, Brooke had full underarm hair (and some around her navel), stomach obesity, and darkened patches inside her elbows. Although I know now that these are signs of an endocrine disorder, all I knew at the time was that other 8-year-olds didn't seem to have them. I took Brooke to a pediatric endocrinologist, who ordered blood tests that turned up abnormally high testosterone, cholesterol, and triglycerides. Despite all this, I was again told not to worry. "Wait until menarche," the doctor said; "then we'll test her again."

When you sense that something is wrong and the doctors tell you that nothing is wrong, all you can do is try to adjust to their reality. And so for the next eight

"I told myself that all girls have irregular periods at first. She developed anxiety and depression–typical adolescence, I convinced myself."

"She was increasingly exhausted and languid, which we attributed to depression, and she began to see a child psychiatrist."

"I imagined that people would look at Brooke's size and assume I was feeding her Twinkies and Coke all day, but nothing could have been further from the truth."

years, I doggedly tried to do just that. Brooke started menstruating at 12, and I reassured myself that this was a normal age for girls "these days." By the time she was 13, her periods had become erratic, with cycles ranging anywhere from 14 days (a spotty, uncertain period) to 50 days (a super-tampon-soaking week of hell).

Her weight continued climbing until, at 14, it was close to 200 pounds, most of it around her middle. I decided that this was because she needed more exercise, and I tried (without much success) to coax her into sports.

One of the strangest things was that Brooke didn't seem to look like anyone in our family. My mother and sisters and I are all slender and athletic, with waists that taper and periods that come like clockwork. On the other side of the family, my husband is angular and muscular, with no sign of a middle-aged potbelly; and his sister is skinny and hyperthyroid.

I wondered if Brook's problems had anything to do with how she ate. From a young age, she had craved carbohydrates, craved them like a starving person. When I limited juice, Brooke drank glass after glass of milk. She would eat three bowls of cereal for breakfast and crave more. She preferred the stuffing to the turkey, the shortcake to the strawberries.

I couldn't figure out why my organically-grown daughter (whose only candy consumption came at Halloween) was so overweight, while all of her friends (who drank soda like water and had pop-tarts for breakfast) stayed beanpole-thin. I'm a granola-head mom who grows her own vegetables, cans her own fruit, and grinds her own whole-wheat flour. I have never let soft drinks pass over my threshold.

I was unwilling to intervene too much and risk adolescent eating disorders. We visited a reproductive endocrinologist who ordered thorough tests of Brooke's insulin, glucose, hormone and lipid levels. His diagnosis was Polycystic Ovarian Disorder (PCOS), and his treatment was to start her on metformin (a diabetes drug to control blood sugar) and hormones.

Unfortunately, every birth control preparation he tried—pills, patches, and vaginal ring—made Brooke violently ill. She was even hospitalized for vomiting at one point. The doctor said that we should hold off for awhile and see if she would outgrow this reaction. In the meantime, he recommended lots of exercise, a high-protein diet, and extra Ibuprofen during her periods to reduce cramping and bleeding.

A year later, I was at the end of my rope. Because she was a conscientious student, her faltering grades made her increasingly anxious and depressed. Her periods were worse; I didn't know it was possible to have such miserable periods. For the first three days, she'd soak through a super tampon every hour and have to wear a super pad to catch the leaks. She couldn't even attend class because the bleeding was so heavy. She suffered severe mood swings—depression to contentment to rage to tears to happiness, all within the span of a couple of weeks.

By this time, I'd been working with Dr. Vliet for several years (having discovered her through her book Screaming to Be Heard*). Because my hormone problems were quite different from Brooke's, it didn't occur to me that Dr. Vliet might also know something about PCOS. But when I mentioned it, I was surprised (and, on reflection, not at all surprised) to learn that Dr. Vliet was in fact finishing a book on PCOS, a kind of follow-up to her book* It's My Ovaries, Stupid*. She said she would elavuate Brooke.*

That visit was a godsend. The detailed blood work that Dr. Vliet ordered showed grim results: Brooke's lipid, insulin, and glucose levels were still too high; her thyroid was low; her iron stores were depleted; her testosterone was elevated; and her estrogen was only 15 ug/dl, the lowest Dr. Vliet had ever seen.

Dr. Vliet explained that her carbohydrate cravings, exhaustion, memory problems, anxiety, depression, and mood swings were tied to her PCOS. The PCOS wasn't limited to "cystic ovaries" but was a more comprehensive endocrine disorder that affected all of her endocrine glands—thyroid, adrenals, pituitary, ovaries, pancreas,

"I decided to concentrate instead on her menstrual problems… maybe there was a doctor out there who would at least take these seriously."

"Brooke was doing poorly in school, falling asleep in class, and complaining of exhaustion and unable to concentrate."

"For the first time, we were given a clear picture of how all of Brooke's symptoms fit together."

and others. Not only did this increase Brooke's risk of heart attack, diabetes, and certain cancers, but if she wasn't already infertile, she was heading there quickly.

"I felt more relieved than scared to get this news."

It corroborated and explained a lifetime of symptoms. I had become almost frantic with worry over Brooke's menstrual bleeding, her psychiatric problems, and her inability to control her weight, but until we visited Dr. Vliet, no one had validated my worries, much less been willing to do anything about them.

As I write this, Brooke is undergoing customized hormone therapy, a regimen of very low-dose estrogen patches increased in tiny, slow increments (with anti-nausea medications on the side) to give her body time to adjust.

"Finally, Brooke and I feel like she's in good hands, taken seriously and treated appropriately. Finally, we have real hope."

To our amazement, she is already developing better tolerance. Soon, she'll be ready for a low-dose birth control pill, the dosage once again tailored to her sensitivity. Brooke is meeting next week with Dr. Vliet's dietician to talk about eating guidelines that make sense for her unique metabolism. Later, we'll look at the other medications she's on and adjust them to the overall plan.

Brooke was elated after our visit to HER Place. "I felt so accepted there," she told me. "No one blamed me for my weight—they understood like no one else does how much you crave food and how awful your periods are and how tired you feel. They knew how hard it is to be me." I felt the same way.

Ovaries and their hormones are intimately linked to all of our other body systems. That's why, when women develop PCOS with its damaging effects on the ovaries, then everything else in the body—from our scalp to our skin and in-between—can be so adversely affected.

Our ovaries are inextricably involved with our entire endocrine system, with the hypothalamus, pituitary gland, parathyroid, thyroid, adrenal gland, and pancreas. Each of these glands secretes its unique hormones that interact with ovarian hormones in many ways.

Our ovaries also have receptors, or docking sites, for chemical messengers that are made in the immune and nervous systems.

Everything is delicately balanced, exquisitely sensitive, and closely intertwined. Our ovaries cycle month after month, year after year, part of a beautifully coordinated hormonal symphony.

So what happens in PCOS to make this symphony so discordant, instead of harmonious? To help you better understand what goes wrong in PCOS, I want to first explain the key hormone "players" in our body, how they work, and what changes take place in a healthy menstrual cycle each month.

What is A Hormone?

Think of hormones as your "chemical communicators" or "connectors" that carry messages to and from all organs of the body and serve to connect one organ's function with another organ's function to keep the body balanced and functioning optimally.

The secretion and interaction of hormones throughout our bodies every day is a highly complex and ongoing process. Each hormone provides a specific set of directions or messages to the target cells to enable the cells to perform certain functions. The cells of the body are like manufacturing plants, making the many chemicals the body needs to function.

Hormones have a variety of functions. Some are similar to those of assembly-line supervisors directing the manufacturing processes, and some are similar to those of team facilitators acting as catalysts for chemical processes to occur in the cell.

The interactions of the hormones with each other and with cells throughout our body is far more complex than most people think. Each molecule interacts in highly specific and complicated ways with docking stations, or receptors. Even small changes in the structure of a hormone can significantly change the way that molecule

Balancing Act
Working with the ebb and flow of our ovaries' hormones can be more "art" than "science."

Connections
Without our hormones to keep the messages flowing smoothly and our organs functioning in an integrated manner, we would die.

Hormones
are very potent molecules. Minuscule amounts, as little as a billionth of a gram (nanogram), are all that's needed.

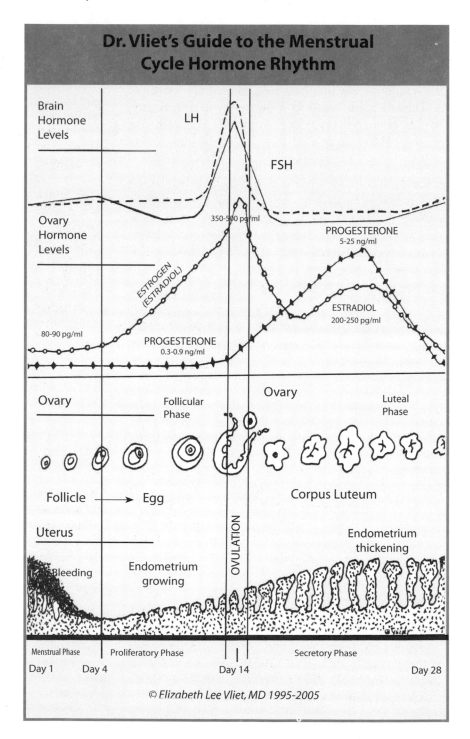

Dr. Vliet's Guide to the Menstrual Cycle Hormone Rhythm

Brain Hormone Levels

LH

FSH

Ovary Hormone Levels

350-500 pg/ml

PROGESTERONE
5-25 ng/ml

ESTROGEN (ESTRADIOL)

ESTRADIOL
200-250 pg/ml

80-90 pg/ml

PROGESTERONE
0.3-0.9 ng/ml

Ovary

Follicular Phase

Ovary

Luteal Phase

Follicle ⟶ Egg

Corpus Luteum

Uterus

OVULATION

Endometrium thickening

Bleeding

Endometrium growing

Menstrual Phase	Proliferatory Phase	Secretory Phase	
Day 1	Day 4	Day 14	Day 28

© Elizabeth Lee Vliet, MD 1995-2005

interacts with its receptors. The receptor sites may be located on cell surfaces or inside cells at the nucleus, which is our cellular "command central."

To simplify it, I have often used the visual analogy of a "key in a lock" image to describe these interactions for hormones to attach to their specific receptor sites all through the brain and body and then trigger their action on the target cells.

Essential Key Each hormone, or other chemical messenger is a specific molecular "key," and each has a receptor site, like a "lock," into which it fits.

As with keys, similar keys may fit in a lock, but not be able to turn it. Some keys fit partially and turn the lock slightly. Only the exact, specific key opens the lock easily and fully, just as the exact hormone molecule binds completely in a good "fit" with its receptor site to trigger the normal actions.

It's actually much more involved than this, based on our current knowledge of the complexities of the hormone-receptor interactions and factors that affect it. This simple analogy helps you see that it is important to have the identical hormone molecules available to attach to their receptors for everything to work optimally.

The Brain
Central Command and Communication Pathways

We have such an array of hormone messengers we need a way to coordinate their action in the body. The brain serves this Central Command role. The hypothalamus, lying at the base of the brain in an area almost between our eyes, serves as the "master conductor" of our hormone "orchestra." Other brain pathways and areas are also involved.

A two-way process: The brain directs the out-put of hormones, and the hormones in turn affect the brain's responses.

In its role as conductor, the hypothalamus directs and coordinates the actions of all these various players (hormones) to produce the "symphony" of our body rhythms and functions. Then the "music" generated by the action of the various hormones is "heard" by a variety of areas in the brain in a feedback loop that allows the brain's conductor to direct the next responses.

In women's bodies, the process is more complex. The menstrual cycle rhythm of changes causes the brain-body systems to continuously adapt to the changing hormonal environment.

The brain has a multitude of ways to direct the orchestra of the body to respond to what it (the brain) perceives, from inside the body physically, from inside the mind's thoughts and feelings, or from outside the body. The brain and body are interconnected by an incredible array of chemical and electrical circuits, each one interacting with and affecting others.

Unlike the male body, which maintains a fairly steady, or *tonic*, pattern of testosterone production all month long, the female body has a predictable, *cyclic* rise and fall in its ovarian hormones every month in the pattern we call the menstrual cycle.

It takes all of the hormones in proper balance, each carrying out their own tasks, yet working together to produce a fertile menstrual cycle and optimal function of a woman's body.

Many women, as well as most doctors, simply don't appreciate all the diverse effects throughout the body and the myriad influences of these crucial female hormonal rhythms.

Effects: Ovarian hormones influence extends far beyond just reproduction, though fertility has been the major focus of their effects in most women's health settings.

When our hormone balance goes awry, we can develop a wide variety of symptoms and health problems that can affect virtually every major system in the body. PCOS is a good example of just how profound—and varied—the effects can be when the ovarian hormones are out of balance, both in actual amounts produced and in their ratios to each other.

Let's look at the hormone players in PCOS and what gets off balance to cause the problems.

PCOS: The Hormone Cast of Characters

Not all estrogens are alike

Estrogens don't all have the same effects, so they really aren't interchangeable. It's important to know which type of estrogen is low or high, and then be able to make decisions about what needs to be done to help relieve symptoms.

That's why in testing, and in discussion, I use the term estradiol more often than the non-specific terms, estrogen. For women with PCOS, it is especially important to understand their differences, because some of the symptoms in PCOS are actually caused by *low* estradiol, even when estrone can be too high from excess body fat.

Many doctors, and lay people writing about PCOS, still call it an "estrogen-dominant" disorder, even though not many physicians have ever regularly checked any of the estrogen levels to see if this is really true.

In searching the medical literature, I found only one report of polycystic ovarian disease with significantly elevated estradiol levels. In this case the plasma estradiol was so massively elevated, it suggested the presence of an estrogen-producing tumor, which is extremely rare.

Estrone (E1)

Estrone (E1) is made in the ovary and fat tissue of our bodies before and after menopause. Androstenedione, which is excessively high in PCOS, can be converted to both testosterone and/or more estrone.

Estrone and estradiol molecules don't activate the estrogen receptors in quite the same way. Women with PCOS have symptoms that are actually due to *low estrogen*, but it is *estradiol* that's low.

Estrone is also higher in postmenopausal women because when there aren't any more follicles to make estradiol, the remaining source of estrogen is made primarily in body fat. Estrone does not prevent the unwanted postmenopausal changes in skin, bone, hair, heart and blood vessels, brain and other organs.

High estrone is also associated with higher risk of breast and uterine (endometrial) cancers. Estrone is associated with a slower metabolism, and you guessed it, more gain in body fat. This is especially a concern for women with PCOS, who have additional risk factors for weight gain such as high insulin and high cortisol.

The 3 E's
Our bodies have three types of primary estrogen: estradiol, estrone, and estriol.

Fact:
Most women with PCOS have higher estrone levels than women who don't have PCOS. This is reason it has been called an "estrogen-dominant" disorder.

Fact:
Higher estrone levels don't necessarily mean you can't have symptoms of low estrogen

17-beta estradiol (E2)

17-beta estradiol (E2) is the primary active form of human estrogen produced by the ovaries before menopause.

Estradiol contributes to our normal fertility, healthy energy, positive moods as well as clarity of thinking, memory, ability to concentrate, normal blood pressure, optimal bone density, better quality of sleep, vibrant skin and hair, normal vaginal pH and lubrication, healthy insulin-glucose regulation, and a healthy, active metabolic rate.

We lose estradiol when ovarian function is disrupted by surgery, or by a disorder like PCOS, or at menopause when we no longer have any remaining follicles to produce the estradiol. That's why women have so many diverse symptoms and problems after a hysterectomy or menopause.

The low estradiol, often with lack of ovulatory levels of progesterone in the irregular cycles of PCOS, is a significant factor causing infertility.

Loss of optimal serotonin, in turn, causes depression, increased irritability, increased anxiety, increased pain sensitivity, eating disorders, increased obsessive-compulsive thinking and increased disruption of normal sleep rhythms.

All of these combined effects can make metabolism more sluggish, so the cumulative result of losing optimal estradiol is that it is now harder for you to lose excess fat.

Even with high estrone levels, hot flashes, night sweats, palpitations, crawly skin, dry eyes and skin, low sex drive, restless sleep, memory problems, mood swings, vaginal dryness, more frequent vaginal yeast infections and many other problems can happen if E2 is too low.

Estriol (E3)

Estriol (E3), the weakest of the human estrogens, is produced by the *placenta* during pregnancy and is not normally present in measurable amounts in non-pregnant women. If you aren't pregnant, there really isn't a reason to supplement estriol.

Estriol is often promoted as a "safe" estrogen because it is a weaker one, but studies show that if you take enough estriol to relieve symptoms, it causes similar stimulation of the uterine lining (endometrium) and the breast that estradiol does. Since estriol does not replace the metabolic functions of the estradiol you lose at menopause, it is not helpful in maintaining the necessary premenopausal estrogen balance to keep you metabolism more active.

The bottom line is that all estrogens are not alike

So it's important that you know where your estradiol level is when you feel good, and how low it drops when you are having unpleasant symptoms. A thorough diagnostic evaluation, including detailed hormone testing of all ovarian hormones, is crucial to get the answers you need to plan approaches to help you feel your best.

Progesterone

Progesterone is the hormone responsible for preparing the body to sustain a pregnancy and nourish the developing baby. It has many metabolic effects on appetite, weight, insulin response and immune function that help the body adjust to the demands of pregnancy.

Progesterone is high the second half of your cycle, and contributes to the food cravings you notice during this time of the month. It isn't all in your head. Under the influence of progesterone, you want to eat more…both during your menstrual cycle to prepare for pregnancy, and when you are pregnant to nourish the developing baby.

Progesterone holds on to more water, and also slows the movement of food through the gastrointestinal tract, which then permits a woman's body to absorb more nutrients from food she eats. This is also why you feel bloated during this phase of your menstrual cycle.

Fact
Estriol doesn't have the same benefits for the body as estradiol (E2) does.

Estradiol has different effects body from estrone. Horse-derived conjugated estrogens in Premarin, or plant-derived conjugated estrogens in Cenestin, don't act exactly the same way as your own body estradiol does. Phytoestrogens from soy and red clover also have different effects from estradiol.

During times of famine, this effect of progesterone is adaptive, and helps women survive and babies be sustained during a pregnancy.

Progesterone and several of its metabolic breakdown compounds act at the "Valium" receptor in the brain to slow down brain activity. In this way, some women may experience progesterone as calming and sedating; other women feel lethargic and depressed when progesterone is high, especially if estradiol is too low.

Testosterone

Testosterone is one of the *androgens* that are usually thought of as "male" hormones, but women make testosterone in the ovaries and in body fat tissue. In women with PCOS, however, there is often *too much* testosterone produced, which can cause the unwanted effects we have discussed earlier: excess body hair, thinning scalp hair, abdominal obesity, acne, oily skin, irritability, anxiety and restless sleep.

Testosterone is an *anabolic* hormone, which means it helps *build* muscle and lean body mass *and* it uses fat for fuel. In the proper balance with estradiol, it helps women maintain a healthy composition of lean body mass and less body fat. In excess, though, testosterone contributes to more insulin resistance and middle body gain in fat that is undesirable.

Women with PCOS, who have lower than optimal estradiol, and higher androgens, often gain excess weight quite rapidly, and they do not respond as well to just diet and exercise efforts alone.

DHEA and DHEA-s

Dehydroepisandrosterone (DHEA), and its sulfate form DHEA-s, are other androgens produced in the ovary and adrenal glands.

DHEA-s is the form more commonly measured because it doesn't fluctuate as much over the day as DHEA does, but I find it helpful to know the levels of *both* forms of DHEA in determining treatment approaches for my patients.

DHEA and its partner, DHEA-s, are made from the basic building block of cholesterol, in a series of steps that initially take place primarily in the adrenal glands, with the final steps in the ovary and adrenal glands making DHEA from intermediate compounds.

DHEA is also synthesized in nerve tissue from cholesterol. Neurosteroids are still present in the brain even if the ovaries or adrenal glands are removed. Neurosteroids play roles in mood, memory, attention, sleep, pain and other functions that we are just beginning to understand.

DHEA supplements are heavily marketed today as over-the-counter weight-loss aids and energy boosters, but excessive amounts can actually cause weight *gain* and insomnia that leads to fatigue.

Thyroid

T3 and T4 are the two primary thyroid hormones produced by the thyroid gland. These are your major metabolic regulators, along with the ovary hormones, since they govern energy use and production in every cell and tissue in the body.

All of our metabolic pathways depend upon normal thyroid function for the chemical reactions to take place at the cellular level. When thyroid function is too low, especially when our ovary hormones are also out of balance, women will gain body fat very easily, even when cutting back to very low calorie levels.

If thyroid function is impaired, it further disrupts ovarian function and adds to the problems of menstrual irregularity, infertility, and weight gain that already occur due to PCOS.

Sometimes, even in conditions of *excess* thyroid hormone production, women will gain weight in the early phase due to the appetite-stimulating effects of overactive thyroid hormones. It is very important to have a thorough evaluation of thyroid function, as I outline in Chapter 8.

Fact: DHEA is also one of a number of steroids made in the brain, called neurosteroids

Warning DHEA levels tend to be too *high* in women with PCOS. I don't recommend taking supplements of this potent hormone.

Cortisol

Cortisol is known as our stress hormone, and it rises in response to immediate stressors as well as longer lasting ones. Short-term or acute stress also triggers a rapid release of adrenaline, known as the "fight or flight" stress response.

Fact

Both acute and chronic stress promote middle body weight gain and storage of fat in the abdomen instead of promoting fat breakdown.

After acute stress you often feel really hungry as a result of the adrenaline outpouring; this can lead to food cravings, especially sweets that make you eat more than normal to compensate. Chronic stress, on the other hand, leaves you feeling fatigued, with low energy levels, general loss of your zip and craving the classic "comfort foods" like carbs and sweets.

Cortisol production tends to be high in women with PCOS for a variety of reasons that I describe further in later chapters. High cortisol can add to the difficult problems of PCOS by further adding to the weight gain, acne, insulin resistance and also increasing the risk of diabetes. Women with PCOS should have thorough evaluation of cortisol, as I outline in Chapter 8.

Insulin and Glucagon

Fact:

Insulin and glucagon have important effects to regulate our blood glucose ("sugar") and govern the amount of body fat and muscle, among other functions.

Insulin and glucagon are called "counter-regulatory" hormones because they have opposite effects on blood sugar (glucose).

Insulin's normal effect is to lower blood glucose levels by (1) moving glucose from the blood into muscle cells, where it can be burned for immediate energy, or (2) moving glucose into fat cells where it is used to store more body fat.

The speed and amount of insulin release is triggered by the type of food we eat, when we eat it, and what other foods are eaten at the same time.

Insulin release is also affected by the balance of our ovarian hormones and vice versa. Reduced sensitivity to insulin action makes us store more fat around the middle of the bodies, and then increased body fat causes more insulin resistance. It's a vicious cycle.

Glucagon has the opposite effect. When the brain senses a falling blood sugar, glucagon stimulates the liver to send the glucose out of storage, into the blood stream to raise blood glucose and deliver it to the cells for fuel.

Too much insulin causes blood sugar to drop rapidly and unpredictably, which in turn causes more glucagon release. It becomes quite a "roller coaster" effect until you can get on the right balance of diet, medications, and exercise to correct the problems.

Fact
In PCOS, there is excess production of insulin, which contributes to the over production of androgens and also causes "Insulin resistance."

Prolactin

Prolactin is a hormone produced by the pituitary that regulates the release of milk during nursing. It rises to its highest level in the third trimester of pregnancy, then slowly decreases in the first few months after delivery. Levels may not return to the normal low baseline until several months after a woman stops nursing.

When prolactin is high, it typically causes menstrual cycles to become irregular and suppresses estradiol levels. Other problems can occur with high prolactin: weight gain, breast enlargement, headaches, low sex drive and depression. Physicians may miss these other clues to high prolactin.

Alert
Prolactin is often elevated in women with PCOS.

Elevated prolactin triggers weight gain by mechanisms similar to the increase in appetite seen in nursing mothers to stimulate increased food intake to support the caloric needs to feed mother and baby.

Prolactin may also trigger gain in body fat by suppressing the ovary production of estradiol and testosterone—both of which keep our metabolism revved up, and help to maintain normal insulin-glucose regulation, boost muscle mass and bone growth.

The problem is if you are not nursing, that you don't need to be eating for TWO, so the extra calories just get stored as more body fat.

In fact, women with high prolactin not only gain body fat, they also lose muscle and bone. Early bone loss leading to premature osteoporosis is one of the complications of untreated high prolactin levels.

If you are already gaining weight because of other PCOS-triggered hormone problems, high prolactin makes the situation worse.

Summary

PCOS causes abnormalities in all of the ovarian hormones, particularly the estradiol to estrone ratio, DHEA and testosterone. PCOS can also cause high LH, elevated cortisol and insulin as well as high prolactin.

Problems with the thyroid hormones aren't typically caused by PCOS, but may co-exist with PCOS. Since there is so much overlap in symptoms and health problems between PCOS and thyroid disorders, it is important to also carefully check thyroid function.

These combined hormone imbalances set women up for many health problems, as I describe further in upcoming chapters.

Chapter 4
The Life Cycle of Your Ovaries

Your ovaries travel a remarkable journey from fetal life to the waning days of our lives, with a number of important stages during their life cycle. To help you better understand what goes wrong in PCOS, it is important to understand the healthy ovarian cycle of hormone change that occurs monthly, as well as the phases of change throughout our lives as women.

At any point along the way, illness, lifestyle habits, and surgical interventions can have a critical impact on the function of your ovaries. Knowing what is happening at each stage will help you to understand how such disruptors affect you, and what you can do to help avoid problems.

Before Puberty

You are born with all the eggs/follicles you will ever make. By puberty you will probably have 300,000 or so left to start your periods. By 40, the average woman has only 5,000 to 10,000 follicles remaining.

A number of follicles are "recruited" each cycle, of which one or two are used. The others are lost, leading to a decrease in follicles with every menstrual cycle. Many factors, such as illness, environment, and stress also contribute to the loss of follicles.

Follicles and maturing eggs produce estradiol, the most active form of estrogen. As you lose more and more follicles, estradiol levels decline erratically, causing disruptions and problems throughout your body. Declining estradiol brings on many of the classical symptoms of menopause. Menopause happens around age 50 on average, but these symptoms can occur in younger women, if follicles are damaged and lose the ability to produce adequate amounts of estradiol.

Sadly Younger women experiencing these problems are often undiagnosed because no one is checking the estradiol levels

Many young women with PCOS have symptoms like menopause, due to lower than normal estradiol production because of impaired follicle development. There are simple, reliable blood hormone tests to measure this crucial hormone.

Puberty: The Awakening of Our Ovaries

American girls generally enter puberty between age nine and fourteen. The average age of 12.8 years for menarche held fairly steady until the 1990s, when we began seeing girls develop breasts and menstruating at much younger ages. If puberty occurs earlier than age 8, it is called *premature (or precocious)* puberty. Girls destined to develop PCOS often enter puberty much earlier than their peers, and may start developing body hair as early as age 6 or 7.

The average time span from the first stage of puberty to the first menstrual bleeding is about 4 years. The first stage is called *thelarche*, or the beginning of breast development. This is followed by *adrenarche*, triggered by the release of adrenal androgens, with the appearance of pubic hair, axillary hair, oily skin, and acne.

Menarche is the beginning of menstrual periods. The first menses usually occur when the breasts are more defined and body fat has reached a critical percentage, which is usually around the age 11.5 to 13.

Menstrual onset also varies due to race, diet, weight, percentage of body fat, light exposure, the presence of certain diseases, and genetics. Recent research suggests it isn't just how many pounds we weigh but the ratio of body fat to total weight that triggers onset of menstruation.

Thin girls tend to get their periods later than heavier girls. Girls with diabetes tend to have a delayed menarche. Ethnic background also plays a role. African-American and Hispanic girls tend to start menstruating earlier than Caucasians. Blind girls, who do not have significant light stimulation of brain centers, tend to have an earlier menarche than girls with normal vision.

Puberty is triggered by a series of hormone reactions. It starts with the hypothalamus increasing secretions that cause the pituitary gland to release increased amounts of gonadotrophins, follicle stimulating hormone (FSH) and luteinizing hormone (LH), into the bloodstream. These gonadotrophins stimulate activity in the ovaries in females, and the testes in males.

FSH and LH together direct the ovaries to produce elevated levels of estradiol, which leads to visible signs of maturing, such as developing breasts, pubic hair, under arm hair, and often a change in the timbre of the voice. These secondary sex characteristics are typically followed by a growth spurt that usually occurs two years earlier in girls than boys, which explains why girls at this age are often taller than boys.

Internal changes are also occurring due to the influence of these hormones at puberty. The walls of the vagina become thicker, and the uterus becomes larger and more muscular. The pH of the vagina also changes from alkaline to acidic due to the increase in estradiol in vaginal and cervical secretions.

Early in puberty, menstrual flow is usually very light, and comes with little warning. Periods may be irregular at first but usually become regular fairly quickly.

Prior to puberty, growth focuses on becoming taller and stronger. Most of the physical changes of growth are fairly well completed during the early years of puberty. With puberty, hormone changes prepare the body to reproduce.

Behavioral changes occur throughout adolescence, the longer span of time of psychological growth, when social adjustment and maturation are added to our physical

We now know— It is not normal to have irregular menses after the first year or so. Fertility, the ability to conceive and bear children, occurs when ovulation begins.

changes. These emotional and social transitions are less defined and less orderly than the physical ones. This unpredictability leads to the "turbulent teens." Thankfully, most of us eventually transition into a mature young adult.

The menstrual cycle is a normal process of being a woman and there is no reason to curtail normal activities during your period. But it is helpful to pay attention to your monthly cycles and patterns of physical and emotional changes such as headaches, bloating, tiredness, changes in mood, body aches, food cravings, acne or minor breakouts, cramps, tender breasts, constipation, cold sores, and even nosebleeds.

I have described the more "typical" onset and stages of puberty. But what about girls who enter puberty far ahead of the average age? Why should you be concerned about early puberty?

Alert!
Paying attention to your body signals and understanding your unique responses during your cycle will help you recognize changes triggered by hormone shifts.

Do it!
Keeping a menstrual response calendar can be helpful in understanding your symptom patterns and getting a proper diagnosis.

Health Risks of Premature Puberty

More girls today are entering into puberty at younger ages. Girls only 5, 6, and 7 are developing breasts. It's as if we have a generation of girls who are *hormonally accelerated*. There are many serious reasons why this is happening.

During the 1800s, girls on average began to menstruate at about age 17. By the mid-1990s, however, about 1 in 5 Caucasian girls *by age* 8 were showing breast buds and pubic hair, the beginning signs of puberty. This is a staggering change.

50% of African-American girls now reach puberty *by age* 8; another 15–20% have hit puberty *by age* 7. In the few studies that have been done to date, Hispanic girls show patterns of early puberty closer to those of African-American girls.

Physical:

There are a number of emerging health risks in girls with early puberty: increased risks of PCOS, adolescent and adulthood obesity, diabetes, endometrial, and breast cancers. Researchers worldwide are looking at these important issues.

Dr. Dimartino-Nardi at Montefiore Medical Center in New York evaluated African–American and Caribbean–Hispanic girls with premature increases in adrenal androgens, and found that both ethnic groups were obese, had high insulin levels with insulin resistance, elevated androgens, and subtle decreases in their "good" cholesterol (HDL). Many of these girls also had a strong family history of type 2 diabetes mellitus.

Dr. Dimartino-Nardi found that girls with premature rise in adrenal androgens (adrenarche) are at risk of developing Polycystic Ovary Syndrome (PCOS) as they go through puberty, if they remained obese. The girls with elevated androgens and insulin resistance before puberty continue to have obesity, insulin resistance, and high androgens after puberty. They developed classic symptoms of PCOS related to the high androgens and insulin: irregular menses, excess facial and body hair, and severe acne.

Premature adrenarche and early puberty can be a risk factor for continued obesity for certain girls, and an early stage in the progression to the adult metabolic disorder we call Syndrome X. These early changes set up a lifetime of health problems, so it is critical that we get better at early identification of girls at risk.

A recent study found that levels of Growth Hormone Binding Protein (GHBP) are significantly higher in girls with premature puberty and middle-body fat. This leads to less free, active Growth Hormone (GH) available to stimulate the building of bone and muscle.

Less muscle mass creates a vicious cycle of more body fat, followed by more insulin resistance that in turn

Important!
If you develop symptoms of PCOS, have your hormone levels checked and start appropriate treatment early to help prevent damage to your ovaries.

Warning!
Future health risks occur when puberty starts too early. PCOS is one of them.

helps store more body fat, and then even less free growth hormone to build healthy bone and muscle. This means overweight children get even fatter.

Early puberty and a high percent of body fat work together to increase a girl's risk of later developing breast cancer through exposure to estrogens, particularly estrone, at an earlier, critical window of time in development.

Fact:
Less muscle mass creates a vicious cycle of more body fat, followed by more insulin resistance that in turn helps store more body fat, and then even less free growth hormone to build bone and muscle. This means overweight children get even fatter.

Other studies over the years have shown that the longer the breast is exposed to abnormal hormone ratios, especially if there are higher than normal levels of insulin, the higher the risk of breast cancer. Breast cancer risk is also increased with environmental exposure to the many hormone-like chemicals (See Chapter 6).

London researchers, Stoll and colleagues said in 1994,

"Earlier onset of menarche and tallness in adult women are mainly confirmed as risk markers for breast cancer. Recent…studies have reported abdominal-type obesity and higher circulating levels of insulin, testosterone, and insulin-like growth factor 1, to be further risk markers for breast cancer. There is evidence that abdominal-type obesity is recognizable in girls even before puberty, and disparate studies have shown it to be correlated with earlier onset of menarche, insulin resistance leading to hyperinsulinemia, and an abnormal sex steroid profile."

Psychological:

Girls (and boys) between ages 6–10 enter the psychological stage we call latency when both sexes retreat into their own world, avoiding the other sex almost like the plague. You remember this time in your life: girls hate "creepy" boys and boys think all girls have "cooties."

This is a critical developmental stage for both sexes. Girls especially need these years to develop confidence and a strong sense of self, separate from a role defined by boys or men. They need this phase of their lives to develop close friendships with other girls, to develop social skills and a sense of mastery in school and activities—especially sports—that help them successfully navigate the turbulent years of puberty.

If the physical changes of puberty come too early, it gives girls confusing signals—their body is attracting boys like flies to honey, but their psyche is still in latency, not wanting anything to do with boys. Their body looks like a young woman, but their mind is still a child.

If girls don't have enough time in the latency years to develop an adequate sense of self before they are pulled into relationships with boys, they have difficulty defining their sense of independent identity. They become further defined by how they look, rather than who they are. It becomes more and more difficult to develop positive self-esteem. This is especially true for girls with PCOS in the early stages.

Our society already pressures children to grow up too fast. When the body too is filling out and accelerating into puberty *before* the psychological "work" of latency has been completed, it can wreak havoc with later psychological, social, and academic adjustment.

Many social pressures already make it difficult for today's kids to feel good about themselves, so the psychological consequences of early puberty compound an already serious problem.

Sociological-cultural:

There are other ominous pitfalls for girls whose sexual development comes too early: these girls are teased by boys their age but get increased sexual overtures from older boys and experience more sexual harassment, increased risk of date rape, and an earlier vulnerability to accidental pregnancy.

Theories about Causes of Premature Puberty

What is happening to cause this widespread problem of premature puberty? Let's look at some of the culprits.

Another Impact:
In girls with PCOS in its early stages, their body changes—excess weight, acne and body hair–leads to teasing by other kids

Warning:
Girls who look 17, but are really 12, have more pressure from older boys to engage in risky behaviors like smoking cigarettes or pot, drinking alcohol, and street drugs.

Environmental Chemicals

The problem is not limited to the United States. Studies done in numerous countries have found that children's normal progression of sexual and reproductive development is being affected by exposure to the hormone-disrupting chemicals that permeate our food chain and water supplies worldwide. These hormone-mimicking compounds or *persistent organic pollutants* (POPs) are *everywhere.*

Many of these compounds also pass through the placental barrier and expose the developing baby in the mother's womb. They are concentrated in our body fat and breast milk because of its high fat content, and are then passed to infants during nursing.

This is a primary reason that breast-feeding infants in various studies show earlier onset of puberty. Most scientists think the benefits of breast milk for the baby outweigh the risk of exposure to these environmental chemicals, but no one can say with certainty because these issues are just beginning to be studied more aggressively.

These chemicals—DDE, PCBs, Bisphenol A and a host of other—have profound effects on the brain centers that regulate everything from sexual development to metabolism and body weight. The number of these endocrine disruptors is increasing rapidly, and they are not limited to just pesticides. Several different compounds used in the food industry, in plasticizers, and in dental restorations, are also estrogenic.

You can no longer afford to ignore the warnings that we see in animal populations all over the world.

Dietary Excess

We live in the age of "super-sizing," not only food and beverage portions but our bodies too. We live in a culture of *excess everything*: excess calories, excess fat, excess sugars and simple carbs that promote more fat, and excess "couch-potato" time in front of TVs and computers.

FYI:
Doctors don't realize the profound degree that chemical pollutants disrupt critical thyroid and sex hormone pathways and function.

Warning!
There are significant concerns for our health, including major disturbances in sexual development, increased risk of obesity, PCOS, endometriosis, infertility and other problems.

How does this contribute to earlier onset of puberty? We have known for a very long time that reaching a certain amount of body fat for girls plays an important role in signaling the brain to begin menstrual cycles. Overweight girls tend to begin to develop breasts and menstruate at younger ages.

Sociological Pressures:

Sexualized messages and images besiege girls and boys at younger and younger ages. Immersion in provocative, erotic images also contributes to changes in brain chemistry that trigger the onset of puberty.

If you think this is a strange idea, just remember that seeing someone eat a chocolate chip cookie can make you salivate, or watching a horror movie makes your heart race—so for all of us, seeing things around us will trigger physiological changes in the brain and body.

We also know that women who live together—in families, in college dorms, in residential high schools, etc. will typically begin to menstruate together. Menstrual synchrony seems to occur from a variety of olfactory and environmental cues that stimulate the brain-ovarian pathways to entrain, or synchronize, menstrual cycles.

Warning! It may not be so far-fetched to think that constant exposure to visual sexual images may also contribute to brain changes that accelerate sexual development

The Ovary Life Cycle: Our Fertile Years

Your menstrual cycle tends to regulate itself by mid-late teens unless you have PCOS in its early stages, which causes continued irregular cycles. Hormone production is more predictable, helping to keep a regular cycle of approximately 28 days. Estradiol levels are high in the first half of the cycle, called the *follicular* phase, then estradiol falls just before ovulation. Estradiol rises again to another peak in the second half, or *luteal* phase of the cycle, about day 20–21. During the first half of a normal menstrual cycle, progesterone is barely detectable.

During the second half of a healthy menstrual cycle after ovulation, progesterone is produced by the developing "egg," or corpus luteum, preparing the body for a possible pregnancy until the placenta takes over hormone production after a pregnancy is established. Progesterone continues to rise until it peaks about day 20–21 of the luteal phase. Then if the "egg" isn't fertilized, the corpus luteum dies, progesterone falls and triggers shedding of the uterine lining to being the next menstrual period.

Testosterone levels remain fairly constant throughout the cycle in women, and don't rise and fall in a predictable monthly pattern like estradiol and progesterone do.

In PCOS, when follicles don't develop normally, and theca cells in the ovaries are over-stimulated by the continuous high LH, there is excessive production of the androgens, especially DHEA and testosterone, all the time.

By 25, most women have reached the peak of their fertility and peak function of body systems to meet the demands of future pregnancy with the least stress on our body.

Misconception
Progesterone declines first, causing "estrogen dominance" and low progesterone. Not so!

By your mid-30s, you may begin experiencing a small change in your menstrual flow. By your late 30s or early 40s flow may become noticeably lighter and last for fewer days. Your cycle length may become either longer or shorter. This is a time when women notice more pronounced premenstrual mood, energy, and appetite changes that we know as premenstrual syndrome (PMS), or as more severe cases are called, premenstrual dysphoric disorder (PMDD).

Also at this stage, women tend to experience a wide variety of other effects from estradiol decline: worsening migraines, fibromyalgia, bladder problems, vulvodynia, loss of lean tissue, increasing fat stores, and other annoying symptoms that get worse as perimenopause progresses toward the end of menstrual cycles at menopause.

In women who have had regular, fertile menstrual cycles, *estradiol is the first ovarian hormone to decline* leading toward menopause. Women in this first phase of ovarian decline typically still have normal ovulatory progesterone levels even though estradiol typically is lower than it should be.

The Waning of Our Ovaries: New Insights on Stages of Ovarian Decline

The climacteric refers to the period of decline in hormone production from full reproductive capability to menopause, but it may also be called "perimenopause."

This decline in estradiol and then progesterone commonly begins between the ages of 35 to 40, as the number and/or quality of remaining follicles decrease.

But it can begin much earlier in some women, especially those who have had follicles depleted by recurring ovarian cysts or from multiple cycles of follicle stimulation during fertility treatments.

Our standard medical teaching is that premenopause begins with anovulatory cycles (a cycle which does not produce an egg), and loss of progesterone rather than estrogen. This standard "wisdom" is primarily based on observations of women's menstrual patterns, however, rather than on actual systematic hormone levels being done to show objectively what is happening at each phase of the process.

It is my contention that there is an unrecognized phase of estradiol decline that is the first step as our bodies move toward menopause.

It is difficult to "observe" if there is no egg being produced each month, so this is why most doctors don't have a good understanding of what is happening to your actual hormone production. Women deserve and need to have more reliable measures of their hormone levels.

I have been tracking and checking cycle-specific hormone levels for many years, in thousands of women, and then correlating them with symptoms. The objective data shows *how incorrect our standard teaching can be.*

In the women I have tested, I find significant decline in ovarian estradiol levels that preceded the onset of anovulatory cycles and loss of progesterone.

I have discussed my observations with many reproductive endocrinologists trying to help infertile women become pregnant. In doing regular checks of ovarian hormone levels to achieve pregnancy, the fertility specialists encounter same patterns of estradiol decline that I find in my patients.

But many women who struggle with infertility also experience some of the problems I see in my patients as a result of declining estradiol and testosterone: increasing PMS, headaches, muscle-joint pain, fatigue, weight gain, insulin resistance, bone loss, immune problems, low sex drive, bladder and vaginal problems, and a host of others.

Here are the STAGES of ovarian decline as I see them taking place in the women I have evaluated over the years:

Stage 1—Declining Estradiol

This occurs when your estradiol level begins to decrease, but you still have normal menstrual cycles. In what we call the "normal" or usual time frame, this stage would generally begin in our late thirties or early forties. In this phase, progesterone is generally within normal ovulatory ranges, but estradiol has declined below optimal levels.

One of the first symptoms of lower estradiol is multiple awakening during the night, with difficulty getting back to sleep. Our dreaming phase (REM sleep) is altered and you may notice that you don't dream as much as you used to.

Early signs of loss of estradiol may include fuzzy thinking, memory loss, mood swings, fatigue, muscle and joint pain, headaches, increasing allergies, more sensitivity to strong smells, vulvar pain, loss of sex drive, etc.

Women are usually able to recognize these as hormonally-related changes because of the cyclic pattern in which they come and go.

But my detective work to find out why my younger patients have these menopause-type symptoms shows that bleeding patterns are not an accurate marker of hormone levels.

I call this phase *Premature Ovarian Decline* (POD).

This is the time during which I find so many women are under-diagnosed, under-treated, and are seeking answers in the alternative medical field because their symptoms are not recognized by most doctors.

Any of you who struggle with infertility know: you can have regular periods, yet still not get pregnant. You have to measure the ovarian hormones at specific times of the menstrual cycle to see if there are optimal levels and balance of all these crucial hormones.

Stage 2— Beginning of Anovulatory Cycles

This is the beginning of classically defined premenopause. In our "normal" model, this phase would generally begin in our mid-forties, but like all the other phases, can occur much earlier.

There will be cycles when ovulation does not occur, because follicles don't develop properly and estradiol is not produced normally in the first half of the cycle. This then means progesterone doesn't rise as expected in the second half of the cycle.

Levels of FSH and LH are typically still low and haven't risen to the menopausal range. Fewer ovulatory cycles result in estradiol levels continuing to decline, and this is the time you may experience hot flashes and night sweats, especially with the drop in estradiol when your period starts. Your periods typically become irregular, or may skip.

Often common symptoms, from mild to more severe, include insomnia, further memory loss, inability to concentrate or focus, feeling depressed or anxious for no clear reason, pain syndromes get worse, you may have urinary leakage, or feelings of urgently having to go to the bathroom, vaginal dryness, painful sex, and feeling that your "get-up-and-go" got up and went.

Part of this loss of energy may be due to declining testosterone levels as well as the loss of estradiol. Lower levels of both hormones can also rob you of your sexual drive and interest and also make it much harder to have an

Often doctors say "You are "too young" to have hormone problems," or "you're still menstruating, so your hormones are fine."

FYI
PMS doesn't usually occur if there is no ovulation or rise in progesterone.

orgasm because clitoral nerve endings are less sensitive as we lose estradiol and testosterone.

Perimenopause

This stage is classically defined by rising FSH and LH levels as the brain struggles to increase the falling estradiol levels. Estrone, produced primarily by body fat tissue, is *rising* relative to the decreasing estradiol, especially in women who are overweight. This is why you may notice more "brain fog" and mood changes, as well as more fat around your waist.

You will still have periods but they now become more erratic and most cycles will likely be anovulatory. You may skip periods now as well. Bleeding is typically lighter, and shorter in duration, but it can also become heavier, and longer in duration some months. The color of your flow changes too; it is more likely to be brown rather than a healthy, bright red.

You may also notice worsening menstrual cramps. Fibroids and ovarian cysts tend to occur more frequently. As a result, hysterectomy is recommended for many women, although there are a number of non-surgical options to help control or prevent many of these problems.

At this phase of your ovary life cycle, your periods will most likely be erratic, with changing bleeding patterns. If menses come more often than every three weeks, or if you have heavy bleeding, you should talk with your gynecologist to discuss options.

And a caution: with such cycle irregularity and erratic ovulation at this phase of life, you could find yourself with an unexpected pregnancy.

Menopausal Stage

This final stage may seem out of place as part of our "reproductive" cycle since we are no longer able to get pregnant, but it is the stage that brings our ovary life cycle to completion.

Approximately 10–13 percent of women experience true

Wrong!
Doctors are taught that women who are still menstruating must have "normal" hormone levels.

Fact:
Estrone doesn't keep your body functioning at your previous level, since it doesn't act quite the same way in the body as estradiol does.

Caution:
If pregnancy is not desired, then you still need to use contraception until you are clearly menopausal, with an FSH greater than 20.

menopause between age 40 and 47. Another estimated 1% will undergo complete menopause, or premature ovarian failure, before age 40. Premature ovarian decline is a gray zone between the two, in terms of FSH and hormone levels, and can occur in women of any age if there has been damage to the ovaries for any reason.

Early onset of menopause has many causes, which we'll discuss later. Certainly our genetic makeup is one factor: studies of women around the world have shown that heredity is a major determinant of when we will reach menopause. It helps to find out when your mother and grandmothers reached natural menopause, (unless they had a hysterectomy that created an artificial menopause) to give you an idea of what you might expect.

We no longer menstruate because our follicle supply has been depleted and we can't make the hormones that trigger our menstrual cycles. The brain senses the decrease in estradiol, and sends out more FSH and LH to stimulate the ovaries to produce more hormones. FSH and LH levels rise above 20 MIU/ml, which is our official definition of menopausal levels.

But the rise in stimulating hormones FSH and LH is useless because there are no follicles to produce estradiol and progesterone. The low levels of ovarian hormones are now present in steady, non-cycling patterns.

With menopause, *we lose almost all of our 17-beta estradiol production, with levels typically below 30–40 pg/ml.* That's a lot lower than the average 100–500 pg/ml of a menstrual cycle, so it isn't surprising you feel so many body and brain changes!

Progesterone levels remain low because there is no ovulation, no corpus luteum, and progesterone is no longer needed to sustain a pregnancy.

Women also lose approximately half of their testosterone production. The ovary still produces testosterone and other androgens, though at lower levels, but it is no longer producing adequate estradiol to balance these male hormones.

FYI: The average age for natural menopause is between 48 and 52 years of age, but this is just an average.

It's a stunner When menopause comes too early, it can come as quite a shock, both psychologically and physically. It is a physical shock to your body to lose these important metabolically active ovarian hormones at too young an age. And an emotional blow of feeling old before your time and feeling the loss of your fertility.

The "pear" shape female (gynecoid) fat pattern around the hips and buttocks suddenly begins moving up toward the middle of the body to become the "apple" shape (male or android pattern).

In official "medicalese," menopause is defined *as one year* from the "last menstrual period," which may seem a little strange that we identify it so long after the fact.

The problem is our periods get more irregular at the end, so we never know which period is the last one for a number of months. We can then look back and realize "that was it."

Women now notice a marked worsening of brain symptoms such as insomnia, memory loss, foggy or slowed thinking and pain symptoms. Hot flashes occur and get worse with lower estradiol levels. For some women, however, hot flashes diminish as the estradiol becomes steady, instead of fluctuating as much as it does in perimenopause.

Changes in appearance also become more noticeable: skin becomes more dry and "crawly," and loses its elasticity leading to more wrinkles. Hair gets thinner and more brittle and you may start losing large amounts. You may notice more facial hair as well as loss of hair on your legs and arms. There is typically more weight gain around the waist, and your breasts become less firm.

The entire process of ovarian decline may take 15 years or more, or it can be a fairly rapid fall, occurring at nearly any age. This transition involves dimensions of our being: physical, emotional, and spiritual. The biological process will happen sooner or later to all women who live long enough.

It can be confusing to determine what changes occur as a result of the loss of our ovarian hormones and what changes occur as a result of just getting older. Women have a lifetime of experience with their cycles and are often able to identify what is hormonal and what is due to age.

Testosterone effects become more pronounced as estradiol is lost. There is a decrease in the good "HDL" cholesterol, and a rise in LDL and triglycerides. These changes combine to increase risk of cardiovascular disease (CVD).

Previous gender differences now become gender similarities. For example, CVD risk for menopausal women is now similar to the risk for men. The rate of CVD increases as estradiol levels decline relative to testosterone levels, as we see in younger women with PCOS.

Risk of diabetes, colon cancer, osteoporosis, and Alzheimer's disease all increase after menopause as you lose the critical estradiol. Breast cancer risk also increases with age after menopause *even if you never take any hormone replacement therapy*.

It is important to keep in mind that symptoms of hormonal decline can occur at any age. When I describe the ovaries' "normal" aging process, I am only giving you age ranges for a relative idea of when these changes can occur.

PCOS and Changes in Your Menstrual Cycle

Now that we have talked about how ovarian hormones and body changes occur in a "normal" progression through the menstrual life cycle, let's look at what happens in PCOS that is different.

Women with PCOS may have some of the symptoms that occur with low estradiol at menopause, but it isn't exactly the same process because you still have follicles and the potential for menstrual periods and your FSH remains in the premenopausal range of less than 20.

Having PCOS means that your follicles don't develop normally each cycle, and become "stalled" in the form of multiple cysts. When follicles fail to mature, they don't produce estradiol or progesterone at levels that allow normal ovulation or maintain "optimal" metabolic function throughout the body.

Fact: The effects of age and hormone loss combine to produce many of our body changes.

Fact: Blood pressure and cholesterol rise in menopausal women, similar to the pattern in men.

Alert: Your ovaries are as individual as you are and may not follow the "typical" timeline I outlined.

In women with PCOS, there is a higher blood level of LH during the entire follicular phase, unlike the normal menstrual cycle with a surge of LH only before ovulation. In addition, there are abnormal pulses of LH production that also stimulate the ovaries to pump out more androgens than normal. The high LH also stimulates excess insulin production, which then also adds to the increase in androgens being made by the ovaries.

In women with PCOS, suboptimal estradiol and the excess androgens are often gradual changes usually occurring over several years. The change in hormone production may be so gradual that you don't realize what is happening day by day until your symptoms and body changes become more severe.

Eventually, the decline in estradiol changes the ratio of estradiol in balance with testosterone, DHEA, and progesterone. This leads to a wide variety of physical changes and psychological experiences. Some of these may occur for the first time, or take a turn for the worse as your hormone balance changes.

There are many clues to declining estradiol. I have shown some of the more common ones I see in patients in the chart that follows. It is obvious from this list that estradiol affects many body functions.

The lower than optimal level of estradiol in PCOS is usually taking place when women are younger than expected for "menopause" so the symptoms get blamed on something else. That "something" is usually labeled psychological, or "stress," and then young women are told they need an antidepressant. Women experiencing these hormone imbalances may spend years searching for answers.

Persevere when you see such changes happening. Be assertive about getting checked for these potential hormone connections and work to get answers and treatments that make sense to you. There are too many health consequences if you don't.

Summary

Your hormones can be both marvelous and maddening: marvelous when they allow us to function at our best and to even create new life with a pregnancy, and then maddening when they are out of balance or declining, and we don't know what's happening to our body.

Our female hormones are at the core of our being, fundamental to every part and every function of our body and brain, mind and spirit.

The patterns of physiological changes that occur each month and throughout the ovaries' life-cycle give us observable cues that help us to then "connect the dots" and see the hormonal triggers related to physical and mood symptoms. We need to look for these patterns, track them, and then find ways to communicate our observations to physicians.

Many of my patients tell me it is often hard to get their physicians to listen to their observations and pay attention to these hormone-related issues. Many of my patients have done so much research to educate themselves, they often know more about these issues than many doctors!

While there are no easy solutions for changing the health care system to be more responsive to women's observations and insights, I have described in later chapters some suggestions to help you get what you need so you can feel well and energetic, and to improve overall vitality and health for many years to come.

Don't focus on just treating or "getting through" symptoms. That's a lot like just putting a band-aid on an abscess instead of treating the cause of the infection. I think it is crucial to have complete tests of your hormones, as I outline in Chapter 8, if you suspect from symptoms or your body changes that you may have PCOS.

Frustration: When you don't feel well and have sought help from multiple doctors only to be told there is nothing wrong, it can leave you doubting yourself. You feel battered, frustrated, and alone.

Crucial! Failing to check levels of all the ovarian hormones I think is one of the most important missing links in PCOS treatment today.

CLUES TO ESTRADIOL BEING TOO LOW

- ✷ Worsening PMS
- ✷ Restless sleep, difficulty sleeping especially prior to menses, multiple awakenings during the night
- ✷ Loss of energy, feeling too tired to get through the day
- ✷ Premenstrual migraines, more frequent migraines and/or tension headaches
- ✷ Rapid weight gain, difficulty losing weight, even with diet and exercise
- ✷ "Spare tire" around waist and middle; increased abdominal fat gain
- ✷ Food cravings, especially for sweets and simple carbohydrate foods
- ✷ Aching joints, cold hands and feet
- ✷ Thinning scalp hair, or increased hair loss on scalp, underarms and legs
- ✷ Facial hair increased
- ✷ Muscle soreness, stiffness, fibromyalgia pain syndrome
- ✷ Memory and concentration problems that are worse before menses
- ✷ Mood swings, episodic tearfulness for no reason, irritability, angry outbursts, and spells of feeling depressed especially premenstrually
- ✷ Palpitations, especially those that get worse a few days prior to menses and during bleeding days when estradiol is low or falling
- ✷ Anxiety attacks, worse around menses
- ✷ "Spiking" blood pressure, higher blood pressure than normal
- ✷ More "irritable bowel" problems prior to menses and during menses
- ✷ Dry, itchy eyes
- ✷ Brittle, dry, splitting nails
- ✷ Skin becomes dry, crawly, and looser, less elastic due to decline in collagen, more wrinkles appear
- ✷ Vaginal dryness, pain with sex
- ✷ Loss of sex drive, difficulty having orgasm
- ✷ Worsening allergies, sensitivities to chemicals, perfumes
- ✷ Bladder changes: more infections, pain on urination, more frequent urination, urinary leakage
- ✷ Posture may become more slumped

©Elizabeth Lee Vliet, MD 2001-2005

Chapter 5

Theories About Causes

PCOS is such a heterogeneous disorder it is difficult to pin down a single cause. There are many proposed explanations and known contributing factors that can lead to PCOS, but the bottom line is that no one is certain what causes it. Because it presents in so many diverse ways, it is likely that there are multiple causes that produce the same end result of the typical hormone imbalances and metabolic disturbances.

Some Proposed Causes of PCOS

- genetic factors
- factors affecting fetal development
- environmental endocrine disruptors
- dietary endocrine disruptors
- autoimmune disorders–ovarian, adrenal, pancreatic and thyroid
- neuroendocrine dysfunction (hypothalamic-pituitary axis)
- ovarian dysfunction
- adrenal-ovarian dysfunction
- disorders of insulin secretion and action
- medications that increase prolactin
- lifestyle factors–smoking, alcohol, drugs, inactivity, poor nutrition

©Elizabeth Lee Vliet, MD 2001-2005

Your Family Tree: Genes Play a Role in PCOS

PCOS is known to cluster in families, and can lead to hormone imbalances, marked weight gain and increased risk of diabetes in both boys and girls.

Studies show the following examples of patterns in families:

- about half of the sisters of women with PCOS have high androgens and irregular menstrual cycles.
- PCOS sisters with high testosterone also have high insulin levels, more insulin resistance, and are more overweight than controls.
- More brothers of women with PCOS have elevated DHEA-s, high triglycerides, insulin resistance and obesity than do boys in control groups.

Interesting
While it seems PCOS can be genetic, a single gene or contributing factor has yet to be isolated.

These observations of family patterns have led to the search for a genetic abnormality causing PCOS. But studies so far have not found a single abnormal gene or chromosome that causes PCOS.

Rather, it appears that PCOS is just too complex to be caused by only one gene. It's hard to see how only one gene could cause everything from insulin resistance to obesity to infertility to high androgens.

We already know that *each* of the major problems seen in PCOS are individually linked to the presence of abnormal genes: obesity, ovarian dysfunction, hirsutism and other signs of excess androgens, insulin resistance. Most researchers today feel that many genes are likely involved to create the array of problems in PCOS.

You can get these genes from your father's side, from your mother's side, or as a combination of both—it doesn't appear that the genetic pattern is only transmitted via the mother's genes.

Evidence so far supports the pattern of inheritance we call autosomal dominant, and that genes involved lie on a chromosome other than sex (X,Y) chromosomes.

A recessive pattern of inheritance means you need to get two of the genes for the disorder, one from each parent, before you would get it.

Several genetic patterns in PCOS families have been described:

Type A Syndrome

Involves mutations in the insulin receptors and/or how they work after they are activated. Individuals with these mutations have severe insulin resistance, elevated androgens, and *acanthosis nigricans* (darkening of the skin in various areas).

It isn't surprising that genetic mutations in the insulin pathway can lead to the findings we see in women with PCOS. We know that excess insulin stimulates the ovaries to make more androgens, which causes the hirsutism, acne, metabolic and mood changes. High insulin also decreases SHBG production, which means there are higher levels of free androgens to do damage.

Type B Syndrome

Antibodies to the insulin receptor. These individuals tend to have elevated androgens but may not necessarily have all the other findings above.

Mutations of PPARγ system

PPARγ is the system involved in insulin-glucose regulation, called the *peroxisome proliferator-activated receptor gamma*. Individuals with these mutations typically have primary amenorrhea (lack of menses), infertility, hirsutism, acanthosis nigricans, and gestational diabetes.

Other Patterns of Genetic Abnormalities in PCOS:

Androgen Receptor mutations

Women with PCOS have a much higher frequency of abnormal sequences in the gene that oversees development and function of the androgen receptors. If the

Genetics 101: A dominant pattern means that you only need one of the genes from one parent to get the disorder.

receptors don't work properly, the body has to produce higher levels of androgens to compensate for impaired receptor function.

Mutations in SHBG formation

Women with PCOS have a higher frequency of abnormal changes in the gene that codes for SHBG production. If SHBG levels are too low, it causes higher free androgens, and more of the androgen excess problems like hirsutism and ovarian dysfunction.

Ovarian hormone pathway

Another possible genetic mechanism involves how hormones are produced by cells in the ovaries. For example, women with PCOS have been found to have an *up-regulation* of hormone production by the theca cells in the ovaries, which suggests that genetic abnormalities in PCOS affects signaling pathways that control how a family of genes gets expressed in the individual.

Leptin

There is current research looking at a possible link between genetic mutations involving leptin and the development of PCOS. Leptin was first identified in 1994 and is a hormone in the hypothalamus that is believed to control appetite and our body's fat stores by telling you when you have had enough to eat.

Low leptin normally triggers the urge to eat and store body fat; high level should turn off the urge to eat. But some obese people actually have high leptin levels, so researchers now think there is a condition of leptin resistance that is similar to insulin resistance. Leptin links with PCOS are still uncertain, but there is a great deal of ongoing research on this connection.

Other pathways

Recent research has found genetic abnormalities in genes affecting formation of *tumor necrosis factor receptor (TNF-R), aldehyde dehydrogenase 6, and retinol dehydrogenase 2.* Over-expression of these genes in the ovarian theca cells of women with PCOS can lead to many of the abnormal metabolic and hormonal problems we see in patients.

Other Genetic Disorders:

Congenital Adrenal Hyperplasia (CAH)

CAH results from inherited deficiencies in several enzymes involved in the adrenal androgen pathway. Many of the body changes that occur in CAH overlap what we see in PCOS, but the necessary treatment approaches may differ. That's why it is important in the diagnostic evaluation to try and distinguish these disorders, although sometimes it isn't a clear-cut distinction. I describe CAH in greater detail in Chapter 9.

CAH: This syndrome results in over-production of androgens by the adrenal glands

Androgen-producing Tumors

These may occur in either the adrenal gland or the ovary, and can be benign or malignant. Women with such tumors typically have markedly elevated androgens, significantly increased LH secretion, and the body changes that occur with these hormone imbalances: irregular menses, excess body hair, acne, middle body weight gain and insulin resistance.

Women who have tumors like this tend to have more rapid weight gain, more severe symptoms, and more rapid onset than is typical of PCOS. While they can be dangerous if left untreated, such tumors generally are treatable and symptoms resolve with proper treatment.

Cushing's Disease

This disorder has many characteristics in common with PCOS, such as obesity, irregular menses, high levels of androgens, insulin resistance, mood changes, diabetes and hypertension. It can be caused by adrenal or pituitary dysfunction or tumors. Cushing's Syndrome (also called pseudo-Cushing's) can develop when people take long-term corticosteroids such as prednisone and others for treatment of asthma, arthritis, Crohn's disease, Lupus, or similar problems. I explain this disorder in more detail in Chapter 9, to help you understand how to distinguish it from PCOS.

Cushing's Characterized by excess production of the adrenal cortical hormone, cortisol.

What advantages could there be for PCOS to be inherited?

At first glance, it may seem strange that a disorder with so many damaging effects could be inherited, particularly in a *dominant pattern*. But if you look at the long history of human evolution, it really isn't so strange. The types of genetic changes that result in what we now call PCOS actually serve to make it easier for human females to be able to store food as body fat very efficiently.

Mother Nature's plan
It was not so bad for early humans' survival... until we interfered with our invention of high fat, high sugar, readily available food!

During early human evolution, food was typically very scarce. If humans did not have an efficient fat-storing system to provide fuel when food wasn't available, then they starved to death.

Women have to have a certain minimum amount of body fat to be fertile and sustain a pregnancy. In earlier times of food scarcity, women who could store more fat would then be able to preserve their ability to become pregnant even if there was a famine.

It is only with modern Western civilizations and plentiful food that these genetic changes are now a *disadvantage* and lead to serious health problems from excess fat storage such as diabetes, high blood pressure, heart attacks, and certain cancers.

Why is it so hard to determine the genetic links in PCOS?

- Researchers and physicians haven't yet agreed upon a set definition of what makes up PCOS. If we can't define it with a universally accepted definition, we can't know what to study as possible genetic markers.
- There isn't any identified, specific genetic marker for PCOS at this time.
- There isn't just one way that PCOS presents in its outward appearance (called *phenotype*): for example. Thus, the appearance doesn't alert us to a specific abnormal genetic makeup (called *genotype*).

In 1999, Dr. Ibanez proposed that possibly one of the very earliest recognizable phenotypes of PCOS is the onset of premature puberty, also called *precocious puberty* in girls younger than 8 years old.

❧ The data we have so far also suggests that even though the genes involved may be dominant, they have low penetration so that not everyone shows up with the disorder.

❧ We do know that many "endocrine disrupting" chemicals that I discuss later in the chapter can cause damage to a baby's developing endocrine system while in the womb. There is strong evidence that these same chemicals can also cause new genetic mutations. This makes it even harder to pin down exact genetic causes, since new ones may be emerging all the time as a result of humans being increasingly exposed to environmental and dietary chemicals.

❧ We don't yet know for certain what all the characteristics are when PCOS occurs in boys and men, so we don't know what genetic markers in the males may be "red flags" for problems in women.

❧ Since PCOS commonly causes infertility and high rates of miscarriages, families with PCOS tend to be small. Genetic patterns show up more easily when there are very large families with many children in each generation to study.

❧ Collecting *accurate* family history information is difficult. I often find that my patients don't know all the health problems of their family members to be able to give me this information.

In Summary:

So you can see that the job of genetic detective is a very difficult one when it comes to PCOS. The bottom line at this point is that we do know that PCOS can be caused by genetic abnormalities, and *it can also be caused by various environmental factors.*

PCOS very likely results from the *interaction* of a primary

Many Facets of PCOS: Women with PCOS can be fat or thin, may have excess or normal body hair, may have early or late puberty, may have difficulty getting pregnant or no problem getting pregnant... the variation is enormous.

genetic mutation in insulin function and/or ovarian androgen production *with* environmental exposure to chemicals that make this worse, or other environmental factors such as stress, poor nutrition, smoking, inactivity, etc. I describe these factors in the rest of this chapter.

What Happens in the Womb Can Affect You Later

I am sure that most readers have heard a great deal about the risks to the baby when pregnant women drink alcohol or smoke tobacco or marijuana. Most of the focus has been on Fetal Alcohol Syndrome causing babies that have later learning problems, or the risks of low birth weight babies and later risk of lung cancer in children of women who smoke.

Did you also know that there are a number of environmental, hormonal and drug related factors during pregnancy that can increase daughters' risks of PCOS and infertility when they reach puberty?

There are many areas of research to explore these connections and risk factors. New information is unfolding rapidly in this field. I have summarized key issues that you need to know if you are thinking about becoming pregnant, or if you are trying to piece together the puzzle of your own health picture to figure out what may have contributed to your own PCOS.

High Androgens During Pregnancy— Infertility and PCOS Later

I explained earlier in the chapter that genetic studies alone don't explain the prevalence of PCOS or the many different ways it can present in different women. This led researchers to look at other mechanisms in the womb that might explain the later health and fertility problems that occur in PCOS.

One area of exciting research is the adverse effects on the fetus when there are high levels of androgens dur-

Warning!
I feel strongly that if you see your daughter showing signs of pubic hair and breast development before age 8, she needs a thorough endocrine evaluation and checks for insulin resistance that can be the precursor to PCOS.

ing pregnancy. The Rhesus monkey is the model used to study these connections because their 28-day menstrual cycle is so similar to humans, and their growth and reproductive life cycle is also similar to humans. I will summarize here the key points that we know at this time.

If Rhesus monkeys have high levels of testosterone, DHEA and DHEA-s during pregnancy, their offspring develop changes that are almost exactly like the characteristic PCOS changes that we see in human females. The types of later changes that occur in the offspring depend on the timing during pregnancy when the baby is exposed to high androgens, and on how high the androgen levels are.

Researchers have looked at early and late effects of testosterone injected in Rhesus monkeys carrying female fetuses. Early androgen excess (days 40–60 of pregnancy) coincides with when the ovaries, pancreas and neuroendocrine development occur in monkeys. High androgen levels cause abnormal development in all of these areas.

Androgen excess later in pregnancy, (after day 100 in monkeys) coincides with development of ovarian follicles and the development of normal sensitivity of the hypothalamus to hormone feedback in regulating the menstrual cycle. If high levels of androgens are present in pregnant monkeys at this time, it causes changes in the hypothalamus that can lead to persistent high levels of LH secretion in the offspring. Over 70% of human PCOS patients also show high levels of LH.

Female offspring exposed to high androgens during critical times in pregnancy appear to have permanent changes in how their androgen receptors work, as well as how many androgen receptors there are. These offspring also have increased abdominal fat deposits, exhibit abnormal insulin secretion and action, and have increased risk of diabetes as they get older—just like we see in women with PCOS.

Read more:
To see more on this, refer to the 2005 review article by Dr. Dumesic and colleagues listed in the Bibliography.

Do IT!
Get *all your family medical history* summarized *now*, while people are still alive and can give you accurate information.
Then keep this information with your own medical history. You never know when it will be needed.

It appears that androgen excess during pregnancy can cause a combination of metabolic and reproductive abnormalities during fetal development in the womb that is capable of also impairing the quality of the oocytes (future "eggs") in the developing fetal ovary, leading to the observed difficulties in ovulation and fertility later in life.

The bottom line is that *high androgen levels at critical hormonally-sensitive times in fetal development can cause a whole cascade of effects on multiple organ systems* in the baby that later lead to the phenotype, or appearance, that we call PCOS: delayed onset of menses, ovarian dysfunction at puberty, loss of ovulatory cycles, enlarged cystic ovaries, excess androgen and insulin production, insulin resistance, and increased risk of diabetes.

These studies of monkeys have provided direct evidence that the hormonal environment of intrauterine life has a profound effect on programming the differentiation—normal or abnormal—of hormone target tissues in the developing baby. This means that it is possible for genetic or environmental causes of excess androgens during pregnancy to lead to abnormal development in the fetus, and cause PCOS later in life.

The following chart shows how excess androgens during pregnancy can have so many different effects on the developing baby and lead to the problems we see in PCOS later in life.

Nutrition During Pregnancy and Later Risk of PCOS

You may have already read that mothers with gestational diabetes tend to have high birth weight babies, and the concern has been that these babies are then at higher risk for diabetes themselves as they get older. It may surprise you that current studies also find that a low birth weight baby can be at greater risk for obesity, insulin resistance and PCOS later. We don't fully understand why both extremes of body weight can lead to insulin–glucose problems later.

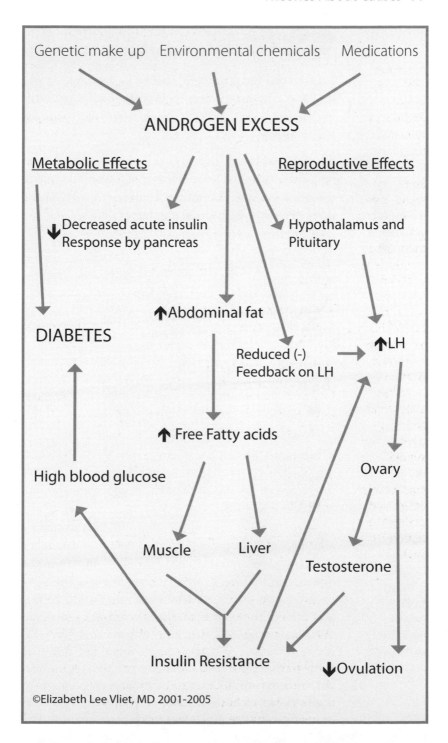

Genetic make up   Environmental chemicals   Medications

ANDROGEN EXCESS

Metabolic Effects   Reproductive Effects

↓Decreased acute insulin
Response by pancreas

Hypothalamus and
Pituitary

↑Abdominal fat

DIABETES

Reduced (-)
Feedback on LH   →   ↑LH

↑ Free Fatty acids

High blood glucose   Ovary

Muscle   Liver

Testosterone

Insulin Resistance   ↓Ovulation

©Elizabeth Lee Vliet, MD 2001-2005

Smoking Affects More Than Lungs... Effects Long After the Womb

I doubt you have thought about the fact that if you smoke during pregnancy, you may be causing infertility later for your children! This is particularly true for female babies.

Heads Up

Smoking makes it even harder for you to get pregnant.

Specialists think this occurs because both tobacco and marijuana contain chemicals that actually kill some of the developing baby's primordial follicles. Since the baby isn't born with the normal number of follicles, she has a harder time getting pregnant later.

These chemicals also appear to cause damage to hypothalamic-pituitary centers that regulate the ovarian cycles when the child enters puberty and can increase the risk for abnormal LH function that in turn can increase the risk of later PCOS.

Lifestyle Factors that Increase Risk for PCOS

- current dietary issues/weight gain
- lack of physical activity
- smoking
- early alcohol use
- other drug use

Heads Up!

Smokers are more likely to have significant fetal growth-retardation, causing smaller babies more likely to be born prematurely.

Most researchers don't think that PCOS *is caused* by poor lifestyle choices, but we do know that a number of dietary and lifestyle habits can make PCOS worse if you already have it, or have a genetic susceptibility to developing it. That's why it's so important to pay attention to these issues and make sure that you make choices that are as healthy as possible.

Cigarette Smoking

For women with PCOS, cigarette smoking is even more deadly than it is for other women. Smoking cigarettes by itself can lead to difficulty getting pregnant and even infertility, as well as causing *premature* menopause in women as young as 30.

In women smokers, most of the problems seen in PCOS can occur independently due to smoking alone. If you are genetically predisposed to developing PCOS, cigarette smoking accelerates the onset of PCOS, increases the damage to your ovaries. Smoking cigarettes makes a bad situation even worse.

The more you smoke, the more follicles you kill off. Women are born with all the follicles they will ever have. When they are gone, they are *permanently* gone. When you lose your follicles you lose your ovaries' main hormone-producing factories too. That means lower estradiol levels, lack of ovulation and rise in progesterone, and more frequent abnormal menstrual cycles.

Loss of follicles also means difficulty getting pregnant, and less chance of fertility treatment being successful. Multiple studies from many different countries over the past forty years have shown the relationship between smoking cigarettes and impaired fertility.

As far back as 1985 one study showed women who smoked cigarettes, compared to non-smokers, were 57–75% *less likely* to conceive, depending on how much they smoked. Women smokers who go through in-vitro fertilization and other assisted reproduction techniques have lower success rates than non-smokers. Many women with PCOS have to undergo fertility treatment. Remember that smoking decreases your chances of success.

Female children born to mothers who smoked during pregnancy have more problems later conceiving their own children, even if they themselves do not smoke. Specialists think this occurs because smoking during pregnancy actually kills some of the developing baby's primordial follicles. Since the baby isn't born with the normal number of follicles, she has a harder time getting pregnant later.

Most patients and many physicians still do not know that cigarette smoking, as well as chronic exposure

Tobacco Warning: Many components of cigarette smoke cause cancer, and are *directly toxic* to the follicles in your ovaries. Smokers have much higher rates of infertility than non-smokers.

Warning: Women who smoke have a greater risk of recurrent ovarian cysts.

to second-hand smoke, causes earlier menopause, five to seven years sooner than nonsmokers. Doctors may say, "I never heard of this problem," but medical studies showing this connection were published over *thirty years ago!* Women smokers have symptoms from the decline in levels of estradiol for many years before periods stop.

Killing off your follicles by smoking cigarettes aggravates the problems of PCOS, and further decreases your hormone production, along with loss of fertility. Lower hormone levels also mean less energy, loss of sex drive, loss of mental sharpness, poor sleep, and an immune system that doesn't work as well.

Alcohol

Over many years, studies from a number of countries have consistently shown that alcohol use can lead to irregular menstrual cycles, lower production of estradiol, and earlier onset of menopause because it impairs the brain's GnRH pulse generator that triggers proper release of FSH and LH. This in turn causes low estradiol and decline in ovarian function. Estradiol and testosterone levels decline earlier in women who drink alcohol regularly, which leads to a rise in FSH at younger ages.

Menstrual cycle length is more variable in drinkers than non-drinkers. Some cycles are long, some are short, and there are more skipped cycles. Women drinkers also have more cycles with no ovulation. Women with PCOS already have these problems. Alcohol makes them worse.

Alcohol acts like a simple sugar in the body, causing a rise in blood sugar level after you drink it, followed later by a drop in blood sugar called *reactive hypoglycemia.* This drop in blood sugar is then a powerful trigger for craving more alcohol to quickly raise blood glucose. So, alcohol makes your body have even more difficulty responding normally to glucose.

All the symptoms from falling or low blood sugar—anxiety, restlessness, low energy, palpitations, etc.—are relieved quickly by alcohol, and you feel better for a short while after you drink. Then as alcohol levels drop, blood sugar falls, the symptoms return, and you crave alcohol (sugar) again. It becomes a vicious cycle, made much worse by the excess insulin produced in PCOS.

Menstrual cycle hormone changes can further increase alcohol cravings and trigger alcohol abuse in a large percentage of women. When progesterone rises, it causes less sensitivity to insulin, blood sugar drops, and you crave more "carbs" and simple sugars.

Then when estradiol and progesterone fall just before bleeding begins, the hormone drop triggers a fall in your "feel good" brain chemicals, endorphins and serotonin. The fall in these chemical messengers causes blue moods, irritability, low energy, anxiety, insomnia.

Alcohol also affects metabolism of the hormones you take in birth control pills, which makes them less effective in suppressing the abnormal hormone production in PCOS. This also adds another factor to the potential for alcohol cravings.

Alcohol intake is an *independent* risk factor for breast cancer, which means the increased risk is not due to other variables, such as total calories, fat, fiber, vitamins or whether you take hormones.

The *age* at which you begin drinking is important; the earlier you start drinking, the greater your risk, regardless of how much you drink later in life. Risk of breast cancer is greatest if regular drinking begins during the vulnerable time of breast development in your teens. Girls with PCOS should avoid drinking alcohol on a regular basis.

You may have heard that alcohol lowers the risk of heart disease. This positive effect occurs primarily in men, *not women*. In women, there was a slight decrease in heart disease risk at the lowest levels of alcohol use

Heads up!
Even just *three or more drinks per week* can increase breast cancer risk from 20 to 70 percent.

Problem:
Many women "treat" these mood changes and low energy with a glass of wine, beer or liquor. The vicious cycle continues.

Warning
To break the vicious cycle, you have to stop alcohol *and* treat the hormone imbalance at the same time.

Don't Smoke! Female children born to mothers who smoked tobacco or marijuana during pregnancy have more infertility, even if they themselves do not smoke.

Warning: Smoking pot only makes the menstrual irregularities and fertility problems of PCOS much worse.

Warning! If you are struggling with the problems of PCOS, don't add pot to the picture!

each week, but a marked increase in deaths from heart disease at higher levels of alcohol use per week. For men, the risk of heart disease decreased significantly even in the higher ranges of alcohol intake.

Women's bodies don't have as much of the enzyme needed to break down alcohol easily like men do, so women are more at risk than men for the damaging effects from alcohol. This is especially true if you have PCOS. With all the negative effects on your ovaries, fertility, mood, sleep, memory and body weight, I very strongly encourage you to minimize alcohol use.

Marijuana

Marijuana disrupts brain centers that regulate hormone production in both males and females. Extracts of marijuana plants contain chemicals that compete with estradiol for binding at the estrogen receptor, which interferes with the normal effects of our own body estradiol.

Women who smoke marijuana regularly also have disturbances in ovulation. Marijuana interferes with luteinizing hormone (LH) so that it doesn't rise at mid-cycle to trigger ovulation. The end result is that marijuana use decreases your own estradiol production, and also competes with the estradiol you do produce for binding space at the estrogen receptor. Women with PCOS that I see in my clinical practice already have low estradiol, so using marijuana makes the situation even worse.

The lower levels of estradiol and progesterone in marijuana users also causes more anxiety and insomnia, so you then smoke more pot to "calm down" and once again, you have a vicious cycle: more pot use leads to more suppression of the ovaries and lower hormone levels, lower hormone levels cause more anxiety and sleep disturbance, so you smoke more pot to help you feel better...and the cycle goes on and on.

Marijuana also increases prolactin, which is already higher in many women with PCOS. High prolactin suppresses normal menstrual cycle and ovarian hormone production. It's another vicious cycle that keeps on going and going unless you stop the pot.

THC and other chemicals in marijuana disrupt normal immune function, leading to more episodes of colds, flu, and chronic "infections" that don't seem to go away. Women with PCOS already have some of these problems due to low estradiol, androgen and insulin excess that adversely affect immune function.

So this "recreational" drug is more damaging than you may have realized. Bottom line? You need to break the cycle by stopping marijuana use.

Medications Making PCOS Worse

Mood Managers

"Serotonin enhancers" (SSRIs) and "mood stabilizers" are doled out to women rather like Lydia Pinkham's Tonic, a popular "women's remedy" in the early 1900s used to treat a host of "women's" ailments like anxiety, depressed mood, irritability, premenstrual problems, headaches, insomnia, low energy, muscle aches, excessive "worrying" and many others.

In women with PCOS, erratic menstrual cycles caused by androgen excess or lower than optimal estradiol or even thyroid disorders may cause "mood swings" that may get labeled "bipolar" illness. "Mood stabilizers" get prescribed without checking hormone levels. Then these medicines can disrupt neuroendocrine pathways that regulate the ovaries and also affect thyroid function.

Lexapro, Celexa, Prozac, Sarafem, Zoloft, Paxil, and Luvox are the most frequently prescribed group of medications for women under 50 in the United States. These mood-altering medicines have a reputation for being so safe and effective that they are commonly prescribed for FDA-approved reasons like depression, PMS, and

Warning: Marijuana use decreases your estradiol and causes loss of ovulation

Too Much? I do not think many of these drugs are really needed as often as they are prescribed for women.

Alert: SSRIs and "mood stabilizer" anticonvulsants further increase release of *prolactin* by action on a brain chemical messenger called dopamine.

obsessive-compulsive disorder, as well as many off-label, non FDA-approved uses, such as chronic pain, bulimia, attention deficit-hyperactivity disorder, borderline personality disorder, hypochondria, fibromyalgia, migraine headaches, and even social shyness.

SSRIs
Widely prescribed for so many problems, women often take them for years and are more likely to develop undesirable side effects.

Many women have symptoms such as those above for a variety of reasons, not purely "psychiatric" in origin. Endocrine problems—for example, low estradiol, high androgens of PCOS, low thyroid—cause many of the same symptoms. You need to know whether your symptoms are caused by hormone imbalance—and need a hormone approach to treatment, or whether you have a psychiatric problem that may need a psychotropic medication.

65%–70% of all SSRI prescriptions are written for women, more often by primary care physicians, gynecologists, neurologists, and rheumatologists. Only about 10% of these prescriptions are written by psychiatrists.

As a result of being used for so many conditions other than depression, and being prescribed by non-psychiatrists, doses are now often larger than originally studied, and medicines are commonly combined with many other prescriptions leading to more side effects from drug interactions.

Their effects can mask other health issues, including other causes of similar symptoms. Used over a number of years these medicines may have subtle side effects on ovarian function that you, and possibly your doctor, haven't realized because doctors don't routinely test for levels of the pituitary hormone, prolactin. If prolactin is too high, it suppresses ovarian cycles and ovulation, already a problem for most women with PCOS.

High prolactin occurs normally during nursing and it serves to decrease the normal FSH–LH regulation of the menstrual cycle, suppress return of ovarian cycles and ovarian hormone production, helping prevent another pregnancy while a mother is still nursing a new infant.

If you have PCOS, and already have irregular periods, any medicine that increases prolactin can, over time, cause more menstrual irregularity, a decrease in the ovarian hormones estradiol, progesterone, and difficulty getting pregnant.

High prolactin also causes weight gain, breast enlargement, milky discharge from the breasts, headaches, fatigue, low libido, scalp hair loss, and depressed mood. All of these symptoms are also caused by PCOS endocrine and metabolic disturbances.

If you are on a mood stabilizer, or a tricyclic antidepressant or a serotonin-booster medication and have any of these symptoms, ask your doctor to do a blood test for prolactin. If your prolactin is too high, talk with your doctor about medication changes.

Lithium is another psychotropic medicine that can cause more problems in women with PCOS. Lithium can cause hypothyroidism by interfering with the manufacture of thyroid hormones, and this causes weight gain, low energy, and depressed mood. More weight gain makes insulin resistance worse. Higher insulin levels trigger more androgen production by the ovaries, and the PCOS gets worse.

Alert: More lithium causes more thyroid dysfunction, more weight gain, more lethargy, and more depression.

If you already have a weight problem from PCOS, taking lithium can be a double whammy because it tends to cause weight gain and thyroid dysfunction that leads to more weight gain…and the vicious cycle spirals out of control.

Low thyroid function then interferes with ovarian hormones, so if you have PCOS, the hormone imbalances get worse. But the hormone levels aren't usually checked, even though the mood symptoms may be actually caused by these hormone swings. Women are typically just given more lithium to deal with the worsening mood problems.

Don't be complacent about these medicines just because they are so widely used. Make sure that you get properly tested for PCOS before assuming that "mood" symptoms are due to a psychiatric disorder alone. Review the potential problems carefully before you turn to these mood pills as a "magic bullets."

Beta-blockers

Beta-blockers are often used for migraine headaches, mitral valve prolapse, some types of anxiety, and to control blood pressure. While these are safe medicines overall, they have some unique problems for women with PCOS, especially if taken for a long time.

Beta-blockers can inhibit the conversion of T4 to T3, leading to symptoms of hypothyroidism that can cause weight gain, fatigue, and depression, as well as disruption in ovarian function. Beta-blockers also impair glucose-insulin pathways, leading to problems with insulin resistance, and even diabetes.

Weight gain, marked fatigue, difficulty concentrating, and decreased sex drive are common with beta-blockers, even if your hormones are in balance. Women with PCOS already have many of these problems, so the medication side effects can make the symptoms and hormone imbalances even worse.

High progestin birth control pills

The progestins in birth control pills, particularly those pills with high progestin-low estrogen formulas, are common causes of fatigue, depression, headaches, low libido, muscle and joint pain, vaginal dryness or vulvar pain. Many of these same problems occur in PCOS, and can be aggravated by high progestin pills.

I think it is important to use birth control pills with the least amount of progestin that will keep the ovaries suppressed. I find it also helps reduce unwanted side effects to use pills that have a better estrogen content relative to the progestin. I discuss this in more detail in Chapter 10.

Remember: Plants can produce potent poisons that humans have used for killing animals (and other people) for thousands of years.

Warning: If you have PCOS, don't take soy or other phyto-estrogen supplements, especially if you are trying to conceive.

Progestin-only contraceptives like Depo-Provera or Norplant are even worse for aggravating depression and weight gain, because they contain only progestin and no estrogen. Progestin-only contraceptives act to further suppress your own estradiol production, and can make the PCOS problems markedly worse.

Soy, Supplements, Herbs and OTC Hormones

Women today are inundated with articles, ads, and multi-level sales schemes pitching a myriad of herbs, soy-containing products, "natural" progesterone-"wild yam" creams, over-the-counter forms of DHEA and melatonin—all touted as other "magic bullets" for PCOS, PMS, and menopause.

Women have the mistaken belief, reinforced by clever marketing, that everything labeled "natural" is automatically "safe" and without side effects. This is not correct.

Many types of herbs and supplements have the potential to cause harmful effects, particularly if you already have hormone problems, or a thyroid disorder, or allergies to plants and pollen, or any problems with liver metabolism.

Taking phytoestrogen supplements does not provide or restore what your ovary made. All of the phytoestrogen chemical building blocks require chemical conversion in the laboratory because our body does not have the enzymes to make these changes.

Even worse, high concentrations of phytoestrogens, such as soy or red clover isoflavones, can overwhelm your declining estradiol at receptor sites and interfere with the action and production of the body's "natural" estradiol. Even though phytoestrogens are less potent than estradiol, if you are taking the high concentrations in supplements, it overcomes the lower potency of the phytoestrogens.

Be aware: All these seemingly innocuous medicines and herbs may affect your ovarian and thyroid hormone balance.

Believe it! Your body cannot make the bio-identical human ovarian estradiol from the phyto-estrogens in soy or yams.

In addition to these receptor effects, studies also show high soy intake in premenopausal women suppresses ovary production of estradiol and progesterone by 20–50 percent. That's a significant loss, especially if you are already dealing with infertility as a result of PCOS.

Summary

Remember, from genes to soybeans and a lot inbetween, there are many hidden saboteurs of ovarian function, particularly in women with PCOS. You can't do much about your genes, but you certainly can do a lot to choose lifestyle habits that don't make you worse!

And you can avoid the tendency to want a "magic bullet" pill for every ailment. Keep your medicines to a minimum, and read carefully about the side effects of new medications that are recommended for you.

Adverse medication effects, as well as drug-drug interactions, and herb-drug interactions are far more common than most people, physicians included, realize.

WARNING: *Always* tell your physicians at *every* appointment all the supplements, herbs or over-the-counter products you are using.

Remember, herbs may be wildly popular today, but many are metabolized by the same liver pathways that metabolize prescription medicines. Taking them together can significantly change the rate of breakdown, and make prescription medicines much less effective.

Women with PCOS have to be even more careful about what herbs and supplements they take. Before you buy more supplements, take time to check a reliable resource for any adverse effects.

In addition, insist on having your hormones properly checked when you start having symptoms, before you start on a lot of medicines to treat symptoms one at a time. I describe in Chapter 8 what tests to ask for, and what optimal ranges typically are.

A good resource is *The Comprehensive Database of Natural Medicines* (www.naturaldatabase.com) available by subscription and published by a team of pharmacists who review the worldwide research to provide an authoritative guide to the safety and effectiveness of thousands of over-the-counter supplements. This is an independent source of information, free of the bias that can be there when people are selling products.

Let your doctor know about any herbal supplements you take, just as you would any other medications, so that if you develop problems, he or she has all the information to properly evaluate your symptoms.

Keep in mind that physicians have many patients to see each day. They may not always remember, or think to ask you, what supplements or herbs you take.

Make a list and take it to your doctor's appointment, and be sure to include what is actually in each supplement, not just the product name.

It is for *your* health and safety that you need to help your doctor have the information s/he needs to be able to help you.

We still don't know all the causes of PCOS. But you can't wait for research to have all the answers. You need to improve your health now, based on what we do know at this point.

Just DO it!

Take steps to reduce the causes of hormone problems I have described here. Then review Chapters 10–12 for additional ways to help you feel better.

You are worth it!

Chapter 6
Environmental *Endocrine Disruptors:* Emerging Causes of PCOS

Environmental and Dietary Chemicals During Pregnancy—Gender Benders for the Children

For many years, I have been interested in the links between environmental chemicals and how they affect our endocrine system. There are many synthetic, man-made chemicals that we call *endocrine disruptors* because of their adverse hormone-like effects in our bodies.

Although these chemicals may have estrogenic or androgenic effects, their effects are consistently negative because they interfere with the normal function of many hormone systems. They disrupt our body systems because they are not the same as the hormones produced by our bodies, and because our bodies do not have the ability to readily metabolize these chemicals, making them difficult to clear out of the body and therefore very long-lasting.

These chemicals can sabotage and disrupt our own hormone systems, which is why they are often called "gender-benders." They damage and distort the reproductive systems of *all species tested to date.*

Endocrine-disrupting compounds increase the risk of a variety of non-cancerous problems like PCOS, infertility, endometriosis. They can also contribute to development of cancers, such as breast and uterine in women, prostate and testicular cancers in men, and bladder cancers in both sexes.

Warning
Environmental chemicals can sabotage and disrupt your hormone balance.

A mother exposed to these chemicals may not have any adverse effects at all, or if there are negative effects, they would not have the same degree of serious damage that can occur in a developing baby, particularly if the exposure comes at the time in pregnancy during which the brain or reproductive organs are developing.

Alarming Trend:

I am convinced that exposure to these endocrine disruptors contributes to the alarming rise in female infertility, ovarian cysts, PCOS, premature ovarian decline or failure, and immune disorders that I have been seeing in my medical practice.

Xenos is a Greek word meaning foreign or different. *Xenobiotics* refers to a whole group of chemical compounds that are man-made, foreign to the body and have generally toxic or damaging biological effects to living organisms.

These chemicals are called *xenoestrogens* if they interact with the estrogen receptors in our body, *xenoandrogens* if they affect the androgen receptors, and *xenoprogestins* if they act at progesterone receptors. Some endocrine-disrupting chemicals have mixed effects, acting at more than just the sex hormone receptors to adversely affect all our hormone pathways.

Some are known carcinogens; some don't seem to cause cancer, but all can damage endocrine pathways. Most have never even been studied to determine any cancer-causing effects, much less toxicity to reproductive, brain and hormone function.

These synthetic chemicals have been found in the body fat and breast milk of humans throughout the world, as well as mammals on land and in the oceans, fish, birds, reptiles and amphibians.

Endocrine-disrupting chemicals adversely affecting health include dioxin, pesticide DDT, its breakdown product DDE, polychlorinated biphenyls (PCBs) and many others.

This is a complicated subject and there aren't clear answers. I feel it is critical to discuss this in a book about PCOS because there are profound implications for you as a woman, and for your children. It may help to think about what chemical exposures you may have had that could be a factor in your developing PCOS.

Endocrine Disrupters—Where They Are and What They Do

These man-made chemicals belong to a group of environmental pollutants that are part of a larger class of both naturally-occurring and synthetic molecules that can act like hormones in the body, although they are not really true hormones. Because these man-made compounds, unlike natural ones, persist for decades or even centuries in the environment without being broken down, they are also called *persistent organic pollutants*, or POPs.

POPs may accentuate or disrupt, or completely alter or even block actions of multiple body hormones, not just estrogen. These compounds may mimic or block estrogen, testosterone, thyroid, insulin or other hormones, so POPs can affect everything in our body that is governed by our hormones…which means just about our entire body!

Whack!
POPs pack a wallop to our endocrine system and hence our bodies

The number of chemicals with this endocrine-disrupting effect seems to grow almost daily; at this writing we know of several hundred, but that's just the ones that have been studied. There are potentially thousands more. Toxicology studies that were done before these compounds are put on the market focus only on cancer-causing effects, so we don't know what other endocrine effects there may be.

In animal studies and cultures of human ovary cells, many of these chemicals kill ovarian follicles: the medical term is follicular toxicants. If your follicles are killed prematurely, it may cause infertility or frequent ovarian cysts, or even premature menopause.

We know men's sperm counts worldwide are lower now, and experts think this is the result of exposure to pollution that includes these endocrine disrupting chemicals. Women's "egg counts" are obviously hard to determine, so we don't have statistics about how these chemicals cause early death of ovarian follicles in women like we can determine sperm counts in men.

Chemicals with endocrine-modulating activity:

1. General categories:

A. Man-made chemicals

- ৶ industrial and household products, such as pesticides, cleaners, plasticizers, solvents (ex. DDT, DDE, PCB, PBB, PAH, TCDD, dioxins
- ৶ DEHA, toluene, xylene, perchloroethylene, etc.), triazine herbicides
- ৶ Pharmaceuticals like DES (diethylstilbestrol), cyclophosphamide (anticancer drug)
- ৶ Dietary supplements and food additives, such as MSG, glutamate, aspartate, cysteine, BHT, BHA (butylated hydroxyanisole)

B. Naturally-occurring compounds

- ৶ phytoestrogens in plants, such as soy and red clover
- ৶ phthalate esters
- ৶ heavy metals (neurotoxins): lead, mercury, arsenic, cadmium, gallium

2. Examples based on types of actions:

Estrogenic

- ৶ o,p'-DDT, Methoxychlor, Lindane (organochlorine pesticides), Endosulfan, Dieldrin, Toxaphene
- ৶ Kepone (estrogenic effects in male factory workers)
- ৶ Nonylphenols (also weak androgen agonist*)
- ৶ Bisphenol A
- ৶ DES
- ৶ Benzylbutylphthalate, dibutylphthalate
- ৶ Genistein, other isoflavones found in soy, clover, grains

Estrogen Blockers (Antiestrogenic)

- ৶ PCBs–(polychlorinated biphenyls)(isomers of DDT)
- ৶ Dioxin and related dibenzo-p-dioxins
- ৶ Dibenzofurans
- ৶ Compounds in cigarette smoke
- ৶ Genistein (both agonist and antagonist actions, depending on concentration), other isoflavones

Androgen Blockers (Antiandrogenic)

- ৶ P,p' DDE (metabolite of DDT), also DDT*
- ৶ Vinclozolin
- ৶ Atrazine
- ৶ Bisphenol A*
- ৶ Butyl benzyl phthalate*
  *based on recent data from Sohoni (see references)

©Elizabeth Lee Vliet, MD 2001-2005

Act By Other Mechanisms:

- ৯৬ Cyclophosphamide
- ৯৬ Benzo(a)pyrene, anthracenes
- ৯৬ Solvents-toluene, xylene, perchloroethylene)
- ৯৬ Methoxychlor
- ৯৬ Nitrous oxide ("laughing gas" anesthesia)
- ৯৬ Ethylene oxide
- ৯৬ Butadiene
- ৯৬ 4-vinyl cyclohexene
- ৯৬ Alkylphenols
- ৯৬ Phthalate esters
- ৯৬ Triazine herbicides (atrazine, simazine, cyanazine)
- ৯৬ Fungicides (Chlorothalonil, Maneb, Metiram, Thiram, Zineb, Ziram)
- ৯৬ Excitatory amino acids (glutamate, MSG, aspartate, etc.)

3. Examples Based on Type of Damage in Women

These are not all of the types of damages caused. I have listed the ones most relevant to women with PCOS:

Health Impact	Chemicals Found to Cause**
Breast Cancer	DDT, DDE, lindane, methoxychlor, PCB, TCDD, possibly DES, triazine herbicides (atrazine, simazine, cyanazine), others likely
Ovarian Cancer	DES, DDE, PCB triazine herbicides (most data is on atrazine), possibly many others
Infertility/impaired fertility	aromatic hydrocarbons in cigarette smoke, Isoflavones (soy, red clover), coumestrol, DES, glutamate, aspartate, cyclophosphamide, PCB, TCDD, PAH, heavy metals, nitrous oxide, organochlorines (DDT, DDE, Lindane, etc.), organic solvents, ethylene oxide, 4-vinyl cyclohexene butadiene
Menstrual irregularity	Isoflavones (soy, red clover), coumestrol, DDT, DDE, DES, glutamate, aspartate, Lindane, heavy metals, PCB, PAH, solvents, TCDD, DES, atrazine,
Increased miscarriages	Isoflavones (soy, red clover), coumestrol, DES, solvents, nitrous oxide, ethylene oxide, possibly others
Early menopause	cigarette smoke, phytoestrogens, DES, PAH, butadiene, 4-vinyl cyclohexene, possibly many others

©Elizabeth Lee Vliet, MD 2001-2005

Health Impact	Chemicals Found to Cause**
Endometriosis	Dioxins (many types), TCDD, PCB, DES
Reduced Lactation	DDE, DES, others not well studied
Osteopenia/Osteoporosis	Cadmium, lead, cigarette smoke chemicals
Thyroid Damage	isoflavones (soy, red clover, others), PCB, MSG, glutamate, aspartate, phytates, iodine deficiency, (iodine metabolism disrupted by a number of these compounds), insecticides (DDT, DDE, Lindane, others)
Immune Damage	PCB, dioxins; dieldrin, may be others. Greater adverse impact on infant with immature immune system when chemicals passed in breast milk
Hypothalamic-Pituitary Dysfunction	heavy metals, PCB, DES, excitatory amino acids (glutamate, aspartate, cystoic acid, MSG), triazine herbicides (atrazine, etc.)

** Based on studies in animals, humans or both

©Elizabeth Lee Vliet, MD 2001-2005

Endocrine disruptors affect the ovarian pathways in another way: many of them cause profound damage to the thyroid, our master metabolic regulator that affects the function of just about everything in the body. Some interfere with iodine metabolism, which can cause hypothyroidism as well as breast and ovarian cysts.

Why NOW?

Current generations of young women are more affected than their mothers and grandmothers because none of these organic compounds existed before the 1930s. Pre-1930s people simply were not exposed to such an incredible array of synthetic chemicals. Most have been invented in the "chemical age" that started just prior to World War II.

The 1940s and 1950s are when the world's living beings were first exposed to these pesticides and industrial chemicals on a wide scale. Subtle disruptions in hormones and reproduction began to appear.

Rachel Carson first warned of these problems in her classic book *Silent Spring* in 1962. She wrote eloquently of the reproductive damage in wildlife from the pesticide DDT. DDT *use* was banned in the United States in 1972 but it is still *manufactured* here for export to countries around the world where it is still in widespread use. Beyond what it does there, DDT then comes back to us on the winds, oceans, rain and imported foods to continue its dirty work in our bodies.

If you were born after 1972, you were exposed to DDT from residues in your mother's body fat that flowed across the placenta. As an infant you were getting DDT residues in either human breast or cows milk, since cattle that had eaten grains and grasses with DDT residues would have the persistent chemical in their body fat to then leach into their milk, just as in human breast milk. Most Americans alive today carry some DDT residues because it is stored in the environment and the body for decades.

In the body, DDT is metabolized to a compound called DDE. Recent research shows that DDE is an *antiandrogen* that blocks testosterone from activating its receptor complex. This receptor blockade causes many adverse affects in males. We don't know all the potential adverse reproductive effects DDE has in women because *no research has been done on women.*

We know that DDE leads to abnormal testosterone production and action, and DDE may also lead to mutations in the androgen receptor. All of these changes in testosterone and androgen function can contribute to the problems of PCOS.

For example, if testosterone can't activate its receptor normally, the body may compensate by producing excess androgens to overcome the block. Then the androgen excess causes the problems we see in other body systems in women with PCOS.

The problem has *not* gone away since *Silent Spring* was published. It has, in fact, gotten far worse and more ominous today. Creative chemists have gone on to exponentially increase the problem by creating even more deadly and persistent chemicals in thousands of common products used daily.

A New Era: From roughly 1970 through the 1990s, the *first human generation ever* exposed to DDT and other POPs during fetal life began reaching their own reproductive age.

DDT Exposure *All* of us born prior to 1972 were exposed to DDT in our diet because DDT was commonly found in dairy products, meats, and vegetables sprayed with it.

What are some of these chemicals?

They make up an alphabet soup of toxic compounds: common ones include DDT, DDE, DES, TCDD, BHA, PCB, PBB, PAH, CCA. There are hundreds more that are not normally found in nature and cause damage to living organisms. Their longer names are all listed in the charts (pages 108–109), grouped by categories of where they are found, type of action, and types of damage they cause.

Sad, but True

We don't know what other endocrine effects there may be. Chemical manufacturers simply don't look into toxic effects on all these other body systems.

I want you to have this information available so you can check product ingredient labels on foods, cleaning compounds, cosmetics, household "pest" killers, dog and cat flea collars, lawn care products and other items you buy and use.

There are also naturally occurring endocrine-disrupting compounds, such as the *phytoestrogen isoflavones* in soy, grains and clover. Many of these are even made into OTC products and marketed to women for treatment of hormone problems like PMS and menopause, even though all may have significant "endocrine disrupting" effects.

Sad, but True

We are the only species with a brain creative enough to make chemicals capable of wiping out our entire race, by insidiously poisoning our hormone and reproductive systems.

High intake of these plant compounds, even though they are "natural," can significantly disrupt the menstrual cycle, reduce hormone production, and impair fertility. This effect to cause infertility was observed decades ago in cattle feeding on red clover, which is rich in the phytoestrogenic isoflavones.

Other endocrine disruptors in the naturally occurring group, such as genistein found in soy, have mixed effects: beneficial at some concentrations, and adverse effects at other concentrations. A few of the naturally-occurring ones have modest positive effects—such as lower cholesterol seen from a diet higher in phytoestrogens.

But it is clear that even naturally-occurring phytoestrogens have the ability to disrupt your own hormone systems, and have a mixed bag of effects.

Where Are Endocrine Disruptors Found?

Simply put, they are now everywhere. Man-made endocrine disruptors, the persistent organic pollutants—POPs—may be found in the water we drink, the food we eat, the air we breathe, the objects we touch around our homes, workplaces and recreational areas. They are found in the plastic linings of canned foods and plastic food wrappers. They are found in common chemicals probably sitting under your bathroom and kitchen sinks or in your laundry room and garage. Heavy metals are found in soils and water naturally and from contamination from computers and other electronic equipment put in landfills.

These chemicals are in widespread use in our daily life. They are found in cigarette smoke, plastics, detergents, pesticides, herbicides, fungicides, hair dyes, paints, solvents, dry cleaning solutions, cosmetics, food additives and preservatives, fabric coatings, wall coverings, carpets, playground equipment, and vehicle exhaust—just to name a few of the sources we encounter daily.

We also unwittingly add these chemicals into the environment: you may not realize that all the things you flush down the toilet or rinse down the kitchen sink can end up in our water supply, bubbling up in rivers and streams!

A US Geological Survey on 140 waterways in 30 states tracked 95 different pollutants, with these surprising results: 74% of the samples contained insect repellants, 48% contained antibiotics, 40% contained reproductive hormones (e.g. birth control pill estrogens and progestins), 32% contained other prescription drugs, and 27% were found to have chemical compounds used for *fragrances*.

These organic pollutants are fat-soluble compounds, so they become concentrated in the fat tissues of fish, animals, and humans. Animals, fish, and humans who are at the top of the food chain because they eat smaller animals and fish accumulate the most POPs in body fat.

Too Scary
From the increase in young women with symptoms of PCOS and other types of ovarian dysfunction that I see in my practice, and from the rising incidence of PCOS reported in worldwide studies, it is clear women are affected too.

Don't!
Don't even think of flushing left-over or outdated pills down the toilet or drain. They do come back to haunt you, eventually. And you are only adding to the problem.

When one animal or fish eats a smaller one that has been exposed to these chemicals, the bigger one adds a little more of the pollutants to its fatty tissues.

Warning
For human women, the fact that these toxic chemicals build up in fat carries a special risk: we have more overall body fat than do men.

Birds that daily eat fish from toxic waters build up more concentrated chemical levels than are in each fish. Larger prey that eat the birds get a little more, and so on up the food chain. Polar bears, for example, have very high levels of DDT, DDE, PCBs and other chemicals in their body fat because they eat high-fat seals that have eaten contaminated fish.

Our breasts actively store these estrogenic compounds, and concentrate these chemicals to a significant degree over our lifetime. Nursing babies then get the full brunt of the mother's chemical storehouse, particularly the first nursing child. As nursing depletes the mother's breast stores of chemicals, subsequent babies receive smaller amounts.

Even though these chemicals are banned in this country, we are still exposed to them everyday because most are still manufactured for export to countries whose laws are less strict. Winds that blow across the ocean to our West Coast carry chemical residues from countries where they are still in use. Fish, vegetables, and fruits from other parts of the world are imported and bring POPs residues to our tables.

Peril:
Although banned in 1975 in the U.S., Aldrin was allowed as a termite killer until 1987, so people are still exposed to it.

Banning their use doesn't help much because these chemicals are so long lasting. Aldrin, a termite killer, is converted to dieldrin in body tissues and in the soil, where it remains for years. Dieldrin suppresses the immune system and causes abnormal brain waves in mammals.

Pregnant women exposed to Aldrin would have daughters in their teens and twenties about now, just about the age we start seeing the reproductive damages, such as endometriosis, PCOS, severe PMS, irregular cycles, immune problems and mood-behavioral difficulties.

Others like chlorpyrifos (Dursban or Lorsban), are still infiltrating our lives and health. It is the active ingredient in over 1000 products surrounding us daily—from flea and tick collars for pets, and roach and ant sprays under your kitchen counter to the sprays used on crops we eat.

Another group of POPs, called *triazine herbicides* (atrazine, cyanazine, simazine), are water soluble rather than dissolved in fat. They are widely used across the U.S. from the cornfields of the Midwest to the fruit groves of Florida and California. When sprayed on vegetable and fruit crops to kill weeds, they are taken up from the soil into *all* the plants and leach from the soil into the groundwater as well. We ingest them via produce we eat and in our drinking water. We also get them in meat, poultry, milk and eggs because POPs contaminate corn feeds for cattle and chickens.

Peril: Atrazine is a known endocrine-disruptor linked to breast and ovarian cancers, as well as other reproductive problems such as infertility.

All of these compounds are possible carcinogens. Atrazine inhibits the ability to make testosterone and alters pituitary response to the hormones that oversee ovulation. Links between the herbicide triazine and ovarian cancer have been found for women farmers in Italy.

These compounds have been in use since the 1950s and yet little has been done to study their link to risk of breast and ovarian cancers, much less investigate the degree of their adverse effects on fertility, reproductive disorders such as endometriosis and PCOS, or hypothalamic-pituitary regulation of our other endocrine systems.

Hidden Endocrine Disruptors in Your Diet

Subtle, insidious dietary "hormone disruptors" are added to our foods and affect our bodies' ability to make the ovarian hormones we need to effectively "run" the cellular engines that make up every organ in our bodies. They lurk "innocently" in the foods we are eating and the soft drinks we are collectively consuming, literally by the gallon, every day.

Scary It doesn't matter how careful you have been, you may have been exposed to these compounds without knowing it.

Some of these hormone disruptors are common everyday elements in our lives—such as soft drinks and flavor enhancers like MSG. Even cigarettes have had these same flavor-enhancer chemicals added, unknown to consumers. Inhaling these chemicals in cigarette smoke gives them greater neurotoxic effect than when we eat additives in foods or drink them in soft drinks.

Let's explore some "ovary damagers" that lie in some foods and beverages you probably eat or drink every day.

The Soft Drink-Fast Food Menace: Excitotoxins and PCOS

How can soft drinks and foods affect your ovaries and risk of PCOS? It happens via the brain effects of food additives and sweeteners that are called *excitotoxins*, or *excitatory amino acids* (EAAs), that cause damage or death to nerve cells.

Excitotoxins, also called *neurotoxicants*, stimulate such intense and rapid firing of the nerve endings that the cells run out of their chemical messengers, and then die a few hours later. The nerve cells in the *hypothalamus*, our master hormone regulator, are some of the most sensitive neurons in our body to this type of damage and cell death from EAAs.

Children typically also consume large amounts of these excitotoxins in soft drinks and other processed foods throughout childhood and adolescence. The damage to the hypothalamus accumulates each day and each year, but the impact and damage doesn't show up until many years later at puberty when menstrual cycles begin and "hormone problems" can begin in earnest.

What Are Excitotoxins and Where Are They Found

Some excitotoxins are natural amino acids that occur in foods and are the building blocks of proteins, such as *glutamate, aspartate*, and *cysteine*. Some excitotoxins are even more potent man-made chemicals.

MSG, or *monosodium glutamate*, is a flavor-enhancer first synthesized in the 1920s. It is widely used in making all kinds of processed foods to improve taste and make us want to eat more, and more! MSG is the well-known

Excitotoxins: Where They Are Found

Some are man-made: Hydrolyzed vegetable protein powder

Some are found in nature as amino acids: glutamate, aspartate, cysteine

Examples:

Name	Where Found
MSG–monosodium glutamate	Many types of prepared foods
Hydrolyzed vegetable protein	Many prepared foods, (contains 3 excitotoxins: diet products, glutamate, aspartate, frozen dinners, and cystoic acid)
Aspartate	Nutrasweet®–found in everything from foods to soft drinks
Glutamate	See above
Cysteine (cystoic acid)	See above

©Elizabeth Lee Vliet, MD 2001-2005

chemical culprit that causes "Chinese-restaurant headache" syndrome.

MSG makes foods taste better, by causing a chemical reaction in our mouth to keep us coming back for "just one more." Manufacturers are not likely to stop using these additives anytime soon—they make too much money selling all these prepared foods and soft drinks.

MSG is made by adding sodium to the amino acid glutamate, and it is the glutamate part of the molecule that does the excitatory damage to nerve cells. That's why I don't recommend your using supplements that contain this amino acid in high concentrations.

MSG-induced damage to the brain has been studied and written about for at least *forty* years, but the food manufacturing industry has effectively managed to keep this research from broader public awareness. George R. Schwartz, M.D. described this critical problem in his excellent book, *In Bad Taste: The MSG Syndrome*, (Health Press, 1999). The concerns about over-use of glutamate that he raised have not been heeded, in spite of continuing research showing more damage than first thought. The problems for us today have only gotten worse as an ever-increasing array of foods and beverages contain MSG-related compounds.

In *Bad Taste* focuses on the role of MSG in learning and behavioral disorders in children, as well as degenerative neurological syndromes that occur later in life, but it didn't address the damage to women's hormonal systems that leads to the health problems like PCOS.

Warning:
Excitatory amino acids have effects like the stimulant cocaine. Inhibitory amino acids have effects like the relaxant Valium.

That's why I am addressing these issues and taking the extensive research on excitotoxins to a new level—you aren't likely to find these connections and effects on PCOS discussed other places. Look at the research that shows possible causative links to PCOS.

Brain research by Dr. John W. Olney in the 1960s and 1970s showed that the amount of MSG in even *one* jar of baby food was enough to cause permanent cell death in crucial areas of the retina and brain during development. He also found that MSG caused even more severe damage to the ultra-sensitive hypothalamus, our hormone regulating area of the brain.

Dr. Olney's studies showed that high dose exposure to MSG in mice caused the pituitary glands and ovaries to *shrink* (*hypoplasia*). High dose MSG also caused a major loss of the normal pituitary secretion of Luteinizing Hormone (LH), and Growth Hormone (GH).

But even more alarming, *low doses* that were well *below* toxic levels, caused abnormally *high* LH and loss of the normal bursts of LH secretion. *This is one of the characteristic findings in women with PCOS.* He also found that these offspring didn't have normal Growth Hormone (GH) production. Reduced GH explained the short stature and obesity. Abnormal levels of LH explained the infertility and irregular cycles.

PCOS Parallels
Dr. Olney found that babies of mothers fed MSG were short in stature, obese, had abnormal cycles, and infertility.

These same changes are seen in girls with PCOS. I am concerned that *food additives* are an overlooked contributor to the rising incidence of PCOS today.

The reproductive disruptions and infertility found in all the animal studies are strikingly parallel to what I see in patients. The combined research evidence suggests to me that excitatory amino acids cause damage to the hypothalamus so that the hypothalamus–pituitary–ovarian pathways can't work properly.

This in turn contributes to the many endocrine abnormalities seen in PCOS and other reproductive disorders as women reach puberty. I am convinced that excitotoxins hitting the brain in the womb, in infancy and childhood play an insidious role in the development of ovarian dysfunction, including PCOS, infertility, and other "hormone havoc" syndromes I see in women.

Unlike animals, human brains have additional development during infancy and childhood, not just while in our mother's womb. That means young children who drink a lot of soft drinks are being exposed to these brain-damaging chemicals while their brains are still developing.

The data became so overwhelming about this hidden health hazard to babies that researchers raised the alarm to Congress, and MSG additives to baby foods were banned in 1970.

This was too late for the generation of children born in the 40s, 50s, and 60s. I am certain this is another factor for the high incidence of subtle forms of "learning disorders" in adults now between the ages of 30 to 60. It may be why we are seeing so many more adult women being diagnosed with "Attention deficit" disorder.

Excitotoxins are still added to baby foods today, in spite of the ban, because the banned MSG has now morphed into other chemicals that consumers don't recognize. Some of these are *caseinate*, *"natural flavorings,"* and *hydrolyzed vegetable protein (HVP)*—all of which are typically made from sources high in these excitatory amino acids.

Hydrolyzed vegetable protein is sometimes shown on food labels simply as vegetable protein or plant protein, so you don't really know what you are getting. It is another man-made excitotoxin, derived from plants that aren't fit to eat, but are high in the excitatory amino acids such as glutamate or aspartate. The plants are processed with acid and caustic soda, dried, and made into a concentrated powder that contains a potent mix of the same **three** known excitotoxins—*glutamate, aspartate, and cystoic acid.*

Fact:
A human infant's brain is *far more sensitive to damage* from excitotoxins than the brains in *all* other species studied.

Fact:
The group we call the "baby boomers" ate baby food laced with large amounts of MSG.

HVP is found in much that you eat today, in spite of the known adverse effects of these excitotoxins. It is hard to find something that *doesn't* have them: protein drinks (an obvious place), cereals, frozen dinners, diet meals, sauce mixes, soups, salad dressings, diet drink powders you mix with milk or water, to name a few. The food industry has fought to keep this hidden from the general public. The research is compelling to show damaging effects of these chemicals, but the FDA doesn't warn us of the dangers of these hidden additives in our foods.

Diet soft drinks are an even worse problem because they contain MSG or aspartate (in Nutrasweet) in *liquid form that is more toxic to the brain because they are absorbed faster* and produce higher blood levels than solid foods.

Since their damage primarily hits the hypothalamus, which oversees the endocrine system, the effects aren't seen until children are much older, so parents don't realize how serious the problem really is.

Many scientists think that the rise in learning disorders, impulse control disorders, behavioral problems, obesity, and premature puberty is triggered, in part, by children's widespread consumption of excitatory amino acid additives adversely affecting the brain.

Adults are hit with the damaging effects of excitotoxins too. Common neurological disorders—such as migraine headaches, some forms of daily "tension" headaches, strokes, and seizures (particularly the more subtle types, such as complex partial, absence-type and petit mal seizures) are now linked to these same excitotoxins.

Current studies link the rising rate of degenerative diseases in older people to a lifetime of excitotoxins consumption in food and soft drinks. Diseases such as Parkinson's, ALS (Amyotrophic Lateral Sclerosis, or Lou Gehrig's disease), Alzheimer's, MS, and other less common debilitating nervous system disorders, may have additional primary causes, but the evidence is strong that excitotoxins increases brain damage and younger onset of symptoms.

Hormones, Chemical Messengers and Your Brain: A Brief Overview

Our hormones affect our brain directly, and our brain regulates hormone production by endocrine glands throughout the body. Our brain has to oversee incredibly complex actions and interactions 24 hours a day, 365 days a year. It has to organize, analyze, direct, execute, evaluate, delegate and coordinate…all day long, and all night long. Our hormones serve as chemical communicators that facilitate the connections between all the body's parts, and help all of these brain functions run smoothly.

Nerve cells have to "talk" to each other for our brain and body to work as a coordinated whole. Chemical messengers called neurotransmitters travel back and forth across gaps between nerve endings so that messages can be passed from one nerve to another and one area of the brain to another.

Our hormones also "talk" to nerve cells and to neurotransmitters like serotonin by way of special "docking sites" that we call receptors, specific for each type of molecule. Neurotransmitters and our hormones also have docking sites on the cells of the immune system, as well as our endocrine glands, the intestinal tract, and other organs all over the body.

> **Hormone Helper:** Hormones also act as messengers, helping nerve cells carry their messages.

There are many chemical messengers in the body, but I want to focus on those most critical to the interactions between our hormones and the brain: serotonin (5–HT), norepinephrine (NE), dopamine (DA), acetylcholine (ACh), gamma aminobutyric acid (GABA), glutamate, N-acetylaspartate (NAA).

These neurotransmitters scurry throughout our brain and body, day in and day out, relaying and modulating information between cells in different parts of the body. They link our emotional and physical health.

We make these information-carrying molecules from "building blocks" called *amino acids,* found in the food we eat. We need various vitamins and minerals as catalysts and cofactors for the synthesizing enzymes to make the neurotransmitters. If you don't eat a healthy, balanced diet, your body can't make neurotransmitters *or* hormones, or make them work properly.

Brain Damage! These chemical messengers and pathways are ones that are seriously disrupted by excitotoxins.

Your brain's chemical messengers have incredibly diverse roles and functions. Serotonin, for example, turns out to be involved in aspects we previously thought were just "psychological"—pain, sleep, memory, mood, anxiety, appetite, thirst and other functions are all regulated by serotonin. The *balance* of brain chemical messengers helps regulates mood.

We need the right balance: insomnia, anxiety, and overeating can each occur when serotonin is either too low *or* too high. Serotonin *imbalances* with other chemical messengers also cause other behavioral problems, from compulsive shoplifting and gambling, to compulsive sexual behaviors, compulsive hand washing, and hair-pulling (*trichotillomania*), violent outbursts, and even suicidal thoughts.

Body Damage! Excitotoxins in soft drinks cause even more damage by interfering with your ability to absorb vitamins and minerals.

The balance of ovarian, thyroid, and adrenal hormones influences the balance of these neurotransmitters, and is one way that the hormone changes of PCOS can cause mood symptoms. Depression caused by endocrine problems is a biological disorder caused by these marked changes in these chemical messengers and an alteration in the receptor numbers and sensitivity. Attention deficit disorders are also affected by the balance between serotonin, dopamine, and norepinephrine. These messengers are in turn affected by the balance of estradiol, testosterone, DHEA and progesterone. So you see, these tiny molecules have powerful effects!

Glutamate is an excitatory neurotransmitter that is used by about 40% of the brain's nerve junctions, along with its acidic amino acid relatives such as N-acetylaspartate (NAA). Excitatory amino acids stimulate nerve cells to fire. Inhibitory amino acids, like GABA, described below, slow down nerve cell activity.

Glutamate plays a key role in learning and memory formation, among other functions. "Learning" results in an immediate release of glutamate, followed later by another release of glutamate during memory processing. We seem to require this increase in glutamate outside the nerve cells in order to properly consolidate, or "store," long-term memory.

It is the balance of glutamate delivered to nerve cells that appears to be critical in how well they can function. Memory loss can occur when too much glutamate causes over-excitation, or activation, of nerve cells.

This is why the concentrated glutamate, glutamic acid-herbal mixtures sold in health food stores as memory "boosters" can actually damage memory pathways—they deliver a large dose all at once, which disrupts the normal functioning of the memory pathways and chemical messengers. In the normal process, glutamate is released from its nerve cells, and then taken up by special cells to be converted to glutamine, which is then returned to the neurons that require it for their function. Glutamine is then used again to make more glutamate. Supplements are even more dangerous because these amino acids are widespread in foods and beverages today.

Balance is Key

If too much glutamate is delivered at one time, short-term memory can be disrupted.

Whenever there is brain injury, high levels of glutamate are released from nerve cells in the area of injury. Concussions, or blows to the head that do not cause a skull fracture, can cause significant short-term memory loss because brain damage from the blow leads to high levels of glutamate in the hippocampus, our primary memory center. Strokes, seizures and high blood pressure also cause extremely high levels of glutamate release in areas of injury as well as a breakdown in the protective blood-brain barrier.

L-aspartic acid, another amino acid in this group, can also block glutamate uptake into nerve cells and interfere with memory processing. Glycine is another amino acid that affects both normal action and the toxicity of glutamate and aspartate. The amount of glycine in the diet or in supplements contributes to glutamate damage.

N-acetylaspartate (NAA, for short) is the second most abundant amino acid in our brain, found mostly in the nerve cells. NAA itself hasn't been found to have specific neurotransmitter effects but it is important to our discussion of excitotoxins because of what it does, and because it can be affected by the amount of aspartate, glutamate, and cysteine in our diets. *Balance of NAA seems to be critical.*

Low levels of NAA have been found in the brains of people with such severe degenerative neurological disorders as Alzheimer's and Huntington's disease. Excessively high levels of NAA, on the other hand, actually disrupt the formation of myelin, a protective fatty sheath around nerves that helps conduct of nerve impulses. Loss of myelin is what causes the loss of nerve function in Multiple Sclerosis.

These deceptively simple molecules have a profound impact on many aspects of our health. Chemicals in our environment and in our diet can disrupt *any* of these hormones and chemical messengers and cause depression, anxiety, insomnia and other brain symptoms. In spite of what current advertisements want you (and your doctor) to believe, depression is not *just* a "serotonin deficiency." Nor is it always "psychiatric" in the usual sense. Many causes are "medical," physical-endocrine-metabolic changes that affect the physical function of brain pathways overseeing our moods.

How Do Excitotoxins Affect the Pituitary and Ovaries?

The **hypothalamus** is the master controller for our hormone systems, body temperature, appetite regulation, body weight, sleep cycles, and a host of other critical functions. The hypothalamus is extremely sensitive to excitatory amino acid damage. The hypothalamus is so vulnerable because, even in adults, it lacks the protective blood-brain barrier found in the rest of the brain. This means high levels of offending chemicals in the bloodstream can bathe the hypothalamus directly. That's one reason that Dr. Olney and other brain researchers have been so concerned about the increasing use of MSG, HVP, cysteine, and aspartate as food additives.

Another study by Dr. Ralph Dawson showed that even low doses of MSG produced profound alterations in sex hormone release via the hypothalamus that it caused marked abnormalities in the onset of female puberty. Mice (remember, they are *less* sensitive than humans) given low doses of MSG had decreased estrogen binding at the hypothalamic receptors, abnormal patterns of LH and LHRH release, delayed vaginal opening, and disturbances in sexual behavior.

Even *subtoxic* doses of MSG can cause severe abnormal changes to the hypothalamus and thereby disrupt our entire endocrine "control center." Put another way, it would be like having a computer virus take over your computer's operating system and change all the settings.

I suspect that these food additives are another reason I see some young women that need much higher than usual blood levels of estradiol to maintain their sense of normal mood, sleep and memory. I think a lifetime of soft drinks and "flavor-enhanced" foods act in the brain to change the way the estrogen receptors respond, much like a computer virus disrupts computer functions.

Caution: EAAs in liquid form from soft drinks is far more damaging than solid food because they are more readily absorbed into the bloodstream and reach higher blood levels.

Damage Beyond the Brain

Large doses of glutamate, still below the toxic doses, given to animals caused *reduced* production of thyroid hormones and *increased* production of cortisol—two other hormone imbalances that are common in PCOS and lead to weight gain and also interfere with the normal function of ovaries.

Since MSG causes both "*miswiring*" of nerve pathways and "*misfiring*" of nerve signals during brain development, then it can affect *all* the endocrine glands the brain oversees. This explains why thyroid and adrenal gland hormones, as well as the ovaries, are altered.

When you consider everything the hypothalamus governs, it isn't surprising that we see such diverse damage throughout the body. For women with PCOS, soft drinks can add to the hormone chaos by affecting the function of the hypothalamus.

Dose Effects: Animals and Humans, Infants, and Adults

Remember the point I made earlier: *human* infant brains are many times more sensitive to damage by excitotoxins like MSG and aspartate than the brains of animals used in *all* the studies. Dr. Olney's studies showed that *human* children get a 20-fold increase of glutamate in blood levels while the same dose causes only a 4-fold increase in mice. That's a huge difference.

Keep in mind too that the human brain continues to develop throughout childhood, not just while in the womb. The foods we eat and the chemicals we are exposed to during infancy and childhood have additional potential for harm. Walk around a mall today and you see children of all ages carrying super-jumbo size soft drinks in their hands.

Dr. Olney found that human children often get MSG doses in the range of 100–150 mg per kilogram of body weight just by eating manufactured foods containing these flavor-enhancers and hydrolyzed vegetable protein, and his work was done 40 years ago when 12 oz. cans of soft drinks were all we had. Today's prevalent 32 and 64 oz. super-jumbo drinks were non-existent then. Think about the cumulative effects of super-sized excitotoxin doses! Parents have no clue what subtle brain damage is occurring when they allow children to drink soft drinks all day.

Critical Timing of Exposure

Mother Nature has carefully choreographed the complex process of egg and sperm uniting and then dividing and dividing to ultimately become an embryo, then a recognizable human infant in the womb. Each day of gestation is important, with certain developmental events unfolding in sequence. Disrupt one step and another cannot occur properly.

That's also why the endocrine disruptors are often called "*gender-benders*." Tiny amounts of these chemicals are so powerful they can completely derail the process of gender development, preventing the full complement of male or female characteristics from being displayed at puberty, adolescence, and adulthood.

All humans start out as embryos programmed to be female with a female cyclic brain pattern of response. The change to a male pattern of hormones and organs only occurs if the embryo gets the proper signal at the proper time to trigger the testes to start pumping out testosterone. If this signal doesn't come, or comes at the wrong time, the embryo stays in the female pattern.

Giggle: Don't you know men will love finding out they *really* started out as female!

This critical day—the day a female brain and body is permanently transformed into a male—is *day* 56 of gestation in humans. This is the day that the embryo has to get a signal activating a gene on the Y chromosome in order for the embyro's testicles to being making testosterone.

The presence of testosterone on day 56 changes the basic primordial female brain pattern into a male one. The male brain pattern is programmed to produce steady testosterone levels (tonic pattern) throughout life rather than the cyclic menstrual cycle pattern of estradiol and progesterone that women have. Fetal tissue that would have become ovaries, uterus, and vagina develops as penis, testicles, and prostate. A similar process occurs in all mammals, just at different times during gestation.

What's the message? Be careful what you eat or drink (or smoke or inhale or spray into and around your body) during these critical early days of pregnancy.

If environmental or dietary chemicals interfere with Mother Nature's plan on day 56 in human gestation, it can alter this exquisitely-timed sequence of hormone messages and permanently skew the male pattern of brain, body, and hormone development. A genetic male embryo can be left in a bizarre gender-bender "limbo"—genetically male, but with his male body and hormone patterns not operating normally for the rest of his life.

Studies on women lag behind. There are similar disruptive effects in female embryos and developing babies, but these are harder to quantify because women's internal reproductive organs are more difficult to directly observe and quantify, unlike males where the penis is visible. The damage, such as PCOS, endometriosis and "un-explained" infertility, due to these chemicals are more subtle in women, and harder to identify early.

Other Diet Risks for Your Ovaries: Excess Fats and Sugars

Warning:
Excitatory amino acids are so incredibly damaging to the brain–they interrupt the normal endocrine developmental sequence.

Diet plays a role in disrupting optimal ovarian function. We often really don't want to know everything we are eating. We enjoy a particular food, we want it, we buy it, it tastes good and we play ostrich to what might really be there and what it "may" do to us later. It's time to take your head out of the sand.

Excess body fat can both cause irregular menstrual cycles, abnormal ovulation, infertility and a variety of other hormone problems. Girls are particularly hard hit: childhood obesity leads to premature puberty, in-creased risk of PCOS and endometriosis, increased risk of infertility, a later risk of diabetes, and a higher risk of developing breast cancer, even before menopause.

Excess Fats and Your Ovaries: What's The Connection?

POPs & Fat
Fat of animals and fish, and your own body fat, become the depository for POPs that subtly permeate your body and damage hormone pathways.

Most women don't realize that the average American diet is about 45% fat, a culprit in many health problems that affect your ovaries, and your overall health. The Persistent Organic Pollutants (POPs) accumulate in fat tissues because they don't dissolve well in water.

Most women have heard ad nauseum about saturated fats that increase the risk of heart disease. Long before that happens, however, you may inadvertently sabotage your fertility or make PCOS worse by eating a lot of fats. Increased body fat increases your load of estrone, an estrogen that can over-stimulate growth of the uterine lining and increase your risk of uterine cancer.

The more you gain weight, the more likely you have insulin resistance, and an increased risk of diabetes. The more saturated fats you have eaten over your lifetime, the greater your risk of heart and blood vessel disease, and the greater your risk of developing breast, colon and/or uterine cancer.

Soft Drinks—sugars that aren't so nice

It isn't just fat that makes you fatter. So does excess sugar. Moreover, sugars in these soft drink beverages add further to the neuron damage of excitotoxins by making you fatter and increasing your risk of insulin resistance.

Too much sugar leads to a type of cell-damagers called AGEs, or *advanced glycosylation end-products*. These AGEs literally age your cells at the same time they fill you with empty calories that make you gain weight. So, ratchet down your sweet tooth a few notches. Your brain and body will feel better and work better for you...and so will your ovaries.

Vegetarian Pitfalls for Ovarian Health

I am not against vegetarian diets per se, but most women don't realize the potential pitfalls of vegetarian diets or how carefully you must plan vegetarian meals in order to make certain you are getting complete proteins, adequate vitamins, and minerals. I discuss these issues in more detail in Chapter 12.

If a vegetarian diet isn't properly balanced, you end up with subtle deficits of essential amino acids, vitamins and minerals that can lead to increased problems with infertility, aggravate the hormone problems of PCOS, and cause more fatigue, muscle aches, and fuzzy thinking.

Plants provide less iron than meats, and provide a non-heme iron that is not as well absorbed. High fiber and phytate content of a plant-based diet also impairs absorption of important minerals. Magnesium, in particular, is a crucial mineral to help defend against the cell damage from the excitotoxins you read about earlier. The richest sources of B12 are all animal foods. Too little intake of iodine impairs thyroid function, another factor in infertility.

Catch-22 The more fat in your diet, the higher your exposure to these endocrine disruptors.

Caution: In younger women soy can suppress the menstrual cycle and decrease fertility.

Grains and vegetables also have high levels of estrogen-like compounds (*phytoestrogens*) that attach to the body's estrogen receptors and impair the ovaries' hormone production. This is another reason for the menstrual irregularities and higher incidence of infertility in vegetarians.

Tip: Start now to eliminate as many of the sources of excitotoxins in your diet as possible—the excitotoxin load builds up every day of your life, reaching critical levels of damage.

Researchers in the UK analyzed the influence of a soy-based diet on the hormonal status and menstrual cycle in premenopausal women with regular ovulatory cycles. 60 grams of soy protein containing 45 mg isoflavones was given daily for 1 month. This caused a significant increase in length of the follicular phase and delayed menstruation.

Midcycle bursts of luteinizing hormone and follicle-stimulating hormone were significantly suppressed while the women were taking the soy protein. We see similar responses with tamoxifen, an anti-estrogen. These effects are due to non-steroidal isoflavones and phytoestrogens that sometimes behave as estrogen "boosters" (*agonists*) and sometimes function as estrogen "blockers" (*antagonists*).

Soy foods in modest amounts may have some potential benefit with respect to lowering high cholesterol. But the flip side is that phytoestrogens can decrease hormone production, which then impairs fertility, especially if you have PCOS.

Studies have shown that "eating vegetarian" has cardiovascular benefits due to a lower intake of saturated fats. That's true. For younger women who may be trying to become pregnant, too *little* fat means less of the building blocks to make ovarian hormones, which in turn increases the risk of infertiliy.

It's trendy to eat vegetarian these days. If this is what you want to do, then pay careful attention to getting adequate protein, combining foods properly to get all of the essential amino acids, and eating the right balance of foods to insure adequate levels of key vitamins and minerals. This is one diet you can't approach haphazardly and expect to stay healthy.

In Summary

Excitatory amino acids. Excitotoxins. Hypothalamic damage. Hormone disruption. These are serious health issues that haven't adequately made it into mainstream medicine.

The bottom line is that excitatory amino acids in your foods disrupt function of the hypothalamus that oversees the pituitary, which in turn regulates ovary cycles and other endocrine organs that produce hormones. PCOS can be made worse if you have too much intake of all these chemicals in your diet. You can see why premature puberty, PMS, and PCOS are all on the rise. I am not saying don't ever eat these things, but be aware of the problems they cause.

When we reflect on all this information and it's collective impact on our *neuroendocrine* system, you can see why premature puberty, PMS, and PCOS are all on the rise.

I don't have space here to go into all the years of world-wide animal studies that raised the red flags for humans, or the history of how we got in such a mess with chemicals that pollute and sabotage our fertility and survival.

Your Health Action Steps:

To keep it simple, you must pay attention to these issues —your health is at stake.

If you are interested in the fascinating detective work done by scientists to identify these health effects in animals and humans, I encourage you to read two outstanding and well-researched books: *Our Stolen Future* by scientist Theo Colborn and her team of Dianne Dumanoski, and John Peterson Myers, and *Living Downstream* by ecologist Sandra Steingraber.

Let their descriptions of the animals' plight and their urgent alarm call to humans be your health wake-up call. If you have PCOS, or symptoms that are similar, you need to be aware of the dangers. Pay attention to ways to clean up your diet and personal environment as much as possible.

Watch how often you have them, and control your portion size. Consider other options that are a better use of your daily calorie and fat allowance. Cut out the diet soft drinks and the flavor-enhanced snack foods Drink water or seltzer instead of soft drinks…they are really *much* better for you! Each positive change you make is a step toward better hormone balance and a healthier body.

Chapter 7

The Deadly Quartet of PCOS: Insulin Resistance, Hypertension, High Cholesterol and Diabetes

Sudden, inexplicable weight gain, feeling so tired that you can't get through the day, overwhelming sleep attacks after lunch, or wicked mood swings, are classic symptoms of PCOS.

It's not at all unusual to see teenagers with PCOS put on 50 *pounds or more* in six months. No wonder they feel so out of control.

The young women I see as patients have described, often in tears, all the efforts they have made to lose weight and yet been frustrated with failure to control it.

What causes such marked weight gain and fatigue? Why is it that you seem to eat less and less and gain more and more?

Other parts of this picture that you *don't see* are even more deadly: high cholesterol, high blood pressure, insulin resistance and early diabetes.

Metabolic effects of excess androgens and insulin in PCOS cause early onset heart disease and diabetes in the 20s, 30s and 40s...far earlier than in women who don't have PCOS.

That's why it is so important for you to understand these risks and how to control your weight with the right diet, exercise, and the right medicines *before disease* develops.

Fact: PCOS women are *seven* times more likely to develop heart disease than women who don't have PCOS

Diabetes and It's Precursor, Insulin Resistance: How PCOS Increases Your Risks

Fact:

You need insulin to live, but too much insulin can cause diabetes, early heart attacks, and even cancer.

Most people already know that Diabetes mellitus, or diabetes for short, is a disease of high blood sugar (glucose). But far too many people are walking around in the early stages of diabetes and don't know it. They suffer from the condition called **insulin resistance**, or *Prediabetes*.

More than half of the women with PCOS have insulin resistance, even if they are not overweight. What happens in the progression from normal to insulin resistance to diabetes? Let's explore this.

What is Insulin and What Does It Do?

Insulin is a major *anabolic* (tissue-building) hormone of metabolism, governing glucose regulation, body fat storage and many other functions. Insulin plays a crucial role in moving glucose from the blood into cells that need glucose to survive. Insulin also carries glucose into fat cells to be stored as triglycerides for your body's later energy needs.

Warning!

Diabetes complications can begin years before the disease is actually diagnosed, so you must watch for early signs of glucose intolerance, get tested and treated.

Insulin has many roles in the body. Some researchers now think it is even one of our "master" hormones that plays a role in many diseases, from high blood pressure to cancers, as well as diabetes.

Unlike the anabolic effects of testosterone that build muscle and bone, insulin is an anabolic hormone that builds *fat*.

Insulin is a potent promoter of fat storage (*lipogenesis*) and a potent inhibitor of fat breakdown (*lipolysis*). Insulin actually works to increase the ratio of *fat* to muscle, so the more insulin stimulation you have, the lower the ratio of your *fat-burning* muscle cells.

Lack of insulin can lead to death. If you didn't have enough insulin, your cells would starve and you would die. This is why diabetics who don't make insulin must take it as shots, or in an insulin pump or new nasal spray.

Excess insulin is also a serious problem. Insulin doesn't

just act to ferry sugar into the cells. Insulin tells the kidneys to hold onto more salt, and more salt means high blood pressure. Insulin also stimulates cells growth, and in the case of cancer cells…that can mean growing into tumors.

Excess insulin can happen no matter what your age. There are a quite a few causes. Some medications can trigger it by causing increased appetite and weight gain. PCOS can cause over production of insulin. Various types of imbalanced diets can cause it.

Common Triggers Of Excess Insulin in Women

- Weight gain, especially around the waist and upper body
- Constant dieting with the wrong kind of foods, especially high carbohydrate foods,
- Consuming most of your calories late in the day, especially if high carbohydrate foods
- Increased stress with high cortisol
- Low estradiol
- High total and/or free testosterone relative to estradiol
- Excess progesterone relative to estradiol
- High levels of DHEA and DHEA-s
- Disrupted sleep and/or altered sleep-wake cycles, such as getting up at noon and staying up until 2:00 or 3:00 a.m.
- Declining thyroid function
- Sedentary lifestyle, without regular aerobic exercise
- Medications that cause weight gain or decrease insulin sensitivity
- Pregnancy
- PCOS and Syndrome X

©Elizabeth Lee Vliet, MD 2001-2005

How Does Insulin Work?

As you eat, food is converted to glucose and the blood level of glucose rises. The brain senses the rise in glucose, and sends a rapid signal to the pancreas to release insulin.

Normally, insulin levels then quickly drop back down to a low baseline level after it has done its job. Glucose is used for fuel, and there isn't any excess fat stored.

But if you have a disorder like PCOS that causes the body to make too much insulin in response to food, or if you gain body fat that makes

Function:
Insulin's main job is to ferry the rising glucose out of the bloodstream and into muscle and fat cells so that glucose can be used for fuel by the muscles and other cells, or be stored as fat for future fuel needs.

Fact:
Women with PCOS are four to five times more likely to develop diabetes than women who don't have PCOS

the body less sensitive to insulin, then insulin stays too high after eating and causes more food stored as body fat instead of being burned for energy.

In addition, as we gain more body fat, insulin receptors don't work as well. The cells become distorted in shape and size and this causes the receptor site (like a lock) for insulin, to get out of proper alignment. As a result, the insulin molecule "key" no longer fits easily into the receptor "lock." This impairs insulin response.

When this happens, glucose levels remain high after you eat because the insulin, even though present, isn't working well. Your brain sensors detect continuing high glucose levels, and signals the pancreas to release even *more* insulin to bring glucose down. Your bloodstream and cells become flooded with insulin.

Then suddenly, when all this insulin starts working, the glucose rushes into the cells, and your blood glucose level plummets. We call this response *reactive hypoglycemia* (low blood sugar).

A falling blood sugar causes you to feel ravenously hungry, shaky, sweaty, nauseous, lightheaded, and causes fuzzy thinking, heart palpitations and a racing pulse. A drop in blood sugar causes intense food cravings, especially for sweets.

As soon as you give in the whole cycle starts over. A rapid rise in glucose makes you lethargic, sleepy, and unfocused. Clues like sleepiness after eating, afternoon lethargy, or feeling shaky, dizzy and fuzzy-brained 3–4 hours after eating can indicate your body isn't regulating the glucose and insulin normally, which may mean you are becoming insulin resistant.

Since the insulin isn't working properly to deliver a steady supply of glucose to working muscle cells, the effect is the same as not getting enough food. The cells are not getting their fuel, so you get hunger signals and eat more, even though plenty of fuel (glucose) is circulating in the bloodstream.

What's worse is that your fat cells are also screaming for

more food. It's like you have a leak in your car's gas line. Even though you keep filling the tank (eating), the fuel never gets to the engine (your cells) so it can work.

The excess insulin makes your body store more fat, and less effective at burning fat stores for energy. Each day this pattern repeats. You get fatter, and fatter and fatter while you eat less and less and less.

Insulin resistance refers to this entire pattern—high levels of both insulin and glucose in the bloodstream and excess insulin causing glucose to be stored as fat instead of used for immediate energy.

Insulin resistance causes a host of body-wrecking effects:

- ❧ impaired immune function making you more susceptible to infections
- ❧ increased build-up of the smooth muscle in artery walls that narrows the passage for blood flow, leading to both high blood pressure and reduced blood flow to critical organs
- ❧ plaque build-up in the arteries also *reduces* blood flow, leading to strokes and heart attacks, even in younger women (as we see in PCOS)
- ❧ more platelet stickiness leading to increased risk of clots
- ❧ increased risk of diabetes and heart attack
- ❧ later, increased risk of breast cancer
- ❧ growth of other cancers

Excess insulin is now considered a risk factor for heart disease and early heart attacks, particularly when estradiol is too low. These may *sound* like problems for older women, but young women are not immune—I see these problems in adolescent girls.

With optimal levels of estradiol, we are less likely to have problems with insulin resistance because the estradiol improves insulin response in the cells. But estradiol loss is not the only way our ovaries are involved in this insulin pathway.

Researchers have found insulin receptors in the ovary. Insulin acts at the ovarian receptors to change the enzymes so they make more *androgens* rather than the normal estradiol-estrone balance.

Fact: Women with PCOS often show signs of early vascular disease in their 20s.

Higher androgens then feed back to the glucose regulating hormones and cause more insulin production. Higher insulin levels stimulate more androgen production in the ovary.

It is a vicious cycle that makes a woman grow fatter, and fatter and fatter. This is a major cause of the marked weight gain in young women with PCOS. A milder form of this imbalance occurs in perimenopausal woman who are losing estradiol and "unmasking" the effects of their androgens (DHEA, testosterone, androstenedione).

As you shift toward more androgens and lower estradiol, more body fat builds around your waist and deep inside the abdomen (visceral fat), similar to males.

Low fat, high carbohydrate diets stimulate more insulin production by the pancreas and make this worse. More insulin pushes the body to store more abdominal fat. More abdominal fat then makes more insulin resistance.

Diabetes Mellitus

Diabetes is a deadly disease. It kills more than 90,000 women each year, double the number of women who die from breast cancer. Yet most women don't know this and are more afraid of breast cancer.

More importantly, at any age, diabetes disproportionately affects women—both in terms of frequency and severity of disease. Some 8 million women of all ages suffering its ravages.

Fact:
PCOS and obesity have independent and additive negative effects on insulin action

Sadly, in spite of the educational efforts for physicians and consumers by the government and advocacy groups like the American Diabetes Association, diabetes is still a woefully under-recognized medical problem, especially in younger women.

The Federal government is so concerned about the staggering rise in Diabetes, that officials recently changed the names "glucose intolerance" and "impaired glucose tolerance" to "Pre-Diabetes" to encourage people and doctors to test sooner, and prevent progression to Diabetes. Doctors still don't take these early problems seriously enough.

Too many people with prediabetes don't get diagnosed.

Diabetes attacks the tiny end arteries throughout the body that provide blood to cells. The arteries become filled with glucose-laden compounds that damage these blood vessels and reduce blood flow, making cells and tissues starve for oxygen and nutrients and they die.

Diabetes robs you of your energy, memory, sight, and kidney function. It can cause nerve damage, severe pain in the hands and feet, depression, dementia, loss of sexual response, amputation of limbs, and early heart attacks, strokes and premature death.

Fact:
Diabetes kills *twice* as many women every year than does breast cancer.

PCOS Accelerates the Damages of Diabetes

Women with PCOS are even more severely affected: they develop diabetes at much younger ages, and have more severe disease and more frequent deadly complications at earlier ages than do women who don't have PCOS.

These complications not only lead to early death, but they cause major disability, pain and impaired quality of life long before they cause death: blindness, kidney damage requiring dialysis, nerve damage requiring amputation, accelerated bone loss causing hip and spine fractures, dementia due to vascular damage.

These are just a few of the ways that women with PCOS suffer a greater burden from the illness of diabetes. Diabetes must be treated early, and aggressively to prevent these very serious, and expensive, complications.

Warning!
Diabetes complications can begin years before the disease is actually diagnosed. You must watch for early signs of glucose intolerance, get tested and treated!

Diabetes is alarmingly more common as Americans get fatter, and I have explained that PCOS causes accelerated weight gain in women. So you can see how women with PCOS have such an increased risk of becoming diabetic.

In earlier generations, most diabetes developed in adulthood as a result of people getting fatter as they got older. That's why it used to be called adult-onset diabetes. But this name is no longer valid today. There is an epidemic of childhood and adolescent obesity.

Diabetes Hits Women Harder

Diabetes is a greater problem for women than men for several reasons:

- More women of all ages get diabetes,
- Women tend to have more severe and more frequent diabetic complications.
- Women have smaller arteries than men, so diabetes damages arteries throughout the body faster.
- Women are more likely to become obese with age than are men. That means Type 2 diabetes, caused by excess body fat, is far more common in women.
- Depression is also more common in women than men in all age groups but women with diabetes are three times more likely to develop major depression.
- Women being treated for depression get another hit: certain anti-depressants, such as tricyclics, can cause higher blood sugars, more memory loss, and a marked increase in carbohydrate craving which means more weight gain—all making the diabetes worse.
- Women with diabetes who need contraception can get another hit from the wrong choice of birth control pill. Those with high levels of progestin relative to the estrogen, such as Mircette, Alesse, or Loestrin can make weight gain worse, further adding to the problems of controlling glucose.
- Yeast infections are more prevalent in women than men, and women with diabetes have a much higher risk of recurrent yeast infections than women who don't have diabetes. In fact, if you have gained weight and are having more yeast infections, it is crucial to have a check for diabetes as a hidden underlying cause.
- Osteopenia and osteoporosis are also more common in women diabetics because high levels of glucose lead to decreased bone-building, decreased response to the parathyroid hormone, and decreased response to a type of vitamin D needed to build healthy bone.
- Unlike men who make steadier levels of testosterone throughout their lives, women lose estradiol abruptly around menopause, which impairs insulin sensitivity.

©Elizabeth Lee Vliet, MD 2001-2005

Obese children and teens are now developing the "adult" form of diabetes.

Adult-onset diabetes is now called *non-insulin dependent diabetes* mellitus (NIDDM) or *Type II diabetes* to distinguish it from *insulin dependent* or *Type I diabetes*, previously called juvenile onset diabetes. People with Type I Diabetes are not able to make insulin normally, and are typically thin, not fat.

Loss of optimal estradiol, for whatever cause, at whatever age, is one more factor that increases the risk of diabetes. Estradiol actually improves women's sensitivity to insulin, and makes us less likely to become glucose intolerant and insulin resistant.

Estradiol also prevents the excess androgen effects that aggravate insulin resistance, and estradiol acts as an antioxidant to prevent the cell-damaging effects of excess glucose.

Excess glucose makes platelets stickier and more likely to clot. Our natural estradiol helps prevent excess platelet "stickiness" and lowers risk of serious blood clots.

When you lose estradiol, and also have elevated glucose, both factors increase platelet "stickiness" and clumping that may lead to clots and stroke.

Eating a high carbohydrate diet makes this problem even worse: one Harvard study found that women aged 38–63 who ate a diet high in refined (simple) carbohydrates had a 40% greater risk of heart attack or stroke than did women with a diet lower in refined carbohydrate.

Fact: Women with diabetes aren't often told how important optimal estradiol can be in helping them control their diabetes.

Fact: Women with PCOS show signs of early vascular disease in their twenties.

How Glucose is Regulated: The See-Saw of Insulin and Glucagon

Glucose and oxygen are such critical fuels for the brain's survival that the body keeps tight control on levels. Glucose changes can have severe consequences so the body has ways to keep glucose from "swinging" to dangerous extremes, high or low.

Insulin and glucagon are the two major regulators of the glucose to keep it in healthy ranges. They act in opposite ways, much like a see-saw, so they are called the "counter-regulatory hormones," as I described in Chapter 3.

When these two hormones work normally, insulin keeps blood glucose levels from rising too high (*hyperglycemia*), and glucagon prevents blood glucose from dropping too low (*hypoglycemia*).

It isn't just the actual high or low blood glucose levels that cause symptoms. The rate of rise and fall in glucose is a crucial factor that can also lead to the symptoms of hypoglycemia, and trigger insulin and glucagon release.

As we get fatter, however, insulin and glucagon don't work as well, so our body has difficulty keeping blood sugar in the healthy range. That's when we develop problems like hypoglycemia (low blood sugar), glucose intolerance (rapid rises and abrupt falls), insulin resistance (excess insulin and decreased sensitivity to insulin), and Diabetes Mellitus (sustained high blood glucose).

Think of all of these "conditions" as actually a series of steps along a path from being normal to becoming diabetic.

The Deadly Progression of PCOS

WEIGHT GAIN
⬇
ELEVATED GLUCOSE & INSULIN
⬇
INSULIN RESISTANCE
⬇
METABOLIC SYNDROME
↙ ↘
DIABETES ⇨ **CVD**

©Elizabeth Lee Vliet, MD 2001-2005

Insulin, Glucose and Menstrual Cycle Hormone Connections

Since the 1930s, and perhaps earlier, doctors have observed that women have more abnormal changes in their glucose regulation during the second half of the menstrual cycle when progesterone is the dominant hormone.

In 25 years of work with PMS and menopausal hormone changes, I have carefully studied how the cyclic changes in estradiol, progesterone, and the androgens affect blood glucose, glucose tolerance, insulin resistance, food cravings, binges, and weight gain.

I have found a strikingly consistent abnormal pattern of glucose and insulin response in the luteal phase of the cycle in women with PCOS.

If you are menstruating regularly, check to see what patterns you notice relative to your usual cycle with regard to when you crave sweets or alcohol.

If you are not menstruating regularly, then notice what symptoms you experience a couple of hours after eating various foods and record these.

If you don't menstruate regularly, or aren't sure about what time in the cycle to do the test, ask your doctor to do it *whenever you are having the most symptoms*.

If your symptoms are worse the week before your period comes, then I suggest that you **ask your doctor to do the insulin response to glucose test on days 20–24 of the menstrual cycle,** or during the time that your symptoms are worse. See Chapter 8 for more information on this test.

This timing shows how the rise in progesterone affects your symptoms and the insulin-glucose response. If you have PCOS and your estradiol is lower than optimal, your progesterone is normal and the androgens are high, then this abnormal glucose tolerance and increased insulin resistance gets worse.

The right testing helps you pick up early "red flags" that suggest insulin resistance before you become diabetic and your fasting glucose is elevated. See Chapter 8.

FYI
Get tested when YOU have symptoms, not when just when you have a doctor's appointment

PCOS and Heart Disease

Heart disease is the leading killer of women, as it is for men. But being a woman puts you at greater risk of dying from your first heart attack because women are more likely than men to be misdiagnosed and not treated.

Women with PCOS are at greater risk for early onset heart disease, and at even greater risk of dying from early heart attacks. It's a very serious picture, and doctors don't really explain this gender difference in risk very well.

Patients are usually told, "You're overweight, so eat less and exercise more." It isn't that simple for women with PCOS. You need more aggressive approaches, and will often need medication to help the diet and exercise work properly for weight loss.

Heart Symptoms or Heart Disease? Understanding The Difference

Have you ever experienced sudden, horrendous palpitations and pounding sensations as if your heart were going to literally jump out of your chest? Maybe you start feeling anxious; your stomach is a little upset; your skin is clammy.

You think, "What's going on? This can't be me? I'm healthy, and I never had these problems before. What is happening? I must be having a panic attack. Maybe I'm having a heart attack. No, that can't be; I'm too young. What is this?"

Tip: A rising insulin in the face of a falling glucose is a hallmark finding of insulin resistance.

So you see your family doctor, who checks you over and says you're fine, but you need to relax more and reduce your stress. With a deep sigh of relief, you leave and go on about your daily routine. Then, a few weeks later, it happens again. What is this?

Many women experience palpitations, heart flutters, or rapid heart beat, sometimes as early as in their teens or twenties, but even more often after age 35. What can cause these problems? Does it mean you have heart disease or are you just anxious, or could something else be going on?

Palpitations may occur in certain types of benign heart disease, such as mitral valve prolapse, or in potentially serious types of heart disease such as atrial fibrillation. Most doctors do a good evaluation of possible heart disease causes.

But doctors typically label everything else as "anxiety"

Look at this summary of the sequence:

Decreased estradiol from the ovary

Decreased estradiol at brain centers

Decreased brain endorphins and serotonin

A release of norepinephrine (NE) in the brain's "alarm center" in the locus ceruleus

Norepinephrine-stimulated cardiovascular responses:

- Increased heart rate
- Disrupted heart rhythm (palpitations, flutters, pounding, etc.)
- Blood pressure rises
- Dilation of blood vessels to critical organs (can cause lightheadedness because heart beating too rapidly doesn't fill with enough blood to pump with each beat)
- Fear about what's happening intensifies the "alarm reaction" which in turn increases all of the above responses

©Elizabeth Lee Vliet, MD 2001-2005

in women if they don't find actual heart disease. They tend to overlook the fact that *a variety of hormone fluctuations can cause palpitations and heart flutters.*

Symptoms are the changes and sensations you experience, such as headaches, racing heart, clammy skin, pain, flushing, tingling, and a myriad of others. These changes may indicate a normal body response to an environmental stimulus or even to your own thoughts. They could also be a potential warning of disease.

But not all symptoms indicate a disease is present, and not all diseases (at least in early stages) produce symptoms. Hypertension and osteoporosis are classic examples of diseases that do not produce symptoms until damage has already been done to the body by the disease process.

One of my tasks in helping patients is to sort out what the symptoms may indicate, and what diseases could be present that are still silent and not yet producing symptoms.

Women with PCOS may often experience palpitations as a symptom of excess androgens and low estradiol even if they don't have actual vascular disease. How does this take place? Look at the chart on the previous page.

It's a whole cascade of responses affecting your heart rate and rhythm from a hormone-triggered release of the brain's fight-or-flight chemical messengers.

In numerous studies, palpitations occur in anywhere from 40 percent to 60 percent of women during times of the menstrual cycle when estradiol levels drop (bleeding days and around ovulation).

This is such a common occurrence, many women don't even notice it until the hormone loss or imbalance become so marked that the body's responses are more intense. When we have a more pronounced physical response, suddenly, we are aware of it and even frightened by it.

Palpitations and flutters tend to become more frequent, and more intense, as women get older, but they can occur at any age if your estradiol is pushed too low with dieting or other causes. For about 15 percent to 20 percent of women, palpitations may be the only symptom serving as a clue to the decline in estradiol.

Women tell me they know "it's a physical, chemical kind of thing," but they have been told that it's "all in your head," their intuitive body wisdom dismissed.

If you have been checked out and do not have heart disease triggering these episodes, then pay attention to the timing of these episodes with your menstrual cycle. Notice where in the menstrual cycle these palpitations or panicky episodes occur. If your physical symptoms (heart flutters, heart racing or pounding, feeling queasy or nauseous, sweating, feeling anxious for no apparent reason) come right after ovulation, a day or so before your period starts, or the first two or three days of bleeding, you may be experiencing one of the brain effects of dropping estrogen levels.

There are lots of causes of falling estradiol that can hit

Tip:
Palpitations are frightening fluttering or pounding sensations in the chest. But they aren't always caused by heart disease.

younger women, long before you or your doctors think you are "old enough" to have hormone problems.

But it isn't just hormones—there are many other causes of palpitations as well. Anemia may produce palpitations. Palpitations may be a side effect of many medications, herbs, allergy and cold products. They may occur when you have had too much caffeine, or when you stopped drinking and alcohol is wearing off, or you have gone too long without eating and your blood sugar falls.

Panic disorder is a biological condition of excess, and erratic, production of adrenaline-type compounds in the brain that may also produce palpitations.

So palpitations as a symptom have many different causes. Some causes are just normal responses, while some causes of palpitations indicate more serious conditions. And the choice of treatments will be different, depending on the specific cause that is identified in a careful, comprehensive evaluation.

PCOS Hormone Effects on Arrhythmias—One Woman's Story

Kerry was a 34-year-old woman I evaluated for PCOS.

She had been diagnosed with ventricular tachycardia (VT, or V-tach, for short), an abnormal heart rhythm manifested by extremely rapid heartbeat that can cause dizziness, lightheadedness, and fainting. These symptoms happen because, when the heart is beating too fast, the ventricles don't have time to fill with blood enough to be able to pump enough blood with each beat. As a result, the brain doesn't get enough blood flow, which can cause fainting episodes (syncope).

It can be quite frightening, but the primary danger of VT occurs if it degenerates into more serious arrhythmias, such as ventricular fibrillation (or V-fib, as you have probably heard on television) that can lead to death. Consequently, when these episodes hit, and

FYI: Most doctors have not been taught to think about these hormone–brain–body connections, so they don't realize these are clues to dramatic hormone shifts in women.

didn't resolve quickly or she had fainting spells, she was admitted her to the hospital for cardiac monitoring until she was stable.

By the time I first saw her, she had been admitted to the ICU on three separate occasions when these attacks were particularly bad. Her doctors were puzzled; the cardiologist had not found an underlying disease causing the VT, nor did she have any evidence of plaque build up in the arteries of the heart that might contribute to rhythm disturbances. The explanation she was given was she was "anxious and stressed" and to take Xanax.

Timing is everything
Chart when you feel awful along with the dates of your period cycles. Keep a calendar handy just for this.

Kerry had a lot of medical experience even though she wasn't a doctor. She worked as a respiratory therapist at a large urban hospital and was part of a team (that included cardiologists) treating many patients. Kerry was trained to think about patterns and connections when people have medical problems. She began thinking about what she had noticed with her VT episodes, and her observations led her to have the consult with me. This is her story, in her own words, at her first appointment:

"I have had a miserable year with 3 hospitalizations for arrhythmias. First time, it was hot and I was taking care of my horse, and I got so dizzy I couldn't stand up. It passed and I didn't think much about it. Then it happened again while I was at work at the hospital. I had a run of V-tach; they called a code (emergency treatment of cardiac arrest), did all kinds of tests, and found nothing wrong."

"I was put on Tenormin, and that really affected me badly. Now I know what low blood pressure feels like, I could hardly get off the couch! I was tapered off it, but I still had very low BP, and then I had another episode of those horrible arrhythmias. I remember it was right before my period was supposed to start, and it struck me as odd, because that's when it happened the last two times, too."

"They checked me out and sent me home, but this time with meds for anxiety. My doctor just told me I was stressed and anxious. I took Buspar, but it kept me up all night, so weaned myself off. Then they recommended Xanax to take as I needed it and that seemed to at least help some."

"The next time it happened, I was having palpitations really bad, so I put myself on the monitor, and found I was in bigeminy, then it started coupling." (Remember, she works with patients who have these abnormal heart rhythms, so she knew how to read her own EKG strip).

"I showed the cardiologist, and they put me back in the hospital, but then another male physician said there was nothing wrong, that I was just anxious. I suffered a lot of humiliation from these male physicians and I was really upset. They should have known I was an intelligent woman and a medically trained person. I knew there was really something wrong. I was on my period again when it happened, and it was getting so that it happened with regularity like clockwork every month right before my period. It always begins right before my period starts and I have these feeling like I am going to pass out."

Vital: I can't emphasize enough the importance of really listening to a woman's observations and insights about her body and hormone patterns.

"This is a miserable way to live; I only have two weeks of feeling good. I am an outdoors person, I love riding, and I want to be active, but I can't do what I want to do when I feel so lousy. I do everything right, I have very moderate alcohol, I don't drink caffeine, I don't smoke, I eat well, and my the stress is no different than it has ever been. I need something to help this. I saw a newspaper article about your work, and then read your book and I can see that my hormones must be a factor in all this, especially since the episodes always happen with my period. I gave it to my cardiologist and told him he had to read it. They have to take this stuff seriously."

So now that you see these connections, what do you think might help Kerry? I suggested she use an estradiol patch beginning two days before her next period was due to start so that the estradiol would remain steadier until she could then start a trial of the low dose BCP. The steady dose hormones of the BCP would suppress her normal ups and downs of the ovary cycles and keep her hormone levels much steadier overall.

Oversight: Kerry's doctors had ruled out more serious causes of the arrhythmias, but had not checked hormone changes with menses that can trigger the same cardiovascular responses.

She was very pleased with that suggestion, and was especially quick to understand the concept of using the BCP. She said "It makes so much common sense to me. I don't understand why no one suggested this before. Here I work at a major medical center with all these top cardiologists and I have to go out of state to get someone to think of something this simple!"

At her follow up, a little over six months later, she said, "I am doing wonderfully, absolutely fine! I have noticed that I sleep better, my skin and hair are better, I don't have the acne I did before. I don't have any runs of PVCs the way I did before. I am feeling really well now."

Her primary physician agreed to continue her BCP, and I didn't hear from her until about 2½ years later when she called to have another consultation because her gynecologist had wanted her to stop the birth control pill.

At this appointment, she said,

Fact: Steady hormones prevent "destabilization" of brain centers that regulate heart rate and stop the arrhythmias triggered by falling estradiol.

"I had been doing great for a long time; I haven't had anything but the pill for all this time—I went off all the cardiac meds—my cardiologist didn't believe me that it was hormone-triggered but once I was on the pill I was able to get off everything else."

"I had been doing so beautifully, and I didn't have had any blood pressure highs or lows either since I have been on the pill. But then I had my lipids checked and my triglycerides (TG) were up. My Gyn scared the hell out of me saying this pill (Ovcon 35) had too much estrogen; she read me the riot act and recommended I take Premarin but she wanted me off everything for a month so she could check my FSH."

"I told her I was terrified about having arrhythmias again, and she said I could just go to the ER if that happened, but I have been there before and it is scary. I thought that was a very cold response. I went through that before three times and I don't want to go there again, it was very frightening."

"No one believes me that my heart problems were hormonally triggered; they think it is all in my head and due to some kind of emotional stress. But I can see that all

this has been completely eliminated by being on the Ovcon for the last three years, so I know it was connected to my hormone changes. And I am worried it will happen again; my resting heart rate was up to 113 yesterday (off Ovcon for 13 days), and I started having hot flashes again."

"That's why I contacted you again; I want more information about how serious this is with the triglycerides because I want to make an informed decision. I don't like going off the birth control pill abruptly when I was doing so well on it for three years. I think I could end up where I was three years ago, I don't want to go there!"

"I am not having any palpitations any more, I am not on any other medications–and before, I was on a ton of stuff before to control arrhythmias. I was able to wean off everything else."

Kerry was medically knowledgeable so we had a good discussion about the various risk issues, and her concerns for maintaining the stability she had achieved in her health and quality of life. I explained that even with her current slight increase in TG, she was actually at low risk of arterial plaque (atherosclerosis) because her HDL was excellent and her LDL/HDL ratio was also quite good. This put her at ½ average risk of heart disease.

She and I both agreed that her risk of having her previous heart problems was actually much greater from estradiol withdrawal. The drop in estrogen from stopping the Ovcon could again trigger her abnormal heart rhythms and vasomotor instability (that caused her past low blood pressure episodes), along with the possibility of coronary artery vasospasm leading to reduced blood flow to the heart as well.

I suggested she restart the transdermal patch form of estradiol to see how this worked, and then we could decide in a few weeks about the birth control pill.

About a month later, we had another follow up and this is her description of what had taken place since our last appointment:

"It has been a weird month. I had a big fight with the insurance company because they only gave me one set of patches. Then about a day before my period I had a run of PVCs; and I couldn't get my patches because the

Plan:
She was having a return of her low estrogen symptoms, and androgens were rising again, so she needed to be back on estradiol to prevent repeat episodes.

insurance company wouldn't refill it. Then I had a run of tachycardia and PVCs while lying in bed and that was it. I knew where it would lead, and I didn't want to end up in the ER again, so I went ahead and took my Ovcon. No one believes this heart problem is related to estrogen, they just tell me it is stress. I have not had any of my heart symptoms all these years on the pills, and then as soon as I stop them I have these heart symptoms back, so there is no doubt in my mind that my heart problems are related to the fall in my estrogen with my cycles or with the patch wearing off. I haven't felt good off the hormones and I know it is what I need. We have some options to bring down the TG with dietary changes and other medicines if I need them, so I would rather go this route than take a bunch of cardiac meds with a lot of side effects."

I agreed to restart the Ovcon, particularly since the Christmas was coming and she really didn't want to have a hospitalization over the holidays.

Success!
Three months later, she reported doing well back on the BCP, and had no further problems with the cardiac arrhythmias after restarting the Ovcon.

She said, "Even if the BCP may be slightly aggravating the increase in my TG, I feel very strongly that I need the stability of the BCP to prevent those arrhythmias I was having, and I will just work to get the TG down by eating better!"

I think Kerry's saga shows us how crucial it is to listen to what the woman herself thinks is most important and wants to do for her health, rather than taking a hard line based on one small piece of her total picture.

Estradiol and Your Cardiovascular System: Important Research Advances

You may have read about the way that estrogen reduces total cholesterol and increases the body's production of the good type of cholesterol, HDL. But estradiol has many other actions in a woman's body that help reduce her risk of heart disease. Take a look at the following chart that shows, some of the more exciting findings from recent research. But for us to have these benefits, we need optimal hormone *balance* before disease develops.

Differences in the way our natural estradiol works and the way a mixture of estrogens like Premarin affect the body may help to explain why studies, like the WHI, do not show as much protective effect from "estrogen" on heart disease as other studies have.

Such research helps to explain why heart disease increases at menopause when we lose 17-beta estradiol, and estrone and androgens are higher. Newer research also helps explain why heart disease hits younger women with PCOS who have excess androgens and low estradiol.

All of these exciting developments indicate the depth of the worldwide research on how our premenopausal estradiol helps maintain healthy heart and blood vessel function throughout the body. For more information, read *The Savvy Woman's Guide to Estrogen*.

PCOS and Breast and Endometrial Cancers

We have already discussed the ways that PCOS leads to marked, abnormal weight gain and obesity. Obesity, plus the abnormal hormone balance in PCOS, create additional risks for development of endometrial (uterine) and breast cancers.

Obesity alone causes a four- to seven-fold increased risk women getting breast cancer and endometrial cancers. Excess body fat contributes to higher levels of estrone and the male hormone, DHEA, circulating in the blood. We are not sure which of these hormones is the culprit but two factors imply that is is estrone.

First, 80 percent of breast cancers arise in women after menopause, when estrone is the primary estrogen present in the body (produced in the fat tissue and the adrenal glands) and there is very little 17-beta estradiol (the premenopausal 'good' estrogen) remaining.

Second, the location of the fat on the body is important—there is about a sixfold increase in risk of breast

Inspiration
I hope Kerry's assertive example to follow her own wisdom and knowledge will help inspire you to do the same in your life.

Fact:
Studies show women are more worried about breast cancer, but they actually suffer far more from heart disease: more disability, pain, loss of ability to be active, and premature deaths.

SUMMARY OF KEY ESTRADIOL (E2) BENEFITS ON OUR HEART AND BLOOD VESSELS

- E2 lowers blood pressure by dilating blood vessels
- E2 increases HDL ("good") cholesterol
- E2 decreases total cholesterol and ("bad") LDL
- E2 improves carbohydrate metabolism, decreasing risk of diabetes, a risk factor for heart disease
- E2 reduces platelet stickiness and clumping that causes clots, artery-clogging plaque, strokes; increased secretion of prostacyclin
- E2 (non-oral) reduces risk of blood clots by decreasing fibrinogen
- E2 has antioxidant effects on artery walls and acts as a free-radical scavenger that helps reduce plaque
- E2 reverses the impaired blood vessel response to acetylcholine in atherosclerotic coronary arteries. Gender specific.
- Estradiol enhances release of endothelium-derived NO (nitric oxide), a potent vasodilator; that helps lower BP
- Estradiol acts as a calcium-channel blocker, which also helps blood vessels dilate, improving blood flow and lowering BP
- E2 alters synthesis, release and response to vasoconstrictive peptides, e.g. endothelin-I and angiotensin-II
- E2 increases endothelial permeability, transport of blood-derived O2
- E2 lowers plastminogin activator inhibitor (PAI-1) and helps dissolve blood clots

cancer in women who have excess upper-body fat (i.e., from the belly button to the shoulders) compared to women whose fat is distributed more around the hips, buttocks, and thighs.

Breast cancer risk may be increased in patients with PCOS due to the effects of insulin resistance making more body fat, which in turn increases estrone levels. The effects of excess insulin cause even more cell growth, which in turn increases risk for breast cancer even further.

News: Current research also implicates excess insulin as a factor contributing to increased risk of breast cancer.

We suspect an increased risk of breast cancers in women with PCOS, but the data is mixed. Some studies show women with PCOS have higher risk of breast cancer, and other studies find PCOS women have the same or lower risk as control groups. Part of the problem causing this discrepancy in breast cancer risk is the whole issue of accurate diagnosis of PCOS, as I discussed in Chapter 5. There is still a lot of research that needs to be done on this question.

We do know with certainty that women with PCOS have higher rates of endometrial cancers, both after menopause, and in younger women. Uterine or endometrial cancer is increased for reasons similar to the ones I just listed for breast cancer. Excess stimulation of the uterine lining by estrone causes the lining to keep growing and growing and growing.

Alert Higher than normal insulin levels during the early stages of "insulin resistance" are just as damaging, if not more so, than high glucose levels.

The growth of the uterine lining means more cell division. Dividing cells have an increased likelihood of taking a turn into malignant, cancerous cells.

Proper dose and duration of progestin or progesterone therapy can help lower the risk of endometrial cancers, but recent research suggests that the opposite may be true for breast cancers. Higher amounts and duration of progesterone (and some progestins) triggers more growth of breast cells than does estrogen alone, and an increased risk of breast cancer over the long term.

That was one of the lessons from the Women's Health Initiative: women who still had a uterus took Prempro, a daily combination of estrogen and the synthetic progestin Provera (medroxyprogesterone acetate). This is the group that had a slightly higher risk of breast cancer than the control group on no hormones.

In considering risks for different cancers that can affect women, we need to consider many factors: excess insulin, low estradiol and high estrone, amount of progesterone and progestins, as well as the effects of high androgens. There is much work still to be done to tease out all these issues.

Summary:

PCOS causes many complex metabolic effects that lead to impaired function of many body systems to increase risks of serious diseases. The abnormal hormone balance of PCOS leads to alterations in function of other endocrine pathways such as insulin, cortisol, thyroid hormones, and the various brain "hormones" that serve as neuroendocrine "regulator messengers" to control body weight, fluid balance, appetite, food cravings, and other functions.

The American Diabetes Association states that we currently have more people in the United States with *undiagnosed* diabetes than people who have been diagnosed. Part of the reason is that in the United States, we don't do the most sensitive tests I have described above, and we wait too late to do those we do!

1998 recommendations from the CDC said that with rise in diabetes, every person should be tested by age 25.

The ADA is still focusing on abnormal fasting glucose test results before doing more extensive testing. Especially for women with PCOS, waiting until fasting glucose is abnormal means you are too late. The disease has already developed and has been doing its dirty work on your body.

If these problems are recognized early and treated aggressively with an integrated approach, it is possible to prevent or at least delay the onset of serious diabetic consequences such as nerve damage, kidney damage, blindness, strokes, heart attacks and premature death. The complications of insulin resistance and Diabetes Mellitus are directly related to how long your glucose and insulin have been out of control, and how high they have been.

Guidelines: The World Health Organization recommends a return to the oral glucose tolerance test as one way of identifying people with insulin resistance sooner.

The PCOS "Triple Whammy"

- (1) Loss of protective effects of estradiol, with higher levels of the "unhealthy" estrone.
- (2) Higher levels of the androgens made in fat tissue that promote dangerous "middle-body" fat storage, high cholesterol, and more plaque in arteries.
- (3) Greater incidence of significant insulin resistance than do women without PCOS, which is an independent risk factor for all types of cardiovascular disease, as it is for diabetes. Diabetes then increases the risk of heart disease, so it is a vicious cycle.

©Elizabeth Lee Vliet, MD 2001-2005

You need to get on top of this problem early and treat it aggressively to get back into healthy ranges. Even if you don't develop diabetes, you will have much more difficulty losing excess body fat if you remain glucose intolerant and insulin resistant.

Pay attention to the warnings I have described in this chapter, get tested, and get going with everything you need to do to be healthy!

Toxic effects of excess glucose and insulin

EXCESS GLUCOSE

Examples of Common Symptoms

- ❧ Weight gain
- ❧ fatigue, low energy
- ❧ excessive sleepiness after eating
- ❧ lethargy
- ❧ headaches
- ❧ food cravings
- ❧ memory and concentration problems
- ❧ excessive thirst
- ❧ increased urination
- ❧ blurred vision
- ❧ mood changes, depression
- ❧ increased frequency of yeast infections

Damages

- ❧ forms AGEs (advanced glycosylation end products) products that damage cells
- ❧ arterial smooth muscle overgrowth
- ❧ increased platelet stickiness–increased risk of clots
- ❧ increased "leakiness" (permeability) of blood vessels
- ❧ loss of blood vessel elasticity–increased risk of high blood pressure
- ❧ reduced clearance of lipoprotein particles=more plaque in arteries
- ❧ increased formation of free radicals that damage cells
- ❧ loss of myelin around nerve cells, death of axons
- ❧ impaired nerve impulse conduction
- ❧ impaired immune cell function
- ❧ impaired enzyme function
- ❧ depletes antioxidant vitamins (vitamin C especially)
- ❧ depletes magnesium, potassium
- ❧ increases bone loss

Toxic effects of excess glucose and insulin

EXCESS INSULIN

Examples of Common Symptoms

- waist measure greater than 33 inches
- overall weight gain, especially waist and upper body
- eating less and still gaining weight
- food cravings, especially sweets, simple carbs
- frequent episodes of reactive hypoglycemia
- mood swings
- fatique
- high blood pressure
- elevated cholesterol and triglycerides

Damages

- promotes fat formation (lipogenesis)
- memory and concentration problems
- Inhibits fat breakdown (lipolysis)
- increases cell division, leading to aging of cells
- vascular damage (see also glucose), esp. endothelial cells
- mades adverse androgen effects on lipids worse (elevated cholesterol, increased LDL, lower HDL, increased triglycerides)
- increased blood pressure
- decreases levels of antioxidants such as vitamin E
- death of nerve cells, leading to cognitive damage, etc
- increases risk of dementia (Alzheimers type, and others)
- impaired immune function
- plays key role in growth of cancer cells
- increases risk of breast, endometrial, colon, liver and pancreatic cancers, especially in women

©Elizabeth Lee Vliet, MD 2001-2005

There are four major ways to correct the problems of excess insulin, getting fatter, and becoming diabetic:

Just DO it!

❧ **Exercise more.** Exercise helps lower blood sugar, and reduce the excessive insulin response after you eat. See Chapter 12.

❧ **Eat a lower carbohydrate, balanced diet** with the right amount of calories for your body build and metabolism. See Chapter 12.

❧ **Restore hormone balance** to have optimal estradiol–androgen–progestrone balance, optimal thyroid function, and reduce excess cortisol. See Chapters 10 and 13.

❧ **Use medications to reduce insulin over-production and excess androgens**. See Chapter 11.

Chapter 8

Getting Diagnosed

In this chapter, I discuss the tests I think you need for a thorough baseline evaluation to see whether you may have PCOS. I think it is critical for you to know what the appropriate tests are, why they are important, and what their limitations may be. In later chapters I describe the various treatment options that can be integrated into an individualized plan to help you control symptoms, feel better and reduce serious health risks.

Even though it can be difficult for women to get their physician to order tests, or insurance to cover all the necessary tests to properly diagnosis PCOS, if you feel strongly that you may have PCOS, be assertive about asking your doctor to help you get them done. Your health is too important for you to go quietly away, and not have the proper tests done.

Ovarian Hormones

I regularly use serum hormone levels to monitor need for and response to hormone therapy, and I have consistently found these to be reliable and cost-effective approaches.

Ideally, a baseline estradiol, progesterone, testosterone, DHEA, and DHEA-s should be done in your 20s or 30s when you are feeling really well. Having your healthy baseline gives you a target range to aim for with any later hormone replacement. Unfortunately, this is rarely done. These same tests are even more important as we get older and start having symptoms, especially acne, hirsutism, or rapid weight gain that could signal the beginning of PCOS.

If you have become menopausal or have don't have regular periods or have had a hysterectomy, checking all of the ovarian hormones once on any day of the month will give you a baseline to correlate with your symptoms. You can have the levels rechecked when symptoms get worse, or when you change your hormone Rx.

Checking levels after starting hormone therapy helps you be certain that you are above the currently accepted thresholds for preserving bone, brain, heart and other benefits of estradiol, and helps insure that you are not getting too much testosterone.

Estradiol

I use the blood test for *estradiol*, not "total estrogens," to help in both evaluation and treatment for women with hormone related problems. If you are still menstruating, I check these levels on Day 1–3 (early follicular phase), and again on Day 20–22 (luteal phase peak).

In my clinical work, I find that women typically have their best energy level, mood, sleep, and memory when serum (blood) levels of estradiol are *above* 90–100 pg/ml. This is the *lower* end of the range for healthy menstrual cycle levels.

Levels up to about 200 or so, are the *normal estradiol levels* reached in the first half of the menstrual cycle before ovulation. At ovulation, estradiol levels are typically in the range of 300–500 pg/ml, and then in the luteal phase of the cycle (when progesterone is produced), a healthy level of estradiol is generally in the range of 200–300 pg/ml.

After menopause, women *not taking any estrogen* typically have estradiol levels of only 10–30 pg/ml, a far cry from the levels we have been used to our entire adult life.

Estradiol levels below about 90 pg/ml are generally too low to provide adequate relief of symptoms from hot

To do–
If you are still menstruating, check estradiol and progesterone levels at cycle day 1 to 3 and check the ratio of estradiol to progesterone in the luteal phase about day 20–22.

flashes to muscle/joint pain, insomnia, memory loss, "middle spread," not to mention helping us achieve our usual energy and zest and having our normal feeling of well-being.

International research has found that bone loss continues to occur with estradiol levels *below* about 80–90 pg/ml. Cardiovascular benefits of estradiol have been found to occur at levels *above* about 80–90 pg/ml as a starting point. Memory, sleep and concentration typically improve the most if estradiol levels are above 100 pg/ml.

It's fairly straightforward to know if you are getting too little or too much estradiol. Your blood tests are a guide, but *how you feel* is also important in deciding what dose or type is best for you.

The blood test for estradiol is highly reliable, and commonly used in infertility settings today. While there is some variation over the course of a day, and throughout the menstrual cycle, the variation is no greater than other tests, such as cholesterol, that we use regularly. We simply learn how to take this variation into account in our interpretations.

Target Levels
I suggest you look for a level of about 90 or better if you are taking supplemental estradiol

Tip:
Correlate this with your symptoms to see whether you have reached an optimal level for your body.

Progesterone

Current blood serum tests for progesterone are also accurate and reliable, and used regularly in fertility centers for cycle management.

If you are having regular 28-day cycles, even if you don't know whether you ovulate, I recommend checking progesterone on about cycle day 20 or 21. This should give the peak level of the luteal phase of the cycle, and if you ovulated in that cycle, it will be typically between 5–25 ng/ml. During pregnancy, progesterone levels rise about 15 times higher than this.

If you are taking prescription progesterone, or using an over-the-counter cream, it's important to know that it doesn't take very much supplemental progesterone to give blood levels equal to those of pregnancy. This is why you need to be careful about overuse of any progesterone *creams* that can also contain more then 25–30 mg of progesterone. Because they are better absorbed than oral forms, high dose compounded progesterone creams can give even higher blood levels that make the weight gain and insulin resistance in PCOS much worse. A good rule-of-thumb for converting oral to non-oral doses is that the *cream or gel should be about 1/10 the oral dose*, or 10–20 mg a day, as the prescription form of progesterone (*Prochieve*) delivers.

If you are using a progesterone cream that is more than this amount, and you are gaining weight or having trouble with more acne, depression or marked fatigue, talk with your doctor. You are probably getting more progesterone than you need.

Testosterone

I usually check the total, free and weakly-bound forms of testosterone circulating in the bloodstream so I can better help my patients make the best decisions on the right dose.

In my clinical experience, women typically experience their optimal normal energy level and libido when blood serum levels of *total* testosterone are between 40 and 60 ng/dl, with the *percent of free testosterone* at about 1–2% of the total. For comparison, using the same pg/ml units we use for estradiol, 40–60 ng/dl would be 400–600 pg/ml.

Men's testosterone levels run about 450–1200 ng/dl (or 4500–12,000 pg/ml). Most men don't experience a loss of libido until testosterone drops down to around 600 ng/dl (6,000 pg/ml) or less.

Women are more sensitive to small amounts of testosterone, so a drop of only 10–15 units can make an enormous difference in whether a woman will feel her usual energy level and sexual spark.

For women, "middle-spread" weight gain, excess facial hair, thinning scalp hair, acne, irritability, agitation, restless sleep, are signs of androgen excess. That's why women with PCOS often have these symptoms—they have high free and total testosterone.

The majority of menopausal women I have evaluated, particularly those who have had surgical removal of the ovaries in their thirties and forties, have had testosterone levels of less than 10…with unmeasurable amounts of free testosterone. No wonder they don't have any sexual desire!

Dehydroepiandrosterone (DHEA)

DHEA occurs in two forms in the body, as I described in more detail in Chapter 3: (1) unconjugated DHEA (or DHEA non-sulfate), and (2) conjugated DHEA or DHEA-sulfate (DHEA-s), occurring in larger amounts than cortisol.

DHEA-s levels in the bloodstream are more constant over the 24-hour day than is DHEA. DHEA shows pulse-type variations in secretion similar to the pattern of cortisol, with higher levels in the morning and lowest levels in the late afternoon. That's why some physicians say that measuring only DHEA-s is more reliable, but *I find that it is important in women to know levels of both forms*, especially if they are having symptoms of androgen excess.

DHEA varies a great deal by age, time of day, and to a lesser extent can also vary by menstrual cycle phase. Be sure that you have the blood serum tests done to give a picture of both total and free hormones.

Urine and saliva tests do not give as complete a picture of the hormone reserve that is available for action in the body, and I don't recommend them.

Androstenedione

This is another androgen that is elevated in PCOS. It

Tip: Testosterone levels much above 60 ng/dl in women may cause androgen excess.

Tip: Testosterone levels below 10–15 ng/dl are generally too low to maintain your usual libido, intensity of orgasm, energy level, and bone mass.

is made by the ovary, adrenal gland, and also in body fat, and then becomes a building block to be converted into other hormones such as testosterone and estrone. Androstenedione contributes to the overall androgen excess in PCOS and causes the same adverse effects I described earlier when testosterone and DHEA levels are too high.

Fact:
FSH levels are less than 20 MIU/ml in premeno-pausal women who have adequate levels of estradiol.

It is another test that can be done to help quantify the degree of androgen excess, but because it is nonspecific as to the source of excess androgens, I don't usually order this test. Levels typically decrease with weight loss and the other appropriate treatments to decrease overall androgen production.

Pituitary Hormones

There are several in this group that are important in the evaluation of women with possible PCOS to help clarify the cause of symptoms.

Follicle Stimulating Hormone (FSH)

Along with LH, FSH regulates the menstrual cycle and ovarian hormone production. As estradiol declines, FSH rises as the brain tries to stimulate the ovary to keep up estrogen production. If your hormone therapy dose is right for you (and your brain), FSH comes back down to the lower level seen prior to menopause (less than 20).

Fact:
High FSH levels (above 20 MIU/ml) indicate that estradiol levels are too low, even if you are on hormone therapy.

Although many gynecologists only check FSH, in my opinion, this is not the most sensitive marker of estradiol decline, so that's why I check both the FSH (brain) and the ovary hormone levels, especially estradiol.

Luteinizing Hormone (LH)

LH is the other pituitary hormone that helps regulate the menstrual cycle. In the normal menstrual cycle, LH rises abruptly at about mid-cycle and triggers ovulation. In the majority of women with PCOS, there are both more "pulses" of LH release than normal, and also higher levels produced. Some women with PCOS have relatively normal LH levels, so this test alone is not sufficient for diagnosing PCOS. High LH concentrations in PCOS stimulate theca cells in the ovary to produce excess androgens. In menopausal women, LH levels rise for the same reasons that FSH does, as the brain tries to stimulate the declining ovary to produce more hormones. It also drops to premenopausal levels if hormone therapy is optimal.

ACTH: Adrenocorticotropin hormone

This is the primary regulator of the adrenal glands and cortisol production. Adenomas in the pituitary gland can produce excess amounts of ACTH, leading to over-stimulation of the adrenal glands to make cortisol. Since tumors like this can produce symptoms that are similar to PCOS, there are times when it may be appropriate to measure ACTH if cortisol remains excessively high, and doesn't respond to the usual treatments for PCOS.

Prolactin

This hormone is produced by the pituitary and can be measured in a simple, reliable blood test that is best done between 7:00 to 8:00 AM in the morning. Elevated prolactin is common in PCOS and can also be an indication of a pituitary hormone-producing tumor. These are usually benign, but may cause problems because (a) the tumor is large enough (macroadenoma) to cause pressure on the optic nerve resulting in visual changes, or (b) the hormone production from a small tumor (microadenoma) is enough to disrupt ovarian cycles, cause loss of menstrual periods, and adds to weight gain problems.

In the third trimester of pregnancy, prolactin levels rise to almost 300 ng/ml. Then it slowly decreases in the first few months after delivery to a normal level if a mother is not nursing. During nursing, prolactin levels remain higher than in non-pregnant women, but typically not as high as during pregnancy.

Fact:
In non-pregnant women, prolactin is normally less than about 15 to 20 ng/ml.

When prolactin is higher than about 15-20 ng/ml in a non-pregnant woman who is not nursing, it typically causes menstrual cycles to become irregular and suppresses estradiol levels.

If prolactin levels are too high, and there are visual changes, generally an MRI of the pituitary is done to see whether the best treatment is medication to bring down the prolactin, or whether surgical removal may be needed to prevent permanent damage to the optic nerve.

Medications to lower prolactin include dopamine boosters (agonists), such as bromocriptine (Parlodel), cabergoline (Dostinex) and pergolide (Permax). High prolactin levels can respond very well to these medications, and this may be necessary in women with PCOS whose prolactin levels remain high after other treatment approaches are used.

Thyroid Tests:

I recommend the following tests: TSH, free T4, free T3 and thyroid antibodies (antithyroglobulin, anti-microsomal)

Other Hormones That Should Be Checked:

Thyroid

The thyroid gland plays a major role in women to help regulate the ovarian cycle and maintain normal fertility. Symptoms of thyroid disorders tend to overlap those seen in ovarian problems, so if you are having "hormone problems" you need a thorough check of the thyroid system as well as checking ovarian hormones.

The tests I recommend are more sensitive indicators of subtle (subclinical) thyroid disorders that may be affecting ovarian function and aggravating the problems of PCOS, especially weight gain.

Thyroid Stimulating Hormone (TSH)

This is the hormone that stimulates the thyroid gland to produce more hormones (T3, T4) when the brain senses the thyroid hormone levels are too low. Thus, if your thyroid is sluggish or failing and producing too little of the thyroid hormones, we call this *hypothyroidism*, and your **TSH rises** to stimulate the gland to make more T3 and T4. This means on the lab test, TSH **will be high** (i.e., greater than 4–5).

Hypothyroidism can cause ovarian dysfunction, infertility, weight gain, memory problems, depression, high cholesterol, high blood pressure and increased risk of heart disease. Since this disorder is so much more common in women than men, it is crucial to detect it early and treat it properly.

Current preventive medicine approaches emphasize earlier recognition, and treatment with thyroid hormones until the TSH has reached a level of about 1.0–1.5.

If you are taking thyroid medicine, and the dose is not enough, your TSH will remain high. Even though the "normal" range on the lab reports will typically go up to about 5.0, an optimal range of TSH for women is between 0.6 to about 2.0.

If your thyroid gland is *over*-producing hormones, called **hyperthyroidism**, the brain senses this, and markedly reduces the amount of TSH, so the **TSH will be low**, i.e., less than about 0.5 on the typical lab reference scale.

TSH will also be too low, or suppressed, if you are taking too much supplemental thyroid medication. Too much thyroid hormone in women causes a more rapid rate of bone loss (osteoporosis), disturbances of heart rhythm (palpitations), damage to the heart, muscle wasting, hair loss, and marked tiredness.

Thyroid Antibodies

Autoimmune Thyroid Disorders (Thyroiditis). There are two types of **thyroid antibodies** that I measure: (1) antibodies to the thyroid gland tissue itself (*anti-microsomal* antibodies, or *anti-TPO* antibodies) and (2) antibodies to the thyroid hormone, thyroglobulin (*anti-thyroglobulin* antibody). When these antibodies are significantly elevated, thyroid function is impaired, and gradually declines. Then later women develop significant abnormalities in TSH and free T3, free T4.

Tip: A normal TSH in the presence of elevated thyroid antibodies may occur in the early stages of autoimmune thyroid diseases.

In the early stages of an autoimmmune thyroiditis, the TSH may be normal when the thyroid gland is actually failing. This situation explains the presence of symptoms of "low thyroid" in the presence of "normal" thyroid tests. If the antibody measures are not done, this early phase of illness can be missed.

Hashimoto's (hypothyroidism) and *Graves* (hyperthyroidism) disease are two examples of autoimmune thyroid disorders that are many times more common in women, and can disrupt ovarian function.

I think it is crucial to check thyroid antibodies in women with ovarian problems and suggestive symptoms (weight gain, fatigue, depression, high blood pressure, high cholesterol) because early treatment may help prevent progression of the thyroiditis and more serious illness.

Adrenal Hormones

The adrenal glands and ovaries are closely inter-connected, and symptoms of ovarian disorders like PCOS can also occur in disorders of adrenal function, such as Cushing's syndrome (cortisol excess). High cortisol (greater than $20\mu g/dl$) may occur in PCOS, and may also be a sign of another underlying serious disease, Cushing's Syndrome, which has many features in common with PCOS. I discuss this in Chapter 9.

It can sometimes be difficult to sort out whether someone has PCOS or Cushing's because the body changes and symptoms are so similar. Tests that help to determine whether the problem is adrenal, ovarian, or both are as follows:

૭❧ Cortisol

Cortisol is a member of the *glucocorticoid group* of hormones produced by the adrenal glands, and it prepares our body to deal with the effects of stress. Cortisol and its fellow glucocorticoids are major metabolic regulators, and have many functions in the body.

Cortisol has a definite daily (diurnal) rhythm to its

secretion, normally beginning to rise for the day about 4:00–5:00 AM, and peaking about 8:00–9:00 AM. We need the effects of rising cortisol to get our biological engines going to start our day. Levels should be gradually falling over the day and be lowest at night. When we are stressed, this normal daily rhythm may be blunted, shifted in time, or even completely reversed.

Other adrenal tests can be done if appropriate: serum ACTH, 24-hour urine for urinary total and free cortisol, and Dexamethasone Suppression Test (DST). If these follow up tests are abnormal, imaging studies (MRI, CAT scans, etc.) are usually ordered to check for tumors causing excess cortisol production.

High cortisol may indicate simply excess stress from physical factors like sleep loss, hormone imbalances, medication side effects (i.e., birth control pills), drug use, and also with situational life "stresses."

Low morning cortisol (less than $7\mu g/dl$ range) is much less common than cortisol excess, but can indicate a serious medical disorder, adrenal insufficiency, also called *Addison's Disease*. Women who have symptoms of PCOS, such as excess body hair and weight gain, are not likely to have adrenal insufficiency, since the hallmark of Addison's is *marked weight loss, hair loss, and muscle wasting.*

❧ 17-hydroxyprogesterone

This is a precursor, or building block, molecule that can be elevated in people with a congenital (genetic) deficiency of an enzyme called 21-hydroxylase. Loss of this enzyme means that the body can't make the rest of the hormones in this pathway, so there is a build up of 17-hydroxyprogesterone to levels that can be more than twice normal. Since 17-hydroxyprogesterone has androgenic effects, it can cause symptoms like those seen from high testosterone and DHEA in PCOS. It is best to do this blood test at between 8:00–9:00 AM in the follicular phase of the menstrual cycle to get the most reliable results.

Tip: I recommend measuring the 8:00 AM serum cortisol as a first step. If this is excessively high, then additional tests can be done to more accurately determine the cause.

Tip: Testing for 17-hydroxy-progesterone helps to rule out congenital adrenal hyperplasia.

Sex-Hormone Binding Globulin (SHBG)

This is a carrier protein in the blood stream that binds the sex hormones, holding them in reserve to release as needed to activate hormone target cells throughout the body.

Measuring this protein in the blood helps us determine whether a hormone imbalance has also affected the production of this protein, which in turn will determine the relative amount of estrogen and testosterone in the free, active fraction in your blood.

Too much free testosterone and too little free estradiol, for example, can cause increased body fat, acne, scalp hair loss, as well as determine the areas on your body where fat is stored.

SHBG is often low in women with PCOS, and contributes to high free androgen levels that cause such unwanted health problems. SHBG can be increased, thereby reducing the excess free androgens, with use of oral birth control pills or oral estrogen and progestin menopausal options.

Fasting blood glucose (sugar)

The healthy range is 70–100 mg/dl. Low blood glucose, or *hypoglycemia*, is a fasting glucose less than 50. Fasting glucose between 100–110 mg/dl should be a warning that your body is changing in a negative direction and you need take steps to improve diet and exercise to bring this down and help prevent the progression to diabetes.

Glucose intolerance is indicated by a fasting glucose of 111–125 mg/dl.

Fasting glucose *above* 126 mg/dl is the new cut-off to indicate diabetes.

Fasting glucose and tests for insulin resistance should be done if you are at high risk for diabetes, based on the following:

* family history of diabetes
* more than 10% over ideal body weight

Tip: Fasting glucose should be checked regularly in women with symptoms of PCOS, since they have a high risk of becoming diabetic.

- ❧ have gained more than 20 pounds in the last year
- ❧ have gained weight around the middle of your body, waist > 33"
- ❧ new onset sweet cravings, increased thirst, increased urination
- ❧ elevated triglycerides, even if cholesterol is normal
- ❧ elevated androgens

Fasting Insulin

Insulin resistance is very common in PCOS, and is increasingly common as women get older. Excess insulin is a significant factor that accelerates the excess androgens in PCOS and makes it harder for you to lose excess fat. Insulin resistance also greatly increases your risk of diabetes.

I think this is important to check if you are seriously overweight, or if you have any of the risks I listed under glucose (see above). It is difficult to give you specific insulin values to look for because there are so many different assays used by laboratories throughout the country and the insulin values are not as well-standardized as are glucose values.

If your levels are significantly higher than this, you may need medication to help lower the insulin excess to decrease your risk of becoming diabetic.

Tip: A normal fasting insulin is less than 10 micro-international units per milliliter (mIU/ml), and a 2-hour postprandial insulin range about 6–25 mIU/ml.

Testing for Insulin Resistance

There are some helpful ways to detect insulin resistance. One is the *2-hour post-prandial glucose and insulin test.* For this, you eat a high-carbohydrate meal, and then blood is drawn exactly two hours later to measure your glucose and insulin. This test tells you how high your glucose and insulin rise in response to eating "regular" food.

If the 2-hour post-prandial glucose is 140 mg/dl but less than 200 mg/dl, you are glucose intolerant, and at higher risk of becoming diabetic.

Tip:
The 2-hour glucose will become high long before your fasting glucose becomes elevated. This is a more sensitive test for insulin resistance than is the fasting glucose test most doctors use.

Rationale:
I am not only looking for diabetes. I am looking for the early change of insulin resistance so that women can be treated *before* they develop full blown diabetes.

If your 2-hour post-prandial glucose is over 200, you meet the new ADA criteria for diabetes and need a thorough evaluation by your physician.

If your lab appears to have a different reference range, and your 2-hour post-prandial insulin is at the high end or above the top of their normal range, then you are likely insulin resistant, and at higher risk of becoming diabetic.

High fasting and post-prandial insulin levels are commonly seen in older women who are gaining middle body fat, and also in women with PCOS, even if they are thin. High insulin levels make it even harder for you to lose those unwanted fat pounds.

A more thorough test of insulin resistance is the "*Insulin Response to Glucose Test.*" It involves drinking a measured amount of glucose, then measuring glucose and insulin at regular intervals over six hours to see the pattern of rise and fall in both of these, correlated with any symptoms you experience with these changes in glucose and insulin.

Other doctors have said to my patients, "You don't need to do glucose or insulin tolerance tests, we don't do those to diagnose diabetes," or "It doesn't matter when in your cycle you do a glucose tolerance test, it's all the same," or "A 3-hour test is fine, you don't need the full six hours." I disagree on all those points.

I am getting objective laboratory data that helps to explain patients' descriptions of uncontrollable food cravings, difficulty losing weight, mood swings and other physical symptoms.

Second, it is clear the women's descriptions that there is a definite cycle-specific characteristic to these cravings, so we must do the testing at the time when women experience these symptoms and cravings or we won't discover the physical changes that trigger them.

If we only do a three-hour measure of glucose-insulin response, we miss the last 2 or 3 hours when the most significant abnormal changes tend to occur, both in the glucose and insulin values as well as in your symptoms.

Most patients are never asked if they had any symptoms during the GTT. It seems to me that this overlooks the most crucial information: What YOU have to say about what you were experiencing as the glucose and insulin levels rose and fell. I also have our patients keep a timed symptom log of everything experienced throughout the test, and my staff makes written observations as well.

It also can help to do a short cognitive assessment (to check memory, attention, concentration, etc.) at each hourly blood draw during the insulin response to glucose test. This helps to show how blood glucose changes can affect brain symptoms that often get misdiagnosed as psychiatric or behavioral problems.

These combined observations are discussed in detail when we go over the test results at a follow-up appointment. I have found this approach has been remarkably helpful in identifying overlooked medical problems, and in helping each woman learn how her body responds, what's contributing to the sensations she experiences, and what will be needed in order to create eating plans designed to help relieve her symptoms—the best spacing of meals as well as the most optimal balance of carbohydrate, fat, and protein.

It also helps me to see whether patients may need adjustments in their HRT or birth control pills, or need to add other medications to improve glucose tolerance and insulin response.

When Should the Test Be Done If You Are Menstruating?

In twenty years of work with PMS and menopausal hormone changes, I have been studying the connections between cyclic changes in estradiol and progesterone and how these hormones affect blood glucose, glucose tolerance, insulin resistance, food cravings, binges, and weight gain.

Reality: Most physicians look at the numbers for each hour. If the numbers fall into the "normal" range, the patient is told "everything's normal," without asking YOU how you felt.

Rationale: Information about your symptoms during the test plus objective lab results allows me to correlate your symptoms with actual fluctuations in blood glucose and insulin levels.

If you are still menstruating, I recommend that you do the insulin response to glucose test during days 20–23 of the menstrual cycle, or about a week before your period is due. If done then it shows how the rise in progesterone affects your symptoms and your insulin-glucose response.

In women with lower than optimal estradiol who still have ovulatory levels of progesterone or who have low estradiol and high androgens, this abnormal glucose tolerance and insulin resistance gets worse as they get older.

The women with PCOS that I have evaluated with a 5-hour insulin response to glucose test typically show the following patterns:

- ❧ Rapid early rise in glucose in the first half hour
- ❧ Higher than expected 1 hour peaks of both glucose and insulin
- ❧ Rapid fall off in glucose (sometimes as early as hour 2), triggering symptoms of the "fight-or-flight" adrenaline response (panic, anxiety, nausea, dizziness, fuzzy thinking, rapid heart beat, palpitations, feeling sweaty or clammy, among others)
- ❧ Insulin levels that are too high, and remain high after the glucose has started falling, or that rise after glucose has already started falling too low and causing symptoms.
- ❧ Glucose levels at the 4th and 5th hour of the test that are lower than normal, and associated with symptoms of adverse brain effects: impaired memory, concentration, dizziness, drowsiness, low energy, increased pain, or tearfulness for no reason, etc.

©Elizabeth Lee Vliet, MD 2001-2005

Hemoglobin A1C

This is a measure of the amount of glucose that has been incorporated into hemoglobin, which is the oxygen-carrying molecule in your red blood cells. If you are developing problems in your body's ability to handle glucose, this test is a sensitive marker that can pick up these problems earlier and gives us a way of seeing whether or not you have had high blood glucose levels over the past three months.

If you already have diabetes, Hemoglobin A1C is used to monitor how well your diet and medications are improving your glucose control.

Additional Tests I Think Are Important

CA 125

This blood test measures an ovarian antigen that may be elevated in both malignant ovarian cancer and several benign conditions such as fibroids, ovarian cysts, endometriosis, adenomyosis, and early pregnancy. I find this a useful component in evaluating women with PCOS because it is a useful clue to the presence of unrecognized benign conditions I listed above that have to be addressed in planning appropriate treatment.

CA 125 is currently the only available blood test that could alert us to an ovarian malignancy and is the best "early warning" test we have at this time even though it is not diagnostic for ovarian cancer. I think it is important to have done if you have a family history of ovarian cancer, or if you have vague abdominal symptoms (gas, bloating, distension, change in bowel movements, pain, etc.) that are not responding to other measures.

> **Normal Range:** Hemoglobin A1C will be **less than 6** if your glucose control is in a healthy normal range.

Ferritin

This is a measure of the body's iron stores. Optimal levels for women are about 60–90 ng/ml. The concern about iron and heart disease is that high ferritin levels indicate excess iron that may increase your risk of heart disease.

Low ferritin levels (generally less than about 50) are much more common in women due to menstrual blood loss over the years, and low ferritin is associated with restless legs syndrome, insomnia, fatigue, muscle pain, poor exercise tolerance, thinning scalp hair and a variety of other problems.

If your levels are low (even without anemia yet showing on your hemoglobin and hematocrit), I suggest taking a multivitamin that contains iron. If ferritin doesn't improve after 6 to 12 months of taking iron supplements, you should talk with your physician about evaluating other causes of iron loss, such as an undiagnosed colon cancer.

High ferritin levels (i.e., over 150–200) are not seen often in women because women lose iron every month in their menstrual bleeding and most women today seem to have drastically decreased their intake of red meat, the primary food source of iron. I check ferritin on all my patients, and I have seen *high* ferritin levels in probably less than 1 out of 10 women.

High ferritin is more common in men who don't have menstrual blood loss and who eat more red meat. Excess ferritin can increase risk of heart disease, and may cause damage to liver, kidneys and brain as well as cause a whole host of other problems such as fatigue, weakness, muscle and joint pain, diabetes, and in men, impotence. If ferritin is high, it is important to avoid taking multivitamins that contain iron, and consider donating blood at the Red Cross to decrease iron stores.

Hemachromatosis is a hereditary iron storage disorder leading to iron overload. Ask your physician about having further tests if you have high ferritin that is not from taking iron supplements. You may request information from the American Hemochromatosis Society website.

Summary: What's "Optimal" versus "Normal" Ranges

Getting your hormones and other labs checked can often be confusing when the results come in and your physician says everything is "normal" because the tests within the lab's "normal" range. This may be quite misleading.

First of all, the reference ranges for women's ovarian hormones in particular are often too broad to be meaningful.

Secondly, you have to consider that a given number is not necessarily the "optimal" number for you to feel best.

If your estradiol or testosterone or thyroid is at the bottom of the normal range, that may not be enough to give your brain and body the "hormone power" fuel it needs for optimal performance.

On the other hands, sometimes your hormone levels may be slightly higher that the "normal" range, but this may be where you feel the best.

My desire is to carefully integrate the lab results with what you describe so together we can make the best decisions about appropriate treatment approaches for you.

What about Saliva, Hair and Urine Tests?

You may have seen ads for testing your hormones, quite inexpensively even, by saliva, hair analysis or urine. There has been quite a consumer marketing campaign for these tests over the Internet, through newsletters, and by direct mail. Based on reputable medical studies, these tests are not reliable enough to properly decide your treatment, particularly with something as critical to your health as your hormones. I believe in offering options to my patients, so I have tried these methods and have found they are extremely variable and not at all helpful.

I stopped using saliva tests over a decade ago because of these problems. Current international research has actually compared the saliva and serum results in the same person, at the same time of day, and found the saliva tests vary so much as to be totally unreliable. Medical references on this issue are included in the Appendix.

I have continued to use the "gold standard" serum tests that are used in worldwide hormone research and are much more reliable and clinically useful in helping women design appropriate hormone strategies.

Benefits of Comprehensive Hormone Testing

Other physicians often say it is too "expensive" to do all the tests I have just recommended to carefully evaluate women for PCOS. My view is that it is too expensive NOT to know this information. Without the hormone levels to show what is really going on, women end up

My approach: Listen to what you say about how you are feeling, and not just treat lab numbers.

Salvia Tests: These have not correlated well with women's descriptions, but I find serum tests correlate very well with my patients' self descriptions.

Food for Thought:
I think it is less expensive to check hormone blood levels than to do all the tests and evaluations women have done because hormone problems are not recognized.

spending money, time, and effort seeing other specialists, getting other tests, and even taking potentially unnecessary medication. Besides, it is difficult to put a price tag on improving someone's quality of life. It also does not make sense to me (in time or economics) for women to undergo a series of psychotherapy sessions thinking that their weight gain is just due to stress or empty nest or a bad relationship.

Clearly, having reliable information about hormone levels has made an enormous difference to the women who had been told their symptoms were "all in their head" and who now have a hormone regimen that is right for them.

Many of my patients have been able to stop expensive medications to lower blood pressure and cholesterol, as well as eliminate a variety of pain or antidepressant or sleeping medications when their estradiol levels were again in the optimal ranges.

More Food for Thought:
There are too many "hidden" medical, psychological and relationship costs if you don't know your physiological measures.

In my opinion, the hormone blood tests are efficient, reliable, cost-effective, and psychologically helpful in identifying endocrine causes of symptoms I have been describing. You may find that it is too costly to your quality of life **not** to have this information as you plan how to best achieve your health goals.

Other Important Body Measurements

Don't just focus on how much you weigh! This is not the most helpful measure of either your health risks or your progress! It is far more helpful and meaningful to track other measures that better reflect your fat to lean body ratio.

Body Composition

This term refers to the amount of body fat you have relative to the amount of lean body mass (muscle, bone, and connective tissues). We all need a certain amount of body fat for stored energy, heat insulation, shock absorption, and in women, to provide a source of estrogen (estrone) that helps preserve bone as we get older. Generally, healthy women have a higher percentage of body fat than do men as a reflection of our biological role to sustain pregnancies.

From a medical, health risk standpoint, we generally define obesity as being more than 33 percent body fat for women and more than 25 percent body fat for men.

Tip
So don't obsess about your weight on the scale!

You know the saying, "You can never can be too rich or too thin?" Well, for good health, you can be too thin if you are a woman over 30. As we get older, women lose bone more rapidly if their body fat percent drops much below 24–25%. So, I don't recommend that you push to get below about 25% body fat, if you are over 30.

How do you determine your percent body fat? Scales that measure body fat are now available to consumers. For general purposes of tracking your progress, skinfold measures with calipers by an experienced person at your health club or the electrical impedance methods are fine. You don't really need the more expensive DEXA or hydrostatic weighing.

Muscle and bone weigh far more than fat tissue, so if you are exercising or taking hormones, which both build muscle, you will not see as much change in pounds on the scale as you will see in body composition changes and with the way your clothes fit. Gaining more muscle and losing fat tends to make your body leaner, more compact, leading to a loss of inches. At the same time, however, you could see an increase in pounds as you build heavier muscle and bone.

Health Alert!
You are at increased health risk because of the middle-body fat distribution.

Waist to Hip Ratio: Are You a Pear or an Apple?

Your health risk from excess body fat is determined by both how much fat you have and where the fat is located. I talked in earlier chapters about women's normal "pear" shape with hip and buttock fat patterns, while men build up fat around their bellies, giving them more of an "apple" shape. Women with PCOS, however, undergo an undesirable transformation: they become apple-shaped with the hormone imbalances I've discussed. The middle and upper body pounds of PCOS are more dangerous to health than pounds around hips and buttocks.

If your fat is concentrated mostly in the abdomen like an apple, you are much more likely to develop the serious health problems associated with obesity, such as diabetes. We have a simple way to measure whether someone is an apple or a pear. The measurement is called *waist-to-hip ratio.*

Calculating Waist-to-Hip Ratio: To find out your waist-to-hip ratio, measure your waist at its narrowest point, then measure your hips at the widest point. Divide the waist measurement by the hip measurement.

Alert!
Waist-to-hip ratios of more than 0.8 for women or 1.0 for men means you have become an "apple."

Example: A woman with a 35" waist and 46" hips would do the following calculation: $35 \div 46 = 0.76$. Your health goal is a WHR of less than 0.8.

Checking your waist measure is an even simpler way of telling whether you are becoming an apple. As a general guideline, your goal for a healthy body should be a waist measure of less than 33 inches. If your waist measure is greater than that, you have increased risks of diabetes and heart disease.

Body Mass Index (BMI)

Body mass index, or BMI, is a term new to many women, but it is the measurement of choice for many physicians and researchers studying obesity. BMI uses a mathematical formula that includes both your height and weight.

BMI is calculated by taking your weight in kilograms divided by height in meters squared. (BMI = kg/m2).

BMI tables are available that have already done the math and metric conversions. To use the table, find the appropriate height in the left-hand column. Move across the row to the given weight. The number at the top of the column is the BMI for that height and weight.

A BMI of more than 30 usually is considered a sign of moderate to severe obesity with increased health risks for developing diabetes, heart disease and other problems.

The BMI measurement poses some of the same problems as the weight-for-height tables and does not provide information on your percentage of body fat. However, like the weight-for-height table, BMI is another useful number to help you track your progress.

The Rule: Above age 35, you are obese if your BMI is 27 or more. Younger than 34 years old, you are considered obese with a BMI of greater than 25.

Summary: Measures to Check and Monitor

Laboratory Studies To Check for PCOS :

- ❧ FSH, LH ratio (abnormal if shifted toward LH)
- ❧ Estradiol, estrone
- ❧ Free and total testosterone
- ❧ DHEA, DHEA-s
- ❧ SHBG
- ❧ 8 AM cortisol, and if elevated, 4 PM free cortisol and/or a 24-hour urinary free cortisol
- ❧ 17-OH progesterone–(to identify Congenital Adrenal Hyperplasia (CAH) or 21-hydroxylase deficiency), possibly androstenedione
- ❧ Prolactin
- ❧ Fasting, 2- and 3-hour post-prandial glucose and insulin; or a 5-hour insulin response to glucose test
- ❧ Thyroid profile, including free T4, free T3, and thyroid antibodies
- ❧ Comprehensive Metabolic Profile that includes fasting glucose, tests of liver and kidney function, fasting lipids (cholesterol, HDL, LDL, TG), complete blood counts, calcium, magnesium, iron and ferritin, and homocysteine.

Body Measures to Monitor:

- ❧ Body Composition–Goal: 22–30% fat
- ❧ Waist to Hip ratio–Goal: less than 0.8
- ❧ Waist circumference–Goal: less than 33 inches
- ❧ Body Mass Index–Goal: less than 25–27

Summary: Beyond the Tests: Putting It All Together

PCOS and its potentially serious hormonal imbalances are commonly not recognized, and are all too often misdiagnosed. There are many incorrect diagnoses given to women who, in fact, have declining estradiol, insulin resistance, and PCOS. Some of the ones I see women being labeled are manic-depressive illness, major depressive disorder, atypical depression, chronic fatigue, chronic candidiasis, panic disorder, anxiety disorder, stress reaction, and others.

But even though low estradiol and the excess androgens of PCOS can cause mood effects, many doctors don't realize that these psychiatric disorders don't cause the excess body hair, facial hair, acne and marked weight gain that are seen in PCOS.

If you are experiencing the kinds of symptoms and body changes I have been writing about, it is important for you to seek a thorough evaluation as I have outlined here. Many sure you have the right hormone tests, using the reliable serum assays as I have described.

The goal of a comprehensive evaluation is also to make certain that you do not have another medical problem causing similar symptoms; and to insure that any previously unrecognized secondary disorders, which may be contributing to your symptoms, are diagnosed and properly treated.

Once you have the results of your various tests, you and your physician should then review this information together, and then explore in the next chapters the ways I have outlined can work to improve your hormone levels to the optimal ranges I have described.

My desire is to give you enough information to get the right tests and then know what treatment options there are to help you restore a healthy metabolic balance and feel your best!

Chapter 9

PCOS vs Cushing's Syndrome: How Do You Tell The Difference?

PCOS can cause many of the same body changes and health risks as another problem called *Cushing's Syndrome—obesity, excess androgens, high blood pressure, mood swings, increased risk of diabetes and heart disease, among others.*

The hallmark feature of Cushing's Syndrome is elevated cortisol, but because PCOS can *also* cause elevated cortisol, it may be difficult to distinguish one from the other and for your or your doctor to know which one you may have.

The treatment needed for Cushing syndrome may sometimes be quite different from what I have described for PCOS, so it's important to understand the two disorders.

In this chapter, I will review what Cushing's is, how it is diagnosed, and some of the treatment options.

Cortisol, It's Daily Rhythms and What it Does

As I described in Chapter 8, cortisol is a member of the *glucocorticoid group* of hormones produced by the adrenal glands, and it prepares our body to deal with the effects of stress. Cortisol and its fellow glucocorticoids are major metabolic regulators, having crucial effects on many pathways in the body, including those that regulate body weight, moods, immune function, ovarian function, and others.

Cortisol has a definite daily (diurnal) rhythm to its secretion, normally beginning to rise for the day about 4:00–5:00 AM, and peaking about 8:00–9:00 AM. We need the effects of rising cortisol to get our biological engines going to start our day. Levels then should be gradually falling over the day and are lowest at night when you are sleeping.

When we are stressed, this normal daily rhythm may be altered, shifted in time, blunted, or even completely reversed. For example, you may have low levels in the morning, rising (instead of falling) as the day unfolds so that you have unusually high levels in the afternoon or evening instead of in the morning. Two brain centers, the hypothalamus and pituitary, govern cortisol output from the adrenal glands via three hormones:

Stress Effects:
I often see an abnormal cortisol pattern in my patients with PCOS who describe, "I wake up tired, and I finally seem to get going in the evening and then I can't sleep."

- *Corticotropin-releasing hormone* (**CRH**)–from the hypothalamus
- *Vasopressin* (**ADH**)–from the hypothalamus
- *Adrenocorticotropin* (**ACTH**)–from the pituitary gland

CRH and ADH stimulate release of the ACTH that in turn stimulates the adrenal gland to release cortisol. Rising blood levels of cortisol feed back to the brain letting the pituitary and hypothalamus know the message was received and cortisol has been made. Then levels of ACTH, CRH, and ADH drop back down to baseline, having done their jobs to increase cortisol output.

When we are stressed, however, levels of ACTH, CRH, and cortisol *all* rise, and these normal daily rhythms are interrupted, leading to excessively high cortisol levels produced over more and more time each day.

When cortisol—particularly the *free, active* cortisol—remains too high over time, it leads to high blood pressure, high cholesterol and triglycerides, high fasting glucose, excess insulin release and resistance to insulin effects, increased risk of diabetes, repeated infections (from cortisol's immune-suppression), thin skin, easy bruising, muscle weakness, and increased rate of bone loss.

Together, these negative changes in the body are called *Cushing's Syndrome*, a medical name for cortisol excess. It doesn't matter whether there is too much cortisol being produced by the body, or from taking cortisol-type medications (glucocorticoids, such as prednisone) for asthma, arthritis, and other medical problems. The damaging changes caused in the body are the same.

If you have been under severe, unrelenting stress for long periods of time, such as many months to several years, the adrenal glands eventually lose their ability to respond properly with increased cortisol, and you enter the phase of adrenal insufficiency or "exhaustion." But there are very characteristic—and very different—body changes that occur with adrenal exhaustion that are not at all like what we see in Cushing's Syndrome or PCOS.

Excess cortisol: Effects are marked fat deposits around the middle of the body, breasts, upper back and arms, as well as a rounded puffy face that is called "moon facies."

Adrenal insufficiency may arise for unclear reasons not related to persistent severe stresses, a condition called *Addison's disease*. True Addison's disease (Adrenal Insufficiency, AI, or low cortisol) is rare. The hallmark of adrenal insufficiency is *marked weight loss* (rather than the weight gain seen with high cortisol), loss of muscle mass, markedly low blood pressure, significant fatigue, muscle wasting and weakness, and loss of pubic and axillary body hair (rather than the excess body hair seen in PCOS). Laboratory studies in Addison's show characteristic changes of **low** cortisol, **low** sodium, and **high** potassium. These are very different from effects of cortisol excess.

I have many patients with PCOS who have been told they have "adrenal exhaustion" based on unreliable tests like saliva levels or kinesiology (muscle testing). Most women with PCOS are gaining weight, not losing major amounts of weight; they have high—not low—blood pressure; and they do not have *low* cortisol. A "diagnosis" of "adrenal exhaustion" is rarely accurate in such women.

So how do you tell whether you have PCOS with high cortisol, or Cushing's Syndrome? Sometimes this is difficult to know with certainty, but there are a number of tests that can help differentiate the two problems. I will describe these tests a little later in the chapter, but first let's look at the cortisol pathways in the body and more about how they respond to various stresses—physical, psychological, situational, and environmental.

How We Perceive and Respond to Stress

Fact:

Stress-induced physical changes and high cortisol *add* to the problems of PCOS and make you even fatter

Stress is a good thing, essential to our survival. Without it, we would die. It's *too much stress* that can have negative or damaging effects on our health.

"Stressor" is simply another word for stimuli inside and outside the body that trigger body responses to help us adapt to changes. Stressors may be *external* situations in our lives, or *internal* changes in our body, or *internal* thoughts and feelings.

Stresses of any form—positive or negative—all share the same brain-body reactions. Our brain constantly perceives and processes information coming to it from the world around us and also from moment-to-moment changes inside the body. The brain uses this incoming information to tell the body how much food to eat and whether to release our fat stores for energy or store fat for future emergencies or whether to slam on the brakes in our car to prevent an accident.

Your brain oversees all your thoughts, feelings, moods and behaviors (including eating), and all of these are affected by both external situations and by internal body fluctuations. This means that all the biochemical changes throughout the body are affected by physical causes and psychological ones. So with prolonged stress of any kind—physical, environmental, situational, psychological, spiritual—the body's balance, or homeostasis, is disrupted.

When you experience symptoms from stress, they are caused by two major factors:

(1) the "acute" stress response of increased activity of the "fight-or-flight" (adrenaline) pathways

(2) the "chronic" stress response of increased

production of cortisol and all its metabolic and immune effects.

Hormonal change is one of those stressors that mean that the body systems must constantly be changing and adapting. These changes themselves may become additional stressors on the body and contribute to yet more stress overload.

These effects of stress can occur in all women at some time in their lives. I know when I am stressed and my estradiol is too low, I certainly don't sleep well, feel my best or think well, and that stresses me even more.

The interconnections and the ways in which hormonal production may be altered by stress on the body are often overlooked when women seek medical care. The two-way nature of these pathways is a critical connection, throughout all facets of women's health, which has been the frequently overlooked "missing link."

The diagram that follows on the next page shows some of the ways that stressors of all kinds require the body processes to change and adapt.

Cortisol and Your Ovarian Hormones

When we are "stressed" by physical changes OR by psychological states, and cortisol goes UP, ovarian hormone production is diminished and cycles are even more irregular. There is typically less free, active T3 so thyroid function is also slowed down. This response is part of Mother Nature's built in protective effect to prevent us from getting pregnant if our bodies are too "stressed" to be healthy enough to sustain a pregnancy and nurse the infant.

World-wide studies consistently show a correlation between *high life stress* and *lower levels of ovarian estrogen, testosterone and loss of the normal cyclic production of progesterone*. If this high stress state continues, it may lead to infertility in younger women or earlier menopause in older women.

The damaging effects are even more pronounced in

STRESS RESPONSES

LIFE SITUATIONS	PSYCHOLOGICAL	PHYSICAL	ENVIRONMENT
✿ finances	✿ fears	✿ hormone change	✿ pollutants
✿ work	✿ worries	✿ diet	✿ allergens
✿ relationships	✿ body image	✿ illlness	✿ weather
✿ community	✿ midlife angst	✿ alcohol,drugs	✿ toxins

STRESS

DISRUPTS BODY BALANCE (HOMEOSTASIS), LEADING TO

PSYCHOLOGICAL SYMPTOM

- ✿ food binges
- ✿ "panic attacks"
- ✿ disrupted sleep
- ✿ irritable, anxious
- ✿ depressed
- ✿ angry outbursts
- ✿ desire for alcohol, drugs
- ✿ allergy flares, skin rashes

"FIGHT-OR-FLIGHT" SYMPTOMS

- ✿ racing heart beat, palpitations
- ✿ sweaty, clammy
- ✿ nausea/loss of appetite or
- ✿ increased hunger, sweet cravings
- ✿ blood sugar swings
- ✿ headaches
- ✿ diarrhea, "irritable bowel"

PHYSICAL HEALTH PROBLEMS

- ✿ weight gain
- ✿ high blood pressure
- ✿ marked fatigue
- ✿ autoimmune disorders
- ✿ insulin resistance, diabetes
- ✿ heart disease
- ✿ infections (viral, bacterial, yeast)
- ✿ malignancies

©Elizabeth Lee Vliet, MD 2001-2005

women with PCOS, and can make PCOS get slowly worse. But if your doctors aren't checking the estradiol level and your other hormones, then you don't have any way to know what's making you feel worse and worse. That's why I think it is so crucial to check all of these hormones together.

The connection between ovarian hormones and stress is two-way:

‣ declining estradiol is itself a "stressor" to the body that causes increased cortisol output and loss of optimal function of norepinephrine, serotonin, dopamine, and acetylcholine. These chemical "communicators" are all involved in regulation of the menstrual cycle, body weight and body fat, appetite, muscle growth-repair, sleep, mood, memory, thirst, sex drive and pain regulation;

‣ Stress leads to poor food and vitamin intake. low energy, and difficulty coping... which then adds further stress...that suppresses estrogen and thyroid function even more.

‣ Stress-induced decline in estradiol then causes further increase in cortisol. These adverse effects on brain chemical messengers and the ovary-adrenal hormone output *add more to* the negative body changes from the high androgens and excess cortisol caused by the underlying PCOS.

These back-and-forth processes feed back on each other and make the stress effects even worse. It's no wonder you sometimes feel caught in a trap. On the next page is a summary of the downward spiral that happens.

Vicious cycle
The combination of PCOS and life stress can make you feel like you are in a quicksand pit and can't get out. No wonder it is so difficult and frustrating to try and figure out what's going on.

High Cortisol From Other Causes

Life stress is the usual trigger as a cause of increased cortisol, but there are many other causes: taking steroid medications, infections, dieting, alcohol overuse, drug use, chronic exposure to pollutants or allergens, as well as the more usual psychological triggers such as fear, worry, anger, and other negative moods.

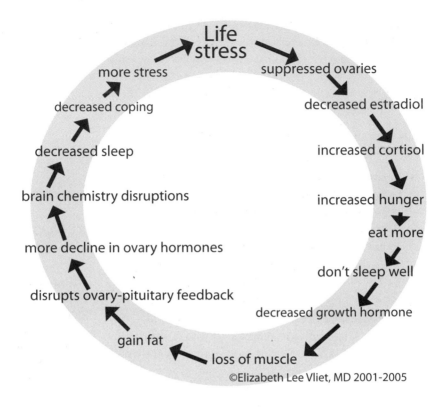

©Elizabeth Lee Vliet, MD 2001-2005

Less commonly, high cortisol can be caused by tumors –benign or malignant—of the adrenal gland or the pituitary gland. The benign tumors are called *adenomas*, and are only damaging because they can produce excess cortisol, or because their size or location causes damage to other structures.

If lab studies suggest the presence of a tumor causing abnormal cortisol or androgen production, then imaging studies, such as an MRI or CAT scan, can be done. These tests can usually identify the presence of these types of tumors if they have reached the size that can be detected (*macroadenoma*). Some adenomas, however, may still be too small to be seen on an MRI or CAT scan. These *microadenomas* too small to be seen are sometimes no bigger than the head of a pin, yet can produce hormones that cause havoc in your body.

For example, if a pituitary adenoma is large, it can cause pressure on the optic nerve underneath the pituitary, and this can cause loss of vision. Such an adenoma would have to be removed even if it is benign. A hormone-producing adenoma may have to be removed to prevent the body-damaging effects of excess cortisol.

Adrenal tumors can produce too much cortisol and they can also produce high levels of the adrenal androgens. So even if they are benign, not cancerous, such a tumor may have to be surgically removed.

Spotting Early Clues

Are there any clues that come early in the process of hormone change that alert you to problems before you gain a lot of weight? I think there are, but all too often these "early warning" symptoms are discounted by doctors, or explained away by patients as "I guess I'm just under a lot of stress."

One clue, often missed by physicians, is that women with PCOS often have food cravings (usually for sweets or rich, fatty foods), "anxiety" or "racing heart" episodes, often right before their periods. They also describe "blood sugar swings," "mood swings," or "horrendous palpitations," and pounding sensations "as if my heart were going to literally jump out of my chest." Often the heart-related symptoms are so pronounced that women don't notice the appetite changes or the connection with food cravings.

Tip: These clues to hormone imbalances are often missed and doctors label these problems "anxiety" or "stress."

A woman who is experiencing this cluster of problems will often get told to relax more and reduce stress. But then it happens again, and again, and again...usually with the menstrual cycles, but doctors still don't seem to pay much attention to this connection. Oftentimes, they simply prescribe medication to relieve "anxiety," it's easy, and they all know that "women have this problem."

So, the "fight-or-flight" symptoms ease up, but food cravings, inexorable weight gain, and PCOS hormone problems continue. If the underlying cause of such episodes was really the brain effects of diminished estradiol, along with beginning glucose intolerance and insulin resistance of PCOS, then obviously anxiety medications won't help very much.

Cortisol starts creeping up, estradiol declines some more without being addressed, and then you start having those torturous nights of restless, disrupted sleep. Sleep disruption adds to over-stimulating cortisol and interrupting the normal daily cortisol pattern, so you wake up tired, hungry, foggy-brained and with muscle aches…and the downward spiral has begun. Meanwhile, the unrecognized PCOS continues to wreak its havoc and make you fatter and less fertile.

Not everyone with PCOS *gains* weight, so there are additional factors that come into play that determine how our body responds to stress: attitudes, balance of other hormones, food choices we make to deal with stress, metabolism, adequacy of vitamins and other nutrients, etc.

Stress is a constant, necessary part of the life process itself, and we can't eliminate it completely. The goal then is to help you be successful in avoiding the traps of the *wrong type* of eating at the *wrong time* of day when you are under a lot of stress so that you don't play into the tempting hands of your fat-storing stress hormone…or its negative effects to decrease the hormone production of the ovaries and the thyroid gland.

Alert: Excess cortisol stimulates more insulin release, which acts like a "partner in crime" to help cortisol store more fat.

How Does Stress Make PCOS Weight Gain Worse?

Eating is a brain-regulated behavior that is profoundly affected by the outpouring of cortisol when we are stressed. Cortisol and other stress hormones affect us both physically (e.g. release of hunger-promoting chemicals) and psychologically (e.g. habits, food preferences). Stress-induced changes affect our weight-regulating neurotransmitters, how fast food moves through our gut, what kind of foods we want to eat, how efficiently our body processes foods, how well our nerve endings respond to food, and all aspects of metabolism.

For example, "anxiety" may be caused by falling blood sugar (internal physical change) *or* by worry (internal psychological feeling), *or* by a car pulling out in front of you (external physical event). Then when we feel anxious, we may have a habit of turning to sweets to calm down.

Decreases in estradiol cause loss of many brain messengers, such as serotonin, dopamine, and acetyleholine, which causes you to eat more of the wrong kinds of foods, like carbohydrates and chocolate (the 'feel good stuff'), which in turn makes the excess cortisol happily pack on more fat!

Then, like adding insult to injury, the excess cortisol slows down the normal production of your thyroid hormones, leading to *less* of the available T3 that is so important for cellular metabolism in skeletal muscle, brain and other organs to use fat for fuel. Excess DHEA and testosterone can make the above picture even worse.

See how the pieces connect? Take a look at the following sequence of events.

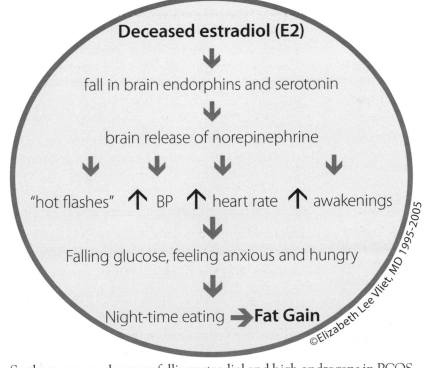

So there you are, lower or falling estradiol and high androgens in PCOS triggers a release of brain chemicals, that leads to a whole cascade of events spreading *throughout* the body, and makes your fat-storing machinery pack on the pounds. This sequence of physical changes is very real, and when it occurs day after day, it contributes to your getting fatter.

Calories count!
It only takes about 50 calories extra each day to add 10 pounds of body fat in a year.

These physical events are so common, and start so gradually, that many women with PCOS don't even notice them. Most doctors have not been taught these hormone-brain-body connections, so they don't realize that there may be something amiss hormonally.

Then there is the decrease in serotonin that occurs due to both persistent stress and to the loss of estradiol. Serotonin helps maintain regular sleep and decrease anxiety, so that drop in serotonin *adds* to the episodes of awakenings at night, and aggravates the adrenaline-induced feelings of irritability, tension, palpitations, and…hunger for sweets.

What you typically eat more of is the carbs, because that's a way the body makes more serotonin. And then, all that cortisol and insulin are lurking around that fat cell, waiting greedily to grab those carbs and make them into more fat.

Intuition knows
Women tell me they know "its a physical, chemical kind of thing," but they have been told that it's "just stress" and no one checks the hormones levels.

Remember, too, that gaining excess body fat is itself a profound stressor on all of the body systems. Obesity makes your cortisol–weight gain problems worse by further interfering with ovarian function, including the way the hormones themselves govern the weight pathways.

Getting Tested for Cortisol and Cushing's vs PCOS

If you've been under a great deal of stress and are gaining weight, or you think you have PCOS, or you wonder about Cushing's Syndrome, then ask your physician to check your cortisol levels.

An 8:00 AM *serum* cortisol level is the most reliable *first* step in checking for low or high cortisol. If this is *higher* than about 20 μg/dl, then other tests can be ordered to clarify the cause. The typical ones for the next step are 4 PM total and free cortisol, cortisol binding globulin, a 24-hour urine for urinary free cortisol, and ACTH.

If these are abnormal, then a next step is usually a Dexamethasone Suppression Test (DST). In this test, 1 mg of dexamethasone is given at 11 PM at night, and tests of cortisol are drawn the next day at 8 AM, noon, and 4 PM. A normal result is to see suppression of the cortisol levels to below 5 μg/dl the day after dexamethasone. If cortisol remains too high the next day, it can be due to major depression or can be an indication that further testing is needed.

If these follow up tests are abnormal, imaging studies (MRI, CAT scans, etc.) are usually ordered to check the adrenal glands and pituitary to check for possible tumors causing the excess cortisol production.

If the 8:00 AM cortisol is lower than 5–7 μg/dl, serum ACTH, and ACTH (Cortrosyn) stimulation tests are generally done next to evaluate the cause of adrenal insufficiency (for example, adrenal destruction or pituitary dysfunction). If the 8:00 AM cortisol is greater than 10 μg/dl, and your serum electrolytes (sodium, potassium) are normal, this makes it very *unlikely* that you have adrenal insufficiency. You should have other hormone systems tested as I describe in Chapter 8 to determine other causes of your symptoms like fatigue, weakness and low energy level.

Remember, marked weight *loss* occurs in virtually all people who have adrenal insufficiency. If you are *gaining* weight, this usually only occurs in excess cortisol production syndromes, not adrenal insufficiency.

Melatonin—Cautions in Women with PCOS

Melatonin has become almost ubiquitous since it became available over-the-counter as a sleep aid. But in addition to being the "night" hormone secreted during darkness, think of melatonin as the hormone of *hibernation*—it triggers the body changes that help Mama Bear *slow* down her metabolism, *store fat* for the long winter, *remain sleepy*, and *slowed down!*

Warning
Melatonin
has a
different
kind of "dark"
side when
it comes to
its effects on
body fat.

Alert:
If you have
PCOS and are
struggling
with weight
gain, I
urge you
*not to take
melatonin*
on a regular
basis.

Researchers have found this effect in studies of melatonin injected into other animals that don't typically hibernate: they overeat, oversleep, are lethargic, and have a slowed activity level. These are NOT effects you want if you have PCOS.

No wonder then that I regularly hear from our *women* patients that they began having an increase in fatigue, food cravings, and drowsiness (not to mention headaches and depressed mood) after starting melatonin supplements.

In addition to this, recent studies have shown an alarming connection in *women* taking melatonin supplements: they had much higher serum levels of cortisol (already high in most women with PCOS, remember?) than did women taking placebo. This effect of melatonin's effect was *not* seen in the *men*.

So when women take melatonin at night to help improve sleep, they have a double whammy: not only does the melatonin itself make you hungrier and *more* efficient at storing fat, but it also *stimulates cortisol production*, which means you have just unwittingly *increased* your fat storage from yet another direction. For women with PCOS, this is a particularly dangerous effect.

All of this just goes to show that studies done in men cannot be applied to women and assume the same effects. It is yet another illustration of the many ways women's bodies respond differently to hormones compared to men.

In studies of seasonal affective disorder (SAD), researchers gave melatonin to women who had been successfully treated with bright light therapy. Melatonin administration did not fully blunt the success of bright light as an antidepressant, but the *women who received melatonin* did have a significant *increase* in other symptoms characteristic of SAD: fatigue, increased appetite, carbohydrate craving, weight gain and social withdrawal. The increase in these symptoms was not seen in women receiving placebo.

The interaction between melatonin and serotonin may help to explain some of these observations. Melatonin is made in the brain from serotonin, and the same area of the brain that regulates melatonin release also regulates serotonin production. Since serotonin is used to make melatonin, it stands to reason that when melatonin levels go *up*, serotonin levels go *down*.

This may help to explain the symptoms of increased carbohydrate cravings experienced by SAD sufferers, since carbs shift amino acid balance in a way that allows the brain to make more serotonin. High-carbohydrate meals enhance all the other amino acids moving into body tissues from the bloodstream, which leaves more tryptophan, serotonin's building block, in the blood so it can be taken up into brain cells to make serotonin.

But what if you are *taking* melatonin supplements? The supplements contain much higher levels of melatonin than the brain normally makes. It appears that these high levels of melatonin end up *suppressing* serotonin production, which in turn triggers the intense carbohydrate cravings, headaches and depressed mood that women describe.

Warning! Melatonin studies quoted in popular books touting melatonin as a powerful "anti-aging" hormone with sleep promoting effects were done in *men* or *male* animals.

SUMMARY

The chart on the following page lists some of the major adverse effects of high cortisol. In Chapters 8, 12, and 13, I describe steps for you to explore on your own and with your physician to help you get cortisol back to healthy ranges.

The higher your cortisol stays, and the longer it is elevated, the more you store pounds around the middle of the body ("apple" shape) that causes you to have high levels of free fatty acids (FFA) that lead to higher cholesterol, lower levels of the good HDL cholesterol, higher triglycerides, high blood glucose, and even more insulin resistance.

High cortisol levels and prolonged stress also uses up our body's supply of important antioxidants, vitamins, minerals that are needed to catalyze the fat-burning pathways in the body. But when we are stressed and don't feel well, we pay less attention to getting what we need in our nutrition, and we may forget to take our vitamins and minerals, so the fat burning pathways get even more sluggish.

Stress and high cortisol have multiple adverse effects. It is a complicated picture, especially in PCOS, and has profound implications for all aspects of women's health. Not only do you have the physical consequences of excess fat, you have the resulting psychological stress and emotional pain of being fat in a culture that idolizes thinness. Then when you feel lousy about yourself, you eat more to ease the pain.

The cumulative effects of persistent high cortisol levels and chronic stress adversely affect practically every pathway in the body. All of these changes together push inexorably toward a higher risk of diabetes, heart disease, and stroke.

For more information about how prolonged stress and high cortisol can damage the body and lead to accelerated aging, I suggest you read *Why Zebras Don't Get Ulcers*, by Robert M. Sapolsky. This will help you better understand why stress management is a crucial component of a sound treatment program for PCOS.

Adverse Health Consequences
Of Excess Free Cortisol

1. Abdominal fat gain

2. Increased risk of heart disease by promoting plaque build-up in arteries

3. Increased total cholesterol, LDL and triglyceride levels, lower HDL

4. Increased risk of diabetes by increasing levels of blood glucose

5. Aggravates insulin resistance

6. Loss of normal collagen metabolism, (the basis of healthy ligaments and tendons) leading to injuries, joint and back pain

7. Disruption in the sleep cycle, leading to less restorative sleep, diminished Growth hormone, and decreased muscle repair at night. These changes all add to the damaging effects of declining estradiol on the same pathways

8. Interference with normal thyroid function, leading to less of the available T3 that is so important for cellular metabolism throughout the body.

9. Immune suppression, leading to more infections and illnesses

10. Increased need for antioxidants, vitamins, minerals as well as proper balance of macronutrients, yet when we are stressed and don't feel well, we often don't get the very nutritional balance we most need

11. Hair loss, thinning skin, easy bruising

©Elizabeth Lee Vliet, MD 2001-2005

Chapter 10
Your Hormone Power Life Plan:
Balance Your Hormones
For Health

I see a lot of women of all ages with PCOS, from young girls already developing the body changes of PCOS at age 10 or 11, to menopausal women with complications from unrecognized PCOS when they were younger.

It is often quite a challenge to find the right combination of hormone and non-hormonal approaches to restore balance. Most of the time, I find it is a process of using a step-by-step approach, and then fine-tuning. Sometimes this can be accomplished in a few months; other times, it may take a year or more to find the right combination and for the body to have time to respond.

Effective treatment for PCOS requires *integrating various approaches*—from lifestyle changes to medication to psychological support. It also requires individualized treatment approaches tailored to each woman.

Although there is no one medication approved by the FDA for the treatment of PCOS, there are many medicines that can help treat the problems it causes.

Clearly, infertility is a big therapeutic issue for many women with PCOS, but pros and cons of the many options for fertility management are beyond the scope of this book. Although I am not a fertility specialist, some of my patients have gone on to become pregnant once I was able to help them improve their metabolic and hormonal imbalances. I have referred others to fertility specialists when they wanted to attempt pregnancy.

Fact: Given the many ways that PCOS can manifest in different women, it is not possible to find one medication that works for everyone.

There are many issues beyond infertility that need to be addressed in designing an effective treatment approach for PCOS. Some of the variables include, for example,

Goal:
Currently available treatment approaches do not cure PCOS. You learn to manage PCOS so you can feel as good as possible.

- How old are you?
- Are you trying to get pregnant now, or preserve your fertility for later on?
- Do you have significant excess body and facial hair?
- Are you losing scalp hair?
- Do you have a lot of acne on your face and/or chest and back?
- Do you have other medical or gynecological problems?
- Are you insulin resistant?
- Do you already have diabetes?
- Has your energy and sex drive disappeared?
- Do you have significant mood or sleep problems along with the other symptoms of PCOS?

Good News!
Don't be discouraged. There are helpful approaches to relieve the distressing symptoms and body changes of PCOS.

It is important to view treatment as a way of managing the troublesome symptoms of PCOS, reducing health risks, and improving your quality of life. This is the same approach used by people with diabetes, heart disease, hypothyroidism, or arthritis. Treatments *reduce* the adverse health impact of having it, but they *don't cure* it. You can feel better and regain your zest and vitality!

Let's look first at some of the hormonal approaches that can help. In Chapter 11, I describe other medications that are also helpful, depending on what problems you are experiencing. In Chapter 12, I describe the lifestyle approaches to help you lose weight and improve your body composition, reduce stress, and improve your outlook.

The combination of these approaches will help you achieve what I think are the key *Therapeutic Goals* to help you manage the wide array of problems PCOS can cause.

GOALS OF TREATMENT FOR PCOS

- Decrease excess androgens
- Lose excess body fat, maintain normal body weight and composition
- Improve insulin sensitivity and glucose balance to lower later risk of diabetes and heart disease
- Improve cholesterol and triglycerides
- Improve ovulatory frequency if pregnancy is desired
- Prevent estrogen-induced stimulation of the uterine lining that can lead to endometrial hyperplasia and later increased risk of endometrial cancer
- Reduce excess body hair and acne
- Reduce hormone imbalances that can cause mood disturbances such as irritability and anger outbursts, anxiety, or depression.
- Restore normal sleep cycle, which is often disrupted by androgen excess and the other hormone imbalances of PCOS

©Elizabeth Lee Vliet, MD 2001-2005

Hormone Approaches:

Oral Contraceptives, or birth control pills (BCP)

Think of combined oral contraceptives as "hormonal stabilizers" for women with PCOS, not just pills to prevent pregnancy. The combined estrogen and progestin hormones in BCP provide an important foundation for treating some of the most bothersome problems caused by PCOS. Let's look at how they work and what they do to provide so many health benefits.

How BCP Work to Improve Hormone Balance

Continuous delivery of the hormones estrogen and progestin gives feedback to the brain that lowers FSH and LH and eliminates the cyclic release of these pituitary hormones that drive the menstrual cycle hormone changes. As a result, BCP *suppress* the abnormal cycling of the ovaries in PCOS, and give you more constant levels of these hormones day to day.

✑ Suppressing the ovarian hormone cycles

This means fewer mood swings from an unpredictable hormone roller-coaster, and less likelihood of PMS symptoms. Sleep and energy levels tend to be more stable throughout the month for women taking BCP, since the hormones aren't changing so much day to day.

✑ Preventing cyst formation

The steady estrogen and progestin of BCP also help prevent cysts from forming. This is a very important benefit to women with PCOS because repeated cysts can add to the hormone imbalance and damage the ovaries over time, leading to more problems with fertility later.

✑ Increasing SHBG levels

All oral estrogen-progestin pills stimulate the liver to make more of the protein called sex hormone binding globulin, (SHBG). This protein is abnormally low in women with PCOS. Low levels of SHBG cause high levels of free androgens that lead to more acne, facial and body hair, and more fat deposits in the male pattern around the waist, chest, back and arms.

ट्ठ Reducing androgen excess

The increase in liver production of SHBG triggered by oral BCP is a good thing, because this keeps more of the DHEA and testosterone in the bound, inactive form in the blood stream.

Stimulating more SHBG is one way the BCP help *reduce the androgen excess* in PCOS. This is one way that BCP work to relieve acne, excess hair *growth* in unwanted places, and the hair *loss* on your scalp.

ट्ठ Improving estrogen balance

Increasing the estrogen-androgen ratio is another way the BCP work to help relieve these symptoms in PCOS. Some progestins can actually aggravate the symptoms of androgen excess, so that's why I find that pills with a little **higher** estrogen content (30–35 mcg) actually work better in PCOS than the very low, 20-mcg estrogen pills.

ट्ठ Preventing hyperplasia

BCP also provide daily progestin that prevents excess thickening of the lining of the uterus that can be caused by the continued stimulation from excess estrone in body fat. Over time, such thickening, called hyperplasia, can lead to an increased risk of uterine cancer.

ट्ठ Preventing ovulation, reducing loss of follicles

Since women are born with all the follicles they will ever have, the more menstrual cycles you have, the more follicles get used up when you are not trying to conceive. Birth control pills can help preserve future fertility by preventing ovulation or loss of follicles at a time when you are not trying to get pregnant, and "saving" them for later on.

Types of Contraceptive Products in the United States

Combined estrogen-progestin options:

Oral pills: There are a few dozen combined estrogen-progestin pills on the market, and all of today's BCP are *low dose* by comparison to older ones used in the 1960s and 1970s.

Non-oral options

In the U.S. we have *Nuvaring* vaginal ring, *OrthoEvra* transdermal patch, and *Lunelle* injection.

Non-oral: These products provide steady delivery of both estrogen and progestin, but since they are not taken orally, they bypass the first pass metabolism in the liver. This means you lose some of the benefit to increase SHBG that occurs with the oral forms.

I find my patients usually like the Nuvaring better than OrthoEvra patch, because the patch is a higher progestin product, and causes more depression.

Progestin-only options:

Oral: The progestin-only pill has been used for several decades when nursing mothers needed contraception in the post-partum months. Brands include *Micronor* and *NorQD*, and there are also several generic ones as well. I don't find this a very successful option in PCOS, because women with PCOS often have *more* weight gain, depression, headaches, and acne when they take only a progestin and already have androgen excess and low estradiol.

Non-oral: The injection *Depo-Provera* is a common one used in younger women because its contraceptive effects last about three months. I don't use Depo-Provera at all in my practice because I have seen patients have so many serious side effects. Some that I see commonly in women who have used this product are marked weight gain and increased risk of diabetes, severe depression, headaches, memory and sleep problems, loss of libido, fatigue, erratic bleeding and cramping, and vulvar pain.

Please note that the above list of options does not include combination products that are FDA-approved for menopause, since the doses are generally too low to provide the suppression of active ovarian cycles that younger women with PCOS need to control symptoms. In Chapter 13, I talk about menopause hormone options and describe appropriate uses for both bioidentical and synthetic hormones.

What Types of BCP Work Best for PCOS?

I find that patients with PCOS often do better on pills such as Ovcon 35, Modicon, Ortho-Cyclen, Yasmin, or Diane 35. In my experience, these have a better estrogen-progestin ratio that is more effective to reduce the acne, hair growth, mood symptoms and weight gain of PCOS.

In my experience, high progestin pills with *less* estrogen (Loestrin, Alesse, Mircette) cause more of the negative progestin effects (weight gain, low libido, hair loss, acne, lethargy, headaches, depressed mood, abnormal glucose/insulin, high cholesterol and high triglycerides) that are already common problems with PCOS.

Pills that have a steady dose formula every day (monophasic) typically have fewer adverse effects, especially on moods, than pills with varying hormone content (triphasic). Examples of triphasic pills include Triphasil, Ortho TriCyclen, OrthoNovum 777 and several generics. Steady dose BCP are also more effective at reducing ovarian cysts than are triphasic pills.

Yasmin and Diane 35 contain the optimal amount of estrogen with a progestin that actually is an "anti-androgen." This means these two pills are especially good for women with acne, hirsutism, and middle body weight gain.

Yasmin is available in the United States. Diane 35 has been a very successful birth control pill in Canada, Mexico, Europe, Australia and New Zealand for several decades. It has been especially helpful for women with PCOS, many of whom have turned to overseas sources, since it is not available in the United States.

Options: Yasmin and Diane 35 are both newer birth control pills, especially designed to help treat the problems of androgen excess that occurs in PCOS.

Pills To Help You Avoid Weight Gain

BCP that are high in progestin (greater than 0.5 mg norethindrone or equivalent), and very low in estrogen (less than 30 mcg ethinyl estradiol) are more likely to cause increased appetite and weight gain.

Hang in There!

Don't give up just because you had problems with one birth control pill—small changes in the chemical make-up can make huge differences in the types of side effects that occur

Pills with a better balance of ethinyl estradiol (30 to 35 mcg) to the progestin typically cause less appetite stimulation and weight gain. I have listed some of these above in the progestin discussion, but three good ones are Ovcon 35, Modicon and Ortho-Cyclen, and Yasmin.

Yasmin is similar to Diane 35 (not available in the United States). It may be an effective option for women who have gained weight with the high progestin content of other birth control pills.

BCP Benefits, Side Effects, Risks and Cautions

"The pill" has long been an effective option for younger women with PCOS but wasn't previously recommended for women over 35. That has changed with results of newer studies. BCP have been found to not only be safe for older women, but to actually provide a number of health benefits.

A June 1999 article in *OB Gyn News* had the following headline: "Prescribe OCs Until Age 52, Expert Advises." Gynecologist Patricia J. Sulak, M.D., of the Scott and White Clinic in Temple, Texas was quoted as follows: "OCs [oral contraceptives] are one of the most important preventive health measures in all of medicine. There's no medicine that offers reproductive-age women more benefits; there's nothing out there that even touches OCs."

Dr. Sulak went on to say, "Women who don't stay on the pill have heavy periods and irregular periods, premenstrual syndrome, functional ovarian cysts, and they get endometriosis and fibroids. If they start the pill and stay on it except when they want to become pregnant and when breast-feeding, they don't have those problems... The pill was really made for women over 35... once you get over 35 your ovaries start acting up; 90% of women will develop irregular bleeding before they get to menopause."

I think this is a crucially important message for women with PCOS, since all these health risks are increasing as they get older and ovarian function becomes more and more erratic.

Previous studies that linked birth control pills with increased risk of stroke and blood clots had two problems that affected the outcomes:

1) they did not take into account the independent risk of cigarette smoking on cardiovascular disease, including stroke, and

2) were based on the older very high dose pill formulations used in the 1960s. None of those high-dose pills are available today. Today's OC formulas are a fraction of the hormone content used when the pills first came out.

After re-analyzing the past data and evaluating current safety statistics from worldwide studies, the FDA found that the potential benefits of BCP for many health problems in women at this age outweighed the slight degree of potential risk.

Many women in this age group still need and want contraception. I had one woman, age 51, whose hormone profile confirmed that she had ovulated during her menstrual cycle, and she said (in a tone of shock and disbelief!) "You mean I could still get pregnant? I thought I stopped ovulating a long time ago. The last thing I need in my life right now is a baby!"

All of the birth control pills in this country are made of synthetic estrogen (usually ethinyl estradiol) and one of several types of synthetic progestins. The natural progesterone and estradiol that we use for menopausal women to restore optimal hormone levels are not po-

Attention: The FDA approved the use of oral contraceptives in non-smoking women over age 40.

Significant Benefits: Birth control pills help prevent osteoporosis as well as uterine and ovarian cancers

tent enough to reliably suppress ovulation and provide contraceptive effects.

Good news about the protective effects of the oral contraceptives is summarized in the chart on the next page. The percentages given are the degree of *reduction* in that health problem when *compared to non-users* of birth control pills.

Warning!
Whatever birth control pill you use, *do not add* St. John's wort if you develop depressive side effects. It can decrease BCP effectiveness by more than 50%!

In addition to this list, studies from Italy first published over a decade ago (1994) along with other confirming studies since that time, have shown significant protective effect on maintaining bone density in women who used the OCs during perimenopause.

If you use an oral contraceptive in the premenopausal years, you typically do not experience the hot flashes and other symptoms that mark the endocrine transition to actual menopause. I often describe BCP to help you sail smoothly over the turbulent waters of PCOS and perimenopause.

Whatever birth control pill you use, **do not add St. John's wort if you develop depressive side effects.** Research at the National Institutes of Health found that St. John's wort can decrease the contraceptive effectiveness of the birth control pill up to 50%. You could be in for a rude surprise with an unexpected pregnancy if you combine St. John's wort with your birth control pill. Talk with your physician about other types of birth control pill products to try if you find that you are feeling depressed with one you are taking.

In addition, St. John's wort increases the liver's metabolic break-down of the hormones and reduces their effectiveness, which means that women with PCOS get less benefit from the BCP they are taking to control the unwanted effects of PCOS. Adding St. John's wort can prevent the BCP from working to suppress the excess androgens, and you are likely to find yourself back in the cranky, irritable, anxious, "perimenopausal panic" mood roller coaster.

BENEFICIAL EFFECTS OF ORAL CONTRACEPTIVES

Condition or Disease	% Decrease Compared to Non-pill Users
Menstrual Disorders	**% Reduction**
♎ dysmenorrhea	63%
♎ menopausal symptoms	72%
♎ menorrhagia	48%
♎ irregular menstruation	35%
♎ intermenstrual bleeding	28%
♎ premenstrual tension (PMS)	29–80% (degree of reduction in symptoms, depends on balance of E and P in pill)
Reproductive Organ Tumors	
♎ breast: fibrocystic/fibroadenomas	60–75%
♎ breast biopsies	50%
♎ benign ovarian cysts	65% (using monophasic pills)
♎ uterine fibroids (fibroma)	59%
♎ ovarian cancer	40%–70%, based on # of years of use
♎ endometrial cancer	50%–75%, based on # of years of use
Other Reproductive Disorders	
♎ endometriosis	50%
♎ pelvic inflammatory disease	10–70%
♎ toxic shock syndrome	60%
♎ uterine retroversion	24%
Other Health Problems	
♎ Rheumatoid arthritis	50%
♎ iron deficiency anemia	45%
♎ duodenal ulcer	40%
♎ sebaceous cysts	24%
♎ acne	20% (better effect to decrease acne if using low progestin pills)

Ref: Richard P. Dickey, MD, Ph.D. Managing Contraceptive Pill Patients, 11th edition, Essential Medical Information Systems, 2002.

As one 45-year-old woman described it to me at a recent follow-up appointment: *"I felt great on the Ovcon 35 for the first few months. My energy was great, my mind was clearing, my memory was getting better, and I felt so good. I even had my interest in sex back. Then the last two months I felt like I was slipping again. I had more crying spells, I felt on edge all the time, like I was going to fly into a million pieces. And I started having spotting almost every day and that had not been happening before."*

When I explored with her what had changed in the last two months, she admitted she had added daily St. John's wort and "a few other herbs" recommended by her homeopathic doctor. She said, *"I didn't think to mention it to you because my homeopathic doctor said herbs are safe and don't have any side effects!"*

Another woman's voice may help you see the some of the potential for feeling better during perimenopause that is possible with the right balance in a birth control pill. RS was 39 when she first consulted me, and these are here words, a year later:

"Finding you was like a Godsend. I went right out and bought your book. It really helped knowing I wasn't losing my mind. I think every woman should read your book. I had sent up a prayer for help and then found your interview on the Web. I have four children and I am a regional director for a large public relations company and it was getting hard for me to even function. My Gyn said I was too young to be going through menopause, but my intuition was telling me that I was in menopause. He said I just had PMS and all I needed was Xanax. Then I went to my GP and he put me on Elavil. All they wanted to do was give me medicine for depression and anxiety and I really didn't like how I felt on all that. Besides, it really bothered me that they said it was just that I was in a stressful job.

"Eleven years ago, I was a single Mom, had just gone through a divorce and my dad died, but I handled all that just fine. But this time, everything in my life was great. I had a husband I loved, a fabulous job and my business was going really well, and I thought to myself why

Vital Info!

Something as simple as grapefruit juice can interfere with the effectiveness of many medications. You need to think about drug-herb interactions as very real possibilities. **Always tell your physician *everything* you are taking.**

is it that now I have these problems and feel like I can't function? My symptoms were getting so bad I couldn't take business trips and I couldn't think clearly to function well. I was beginning to think I would have to give up my business, but then I realized I didn't want to do that so I kept looking for help. That's when I found about your work and made the appointment with you.

"After you started me on the patch, I started sleeping better right away. It was amazing. I could sleep, I didn't have the anxiety attacks or the palpitations—they were gone! Then I started on the right birth control pill a couple months later. At first I felt a little nausea with those, but that went away. After being on the pill about 3 or 4 months, I felt 90% back to my old self. My mind cleared, I could remember things again, I could focus at work, and I felt like my moods were much more even. It was like a miracle."

Fact:
FSH above 20 is considered menopausal.

Transitioning: BCP to Menopause HRT Options

If you don't have hot flashes and other symptoms that mark the endocrine transition to actual menopause, how do you decide when to change from a BCP to postmenopausal hormone options?

I suggest you seek help from a knowledgeable health professional to guide you in this so you don't experience any unwanted effects from stopping oral contraceptives abruptly or from differences in potency of the birth control pills and the natural hormones.

I recommend that you have an annual blood test to measure FSH, beginning at age 50 or so. Take this test on the 5th to 7th days off the active birth control pills, during the "placebo" week when you menstruate. If the FSH is checked at the end of the week of placebo pills, you are off hormones long enough for FSH to rise and show whether you are in menopause.

You do not have to stop the oral contraceptives for several months in order to check the FSH, as many women

Note:
If you have not yet reached menopause, FSH measured on the days off the BCP will still be in the premeno-pausal range of less than 20.

Alert:
You do not have to stop the oral contraceptives for several months in order to check the FSH. Six or seven days is long enough.

are told. Your physician may not yet be aware of how and when to check FSH, since it is still relatively new to use oral contraceptives for perimenopausal women into their early 50s.

Just don't do the blood tests for FSH when you are taking the active hormone pills in your pack, because if you check FSH then, it will be very low due to the hormones you are taking those days, and will not give you an accurate determination of your menopausal status.

If the FSH is less than 20, you could possibly still become pregnant, although it is uncommon. You may want to stay on the oral contraceptives until your FSH is higher than 20 on the 6th or 7th day of placebo pills. Doses of hormones for menopause are not enough to provide contraception for the premenopausal women who still ovulate and could become pregnant.

If your FSH is greater than 20 mIU/mL on the days off the hormone-containing birth control pills, then you have reached the endocrine stage of menopause and I suggest you talk with your doctor about a switch to one of the postmenopausal hormone options.

Why is it necessary to change to another hormone regimen if the oral contraceptives are working well? That is done because even the low-dose oral contraceptives contain more estrogen and progestin than is generally needed for postmenopausal use.

My opinion—
Waiting until TSH is 8 or so is too long, and allows symptoms to get worse unnecessarily.

After menopause, your follicles have been depleted, you no longer ovulate, so contraception is not an issue. You can use the FDA-approved bioidentical human hormones that are more "natural" and have fewer side effects than even low-dose birth control pills.

PCOS and Hypothyroidism— Suggestions for Thyroid Options

Women with PCOS may also suffer from hypothyroidism and from autoimmune thyroid disorders, such as

Hashimoto's and Graves thyroiditis. This is a particularly critical issue for women with PCOS who are trying to become pregnant, since the thyroid pathway is intimately linked with ovarian function. Even subtle disturbances in thyroid function can cause infertility. It can be a challenge to find hormone options to control the ovarian problems, and at the same time, address the thyroid issues for optimal thyroid hormone management.

I hear a great deal from my patients that their doctors feel TSH is still "normal" at 4 or 5. TSH values greater than about 5 on most laboratory reference scales indicate hypothyroidism, although many physicians don't treat with thyroid medication until the TSH rises over 8.

I prefer to begin treatment earlier in the process of a failing thyroid gland to avoid having the person get sicker and have more difficulty regaining optimal health. I generally will start medication when TSH is about 4 or 5, occasionally a little sooner if the antibody levels are quite high and/or there are indications that thyroid is needed to help restore normal muscle and nerve function, metabolic regulation, regular ovarian cycles, and/or to improve memory and mood.

On the other hand, it isn't wise to take thyroid when you don't need it. This is another reason I think it is so important to check both ovarian and thyroid hormones carefully before making treatment decisions. Symptoms of estradiol loss can be quite similar to symptoms of low thyroid function. But if you start thyroid hormone when you don't need it, and your estradiol is low, it will accelerate your rate of bone loss.

Obviously, thyroid hormone replacement is a complex topic and I can't give you all the "specifics" in this short space. You may want to read more about thyroid issues in my earlier book, *Women, Weight and Hormones.*

Caution: If women are given too much thyroid, however, it can cause more bone loss and possible heart rhythm disturbances.

Caution: "Natural" can mean "bioidentical" or it can mean coming from a biological source and chemically different from the molecule made by your body.

Alert There aren't really valid reasons to still use the animal-derived product today, when better options are available.

Which is Best, Natural or Synthetic?

The "natural" buzzword has also hit the thyroid hormone therapy arena as well as the menopause field. The question centers around what type of thyroid hormone to give: synthetic pure T4 (Synthroid, Levoxyl and other generic forms of T4) or a mixed T4–T3 blend that is called "natural" because it is derived from dessicated (dried) animal thyroid tissue (such as Armour thyroid).

"Synthetic" can simply mean "made in laboratory" to be identical to what your body makes, or it can also mean "chemically new" and unlike what your body makes. It is crucial for you to know the difference and not get caught up in the marketing ploys.

Fact:

The earlier treatment is begun, the less likely the person will have other adverse effects of low thyroid such as hypertension and elevated cholesterol.

One of the reasons some practitioners recommend Armour thyroid is that it contains T3 as well as T4. The pig-derived thyroid doesn't have the same ratio of T4 and T3 found in humans, so you can end up getting too much T3 when you use Armour. This can make you feel jittery, nervous, and have trouble sleeping—rather like a "tired but wired" feeling.

In addition, most people given thyroid medication will be able to take the T4 products and then have the body do normal conversion to the more active form of thyroid hormone, T3. For those people who don't convert enough T4 to T3, and still have low T3 levels even on the right amount of T4, I will consider adding a pure, hypoallergenic, sustained release form of T3 compounded by a specialty pharmacy.

I use the compounded product instead of the commercial ones such as Cytomel and Armour because (1) it isn't animal derived, so it isn't antigenic, (2) I can get it made in a longer-lasting preparation, and (3) I can better individualize the dose of both T4 and T3 if they aren't "fixed" in one tablet.

I typically will add T3 after I have observed a person's response to T4 replacement, and have checked the lab results for TSH, T3 and T4. I typically start T3 in much lower doses than the commercial products (Thyrolar, Armour, Cytomel) contain. So I really haven't found it necessary to use the animal-derived thyroid products.

Animal-derived hormones (whether thyroid, insulin, or ovarian, and whether they come from cows, pigs, or horses) have the potential to be antigenic in humans. They can cause our bodies to form antibodies to the hormones, and to our own endocrine glands.

This was one of the early problems recognized decades ago with the animal-derived insulins given over long periods of time to diabetics, and also with the allergies to horse serum when this was used as a base for many medicines in the past. Most of these problems have been resolved with the development of synthetic human insulin and medicines not given in a horse serum base.

Similar problems occurred with animal-derived thyroid products when they were all we had and used more widely. Then scientists created the bioidentical molecule of T4 in the laboratory to produce a synthetic human form of thyroid hormone that did not cause these problems of stimulating antibody production.

Warning: Don't be mislead by the word "natural" when looking for remedies for PCOS.

I have seen too many women develop high levels of thyroid antibodies when they take animal-derived thyroid products long term, so I prefer not to use them. This is an especially serious problem for women with PCOS who need optimal thyroid balance in order to have optimal ovarian function.

Getting the Care You Need: Suggestions to Guide You

There is such an explosion of health information, you need to scrutinize your sources very carefully. Some of it is very helpful and reliable, some of it terribly out-of-date, and some of it blatantly wrong.

I find that many articles and books still perpetuate old myths about PCOS, progesterone creams, and misinformation about the potential benefits of BCP.

You should be very selective about the resources you use—books and articles, as well as the health professionals you choose. Not everyone is interested in, or knowledgeable about PCOS, and you deserve to work with someone who will help you find medically sound ways to feel better.

A variety of herbs are documented to have toxic effects on the liver, and may cause a variety of other problems. Just because compounds are natural to plants does not necessarily they are natural for humans (same reasoning I used in talking about horse-derived estrogens, remember?).

Caution: Herbs have potential downsides, just as taking hormones has potential downsides to consider. There is no one right answer for everyone.

The current research on the human hormone receptor system is revealing incredible complexity of the estradiol, progesterone, and testosterone receptors in various tissues. It is too simplistic to say that herbs with "estrogenic" effects at some receptor sites will do *all of the jobs our own hormones are designed to do.*

For example, even though a high soy diet has been shown to have modest effects to reduce cholesterol, there are also now studies from several countries that show soy isoflavones compete with our own body hormones at the estradiol and progesterone receptors. This competitive inhibition with phyto-estrogens leads to a 20–50% reduction in production of estradiol and progesterone in premenopausal women.

For young women who still want to become pregnant, high soy intake can have a profound negative impact on your fertility, particularly if you already have impaired hormone production due to PCOS. For women after menopause, when their own ovarian production of hormones has decreased, higher soy intake may not be as potentially serious. It really is a complex issue.

You may not be able to get all of your questions answered in one place, because the specialists in different areas tend to know their own field well but may perpetuate inaccurate information about other areas. None of us can know everything about other fields of specialty.

For example, I have an area of interest and expertise in the neuroendocrine issues and know a great deal about nuances of hormone therapy, psychotropic medications, approaches to help high cholesterol, insulin resistance, osteoporosis, and other common problems women with PCOS have to face. I also know how to incorporate a variety of other modalities and lifestyle changes to maintain good health.

But I am not a surgeon and cannot take the place of a gynecologist when my patients need these services. I am not a fertility specialist, and so I refer patients when they need these services. I know about herbal remedies and some basics about their use, but I am not a specialist in the use of herbs so I don't try to prescribe them extensively.

Likewise, you can't expect a non-medically trained herbalist to be as knowledgeable as I am about the current information on hormones. Many gynecologists don't have the time or interest to work with the variety of problems and treatment approaches needed for PCOS.

Caution:
Try to avoid those that are obviously focused on selling products promoted by the author.

If you purchase a book on herbs for menopause, don't expect it to also provide current information on estrogen. In fact, most of these sources I have reviewed are seriously incorrect in the content on both estrogen and progesterone. By the same token, don't expect my book to go in depth about herbs, since that was not my primary focus in writing it.

Remember to keep your expectations to the expertise expected for the person's area of specialty. You will have to do your homework to select a variety of current, reputable, accurate books and other resources to help you develop your "health plan."

Look to reputable sources, such as the *Harvard Women's Health Watch Newsletter*, that aren't trying to sell you a bunch of expensive supplements and "hormone balancer" products.

Keep in mind as well that we have different health needs at different stages of our lives. Women with PCOS have many complex health challenges not likely to fit exactly into any one specialty "box" based on our old models of health care. You need and deserve a variety of integrated approaches and knowledgeable professionals to help you achieve your goals.

When our financial goals and needs change, we change financial advisors. As you get older and experience health changes that have many different ramifications physically, psychologically, socially, and spiritually, you may need to change your thinking about the best health provider to meet your needs.

Keep an open mind, and be prepared to invest time, effort and money to find someone right for you, someone who is really interested in mid-life and the integration of these important dimensions of your health.

The Poignancy of PCOS: Women's Stories

Jodie was 39 when I first saw her. Her hormone evaluation showed abnormal levels characteristic of PCOS. We worked with her over a number of months to restore a healthier hormone balance. But there is a part of her story before I saw her that gives me goosebumps every time I think about it. If you think people are silly to believe in God and guardian angels, her experience may convince you otherwise.

Her first heart attack was at age 36. She was 39 when I saw her, she had already suffered three serious heart attacks and almost died during the third one. In fact, the cardiologist had told her husband she would not likely come out of the coma because her heart simply wasn't pumping enough blood, she wasn't responding to medications, and there was nothing else to try. What happened next was quite touching, and very meaningful to me. Two friends of Jodie's, one a patient of mine

Hormonal Connections

Jodie's heart attacks always happened at the start of her menstrual period, a time when estradiol drops sharply, which can cause spasm and reduced blood flow in the coronary arteries to the heart.

took a copy of my previous book which described the effects of estradiol on the heart, to Jodie's husband at the hospital where she was in ICU, in a coma. The doctors had told Jodie's family that it was "only a matter of time" before she died.

The two women showed the page in *Screaming to Be Heard* to Jodie's husband. He immediately said, "She always thought her heart attacks had something to do with her hormones, and asked many doctors about it, but they always told her it couldn't be. This is amazing."

Right away, they went to the cardiologist and showed him the page describing estradiol's effect on the arteries to improve blood flow. They asked if he was willing to put an estradiol patch on Jodie. The cardiologist read the material and said, "Nothing else is working, we have nothing to lose. We may as well try it. It certainly won't hurt her."

To everyone's surprise and relief, including the doctor's, Jodie's condition improved. Her "ejection fraction" (a measure of the blood being pumped by the heart) was critically low and not improving on the other medicines. Slowly she came out of the coma as her heart function improved. Her doctor continued the estradiol patch during the rest of her hospitalization, amazed at the changes. She was finally discharged, though she still had a long recovery from the damage to her heart.

She wrote her story as she scheduled her first consult with me. I was amazed at the progress after her near-death experience. I reviewed her serum hormone levels and showed her why the estradiol patch had helped so much. Her own menstrual Day 1 estradiol was barely detectable, and her free and total testosterone and DHEA were all quite high, as were her total and LDL cholesterol, triglycerides and insulin.

The low estradiol, coupled with high androgens, high cholesterol with a high LDL and low HDL and her high insulin, set her up for heart attacks. I explained that

Estradiol helped
Within a few hours after the Climara estradiol patch was put on, the ejection fraction began increasing significantly.

Take note:
Low estradiol leads to coronary vasospasm that can seriously decrease blood flow to the heart muscle.

our goal was to keep her estradiol as steady as possible using an estradiol patch during bleeding days, and then decrease the androgens, improve her cholesterol profile, and decrease the excess insulin.

Four years later, she was doing well on her hormone and dietary plan to correct these hormone imbalances. She was able to be a more active Mom, involved with her children and her life again. She gradually lost the weight caused by PCOS, through changes in her diet and a regular walking program. She became an avid spokesperson in Internet support groups for PCOS, and said, "I want to help other women understand PCOS and get proper evaluation before someone else goes through what I did."

Summary

The synthetic hormones in the BCP have gotten a bad reputation, but this is not always deserved. There are many medical situations, beyond need for contraception, in which these synthetic hormones can do a world of good, and prevent serious health problems from getting worse—such as endometriosis, fibroids, heavy bleeding, ovarian cysts, PCOS, severe PMS, menstrually-triggered migraines, severe anemia, recurrent breast cysts—just to name some key ones.

In addition, many women may not ovulate regularly in the decade before menopause, but the very erratic nature of ovulation means that you still need, and may want, contraception.

So don't throw the baby out with the bath water. Give some consideration to the possibility that the BCP can help you with the problems caused by PCOS. The trick is to find ones with the right balance of estrogen and progestin so they don't make headaches, low libido, depression or weight gain worse.

Chapter 11

Other Medication Treatment Options and Surgical Approaches for PCOS

You read in the previous chapter about the use of combined estrogen-progestin contraceptives to help relieve many of the bothersome symptoms and metabolic problems of PCOS. For many women with PCOS, however, the OCs may not be enough to address all the symptoms, or may cause side effects that add to the difficulties caused by PCOS. Other women are trying to become pregnant, and may not want the contraceptive effects of BCP.

Heads UP: PCOS often requires an integrated treatment approach.

For all these reasons, it is important to know what other treatment options are available, and how they can be used alone or in combination to help alleviate PCOS problems. Let's look at the various categories of medicines available. Then later in the chapter, I will review some of the surgical approaches that have been used for PCOS.

Approaches to Treat Androgen Excess

Excess androgens cause a lot of anguish and unwanted body changes in PCOS. Oral contraceptives are a good way to treat this problem, but sometimes that is not enough to block the excess production or the adverse effects of androgens on skin, hair, weight and mood.

There are several other medicines that can be used as effective "androgen blockers." PCOS often requires an integrated treatment approach using several different medications that complement one another and work on several pathways involved in the problematic symptoms.

Spironolactone (brand name: Aldactone)

Spironolactone is an older potassium-sparing diuretic that has been used for several decades to treat hirsutism and acne caused by excess levels of DHEA, testosterone, and androstenedione.

Good option: Spironolactone generally has very few side effects and is well tolerated, often used in combination with birth control pills.

Spironolactone is a good choice, because it blocks activity of the androgens at their receptor sites and also interferes with the body's ability to make androgens. Over time, it causes reduction in the androgens and improvement in acne and excess hair. Another benefit of this medicine is that spironolactone also helps treat scalp hair *loss and thinning* that can also be caused by androgen excess.

Spironolactone is also an antagonist of the fluid regulating hormone, aldosterone, so it functions as a diuretic to relieve water retention and bloating, a nice plus during those "PMS" weeks.

Most doctors feel that the usual effective dose range is 100–200 mg a day. I like to start my patients on just 25-50 mg a day and work up gradually, which helps reduce side effects. Doing it this way, I have found that many women can benefit from doses in the range of 25 mg taken two or three times a day and they often do not have to take the maximum dose of 200 mg daily. But if you are not seeing a response at the lower doses, don't give up. Try increasing gradually, working with your doctor, up to the higher dose ranges that have been found to be effective. At higher doses, fatigue or weakness can be side effects but at low doses I don't find that patients experience these problems.

I have many patients who had major improvement in their acne, facial and body hair when spironolactone was added to their oral contraceptive regimen.

OCs suppress production of androgens by decreasing the high LH that overstimulates the ovaries, OCs stimulate increased liver production of SHBG and bind up the excess free androgens. Spironolactone inhibits androgen binding at the receptor level. Adding all these together really helps decrease acne and excess body hair.

But keep in mind that acne, scalp hair *loss*, and *excess* facial and body hair often take a long time to improve once you start spironolactone. Plan to give it at least six months at a therapeutic dose of spironolactone before you assume it isn't working.

The progestin, *drospirenone*, in the oral contraceptive Yasmin, is derived from spironolactone and like its parent compound, acts to block the androgen receptor as an additional way of relieving symptoms of androgen excess. Drospirenone is approximately equivalent to 25 mg of spironolactone, a very low dose compared to what is generally considered therapeutic at 100–200 mg of spironolactone a day.

Both drospirenone and spironolactone help to relieve fluid retention and bloating, and also help keep the body from losing potassium, one of the problems with other diuretics.

Don't take potassium supplements when you are taking either spironolactone or drospirenone. Although it is important to have enough potassium in your diet, it can be dangerous to overdo it. Excess potassium can cause potentially deadly disturbances in heart rhythm.

The package insert for Yasmin says not to take it with spironolactone, but I have found that using a *low dose* of spironolactone can often enhance the benefits seen with Yasmin alone. The concern about using them together is that you may get too much potassium sparing effect, and have excess potassium.

The important thing to keep in mind for someone on Yasmin, is that if you use *less* than the maximum therapeutic dose of spironolactone, and if you do *not take potassium supplements*, you aren't likely to have these problems.

Watch for side effects such as muscle weakness or severe fatigue that might be clues that you are getting too much diuretic effect from the combined medications. And ask your doctor to check your electrolytes (sodium,

Combined Therapy: Oral contraceptives and spironolactone used together often work much better than either one alone because of the different ways each medicine works to decrease androgens.

potassium, chloride) regularly to make sure you are not getting too much.

Flutamide

This is an *anti-androgen* medication originally developed to treat men with prostate cancer. It has been used to treat women with hirsutism, although not formally approved by the FDA for this purpose. Flutamide is effective but it has the potential to cause fatal liver toxicity. So even though this side effect is infrequent, because it is potential deadly, most physicians don't use flutamide for women with PCOS unless nothing else has worked. If you are taking flutamide, you need to be sure your doctor is frequently checking reliable blood tests of liver function.

Warning: Flutamide is contra-indicated in pregnancy due to risk of damage to the fetus. Use a reliable form of birth control when taking this medicine.

The typical dose of flutamide is 125–500 mg daily, usually starting at 125 mg and working up gradually to taking 250 mg twice a day. More recent data suggest that a dose of 250 mg once a day may be as effective as taking 250 mg twice a day. This lower dose also helps decrease side effects.

Finasteride

Finasteride was also developed to treat men with prostate cancer, but has been used to treat women with hirsutism and acne even though it also is not formally approved by the FDA for this use. This medicine acts to inhibit the enzyme *5-alpha reductase*, which converts testosterone to the more potent compound, dihydrotestosterone, that acts to stimulate hair growth at the hair follicle.

Finasteride also blocks the form of 5-alpha reductase that is involved with the activity of sebaceous glands in the skin. This means it can also be effective in reducing acne.

The dose used is typically 5 mg daily, but sometimes women may see some benefit at half the usual dose. Finasteride doesn't seem to change the menstrual cycle. Women taking finasteride must use reliable methods of contraception while taking it. Both flutamide and finasteride are much more expensive than spironolactone.

Since they also both have significant side effects, they are typically aren't used in PCOS except when a woman has not had improvement using oral contraceptives and spironolactone.

Cyproterone Acetate (2–50 mg daily)

This is an androgen-blocking progestin that has not yet been approved by the FDA, but is available overseas for hormone therapy and for treatment of androgen excess. It is also used with ethinyl estradiol in the birth control pill, *Diane 35*.

In studies from other countries, this progestin is equal to or slightly better than the combined estrogen-progestin contraceptive pills available in the United States. Even though symptoms of androgen excess typically get better with cyproterone acetate, some women still have difficulty tolerating the progestin side effects of weight gain, depression, low libido and headache.

Warning! Finasteride cannot be used in women trying to become pregnant because it can cause malformation of the genitals in a male baby.

Dexamethasone and Prednisone

These medicines belong to a class called *glucocorticosteroids* (also called *corticosteroids*). They may be useful if the excess androgens are produced by an over-active adrenal gland. But it is very important to have a careful and thorough evaluation to determine whether you really do have an adrenal disorder that requires use of these medicines because their side effects can mimic problems already happening in PCOS.

Over time, use of corticosteroids can cause weight gain, mood changes, increased risk of diabetes, immune suppression, and other potentially serious problems. The side effects can be the same whether you are taking "natural" or synthetic forms of corticosteriods.

Because of the potential for making the problems of PCOS worse with these medicines, I don't recommend the increasingly common practice of women being tested using saliva tests, given a "diagnosis" of "adrenal fatigue" and then started on corticosteroids.

I suggest that women seek evaluation and treatment

from an endocrinologist or reproductive endocrinologist if it appears that the excess androgens are due to an adrenal disorder. Then the appropriate treatment can be decided and you can have the proper monitoring to help avoid unwanted side effects.

If prednisone or dexamethasone are used, generally they are given in low doses for about 2–3 months, and then doses tapered down until the medicines can be stopped. This approach usually decreases androgen production to normal levels, which leads to improvement in acne, slowing of the rate of growth of excess body hair, and may also even improve ovulatory function and fertility.

Androgen levels will often remain suppressed after treatment with corticosteroids is stopped, but sometimes levels start to rise again and symptoms return. This is more common with testosterone than with DHEA, but levels of both should be rechecked every 3-4 months for about a year after stopping corticosteroids to be sure that levels remain in the normal range.

Ketoconazole

This is an antifungal medicine that has been reported to be somewhat effective to help improve symptoms of androgen excess. Although you may sometimes see references to its use for PCOS, it is not widely used now.

My medical opinion is that it doesn't provide enough reliable benefits to offset the risk of serious side effects and damage to the liver. I think there are better options available with much less risk of problems.

Leuprolide (Brand name: Lupron)

This is a medication called a *GnRH agonist* because it mimics the action of gonadotropin-releasing hormones (GnRH) in the brain, which in turn results in shutting down the ovaries to stop the production of all the ovarian hormones and eliminate the ovarian cycles.

Lupron and other medicines in the GnRH class have been used to treat refractory PMS, severe endometriosis, to shrink large fibroids prior to surgery and to treat severe androgen excess in PCOS. These medicines are also used for cycle control in fertility treatments.

Since GnRH agonists shut down the ovaries and cut off estrogen and progesterone production in addition to shutting off androgens, they have the drawback of causing sudden and full menopausal symptoms like hot flashes, fragmented sleep, depressed mood, memory problems, loss of sex drive, and many others. GnRH agonists can cause marked loss of bone if they are used for long periods of time.

To eliminate the hot flashes, sleep problems and prevent bone loss and other negative side effects of GnRH agonists, physicians often use "add-back" therapy with estradiol. If you have a uterus, you cannot take estradiol alone for an extended period of time without also taking progesterone or a progestin to oppose the estrogen effects on the uterine lining and prevent bleeding problems or hyperplasia (abnormal thickening).

Because of the expense (approximately $500–$800 per month) of these medications and the careful monitoring needed, I generally don't recommend such a major step for treating PCOS unless it is extremely severe, and you have found *nothing else* that worked.

A trial of GnRH agonists may be particularly helpful if the PCOS is so severe and incapacitating that your physician has recommended surgical removal of the ovaries (*ovariectomy, oophorectomy*) and uterus (*hysterectomy*). Ovarian suppression effects of GnRH agonists wear off after a few months. In this situation, it may be worth a two or three month trial of medical therapy with a GnRH agonist along with add-back estrogen to see whether eliminating the ovarian androgen production and hormone cycling alleviates your symptoms.

Then once you see how you feel, you may be more confident that a surgical approach would help for the long term.

Caution: If using Lupron, add-back therapy is needed to prevent severe menopausal symptons and bone loss!

Option: GnRH agonists allow you to see what is helped with a *reversible medical ovariectomy,* before you have to decide about permanent surgical removal of the ovaries.

Approaches to Reduce Insulin Excess

Metformin and Glitazones: What They Do

Excess production of insulin is one of the cardinal problems in PCOS that stimulates the ovaries to make excess androgens, and also causes marked weight gain.

The more insulin there is, the more glucose is stored as fat, instead of burned as fuel, the fatter you get, and the harder it is to lose weight. Then the more body fat you have, especially the "middle-spread" that makes you more apple-shaped, the more insulin resistant you become. The medicines to improve insulin sensitivity help to break this vicious cycle.

Medicines that lower insulin and improve insulin response, often called "insulin sensitizers," have been used for many years to treat diabetes. For the last twenty years or more, there have been numerous studies and clinical reports to show that these same medicines can be very helpful in PCOS.

Medicines such as m*etformin* (brand name: *Glucophage*) and the *thiazolidinediones (also called glitazones; brand names: Actos, Avandia)* work to reduce excess insulin, decrease the excess androgen production, help restore ovulatory cycles and fertility, and help improve the metabolic imbalances such as elevated cholesterol and triglycerides.

Glucophage and the Actos and Avandia are FDA-approved for the treatment of diabetes. None of these medicines have yet been approved by the FDA for PCOS, but many studies are underway and physicians treating PCOS have seen much success using these medications as part of an integrated treatment program.

Recent Studies and What They Show

Some of the most recent studies are very encouraging about the benefits of medications that act to improve insulin sensitivity. Here are a few of the many that have been done. For those readers who would like to read the original papers, the complete references are listed in the Bibliography in Appendix II.

In 2004, gynecologists at the All India Institute of Medical Sciences in New Delhi, India reported encouraging results from their study of metformin therapy in 50 Indian women followed for 6 months. The women lost a mean of 4.7% in weight, and showed an 80.5% improvement in menstrual cycle regularity. After metformin therapy, there was a significant rise in FSH, decrease in LH, and improvement in LH/FSH ratio. Metformin also resulted in a significant decrease in total cholesterol and rise in the "good" HDL cholesterol. These physicians concluded that the beneficial effects, with few adverse side effects, for metformin supported its being used more widely for women with PCOS.

India: Metformin achieved an overall 66% increase in ovulatory rate, and a 28% pregnancy rate.

A 1998 study published in *The New England Journal of Medicine*, found that 90 percent of the women who took metformin either ovulated spontaneously or with help from the fertility drug Clomid. Only 12 percent of the women taking a placebo pill had ovulatory cycles, even if they also took Clomid. Studies since that time have continued to show metformin's benefit in restoring ovulatory cycles and improving fertility.

What About Metformin in Normal Weight Women?

In a 2004 study published in *Fertility and Sterility*, Baillargeon and colleagues reported on their double-blind study of 100 non-obese women with PCOS who had normal measures of insulin sensitivity. This study evaluated the effects of metformin and rosiglitazone, each given alone and the two given together. The women ranged in age from 17 to 40 years old, and had normal body mass index (i.e. less than 27 kg/m2).

The study looked at four groups of women for six months: Group I had combined therapy with metformin 850 mg twice a day and 4 mg of rosiglitazone 4 mg, Group II was given just metformin alone in the same dose, Group III was given 4 mg rosiglitazone alone, and Group IV received placebo.

2004 Study:

All three groups given the active medications had a 6- to 8-fold increase in frequency of ovulation compared to the PCOS group taking only placebo.

Studies show:

Even women who don't have abnormal measures of insulin may benefit from these medications, especially with regard to improving ovulation.

The results were striking. The 60–70% higher rate of ovulatory bleeding rate was accompanied by a decrease in total and free serum testosterone. In this study, the improved ovulation frequency was seen across the board, whether the women took both medications or just one.

Some women with PCOS may have an overactive insulin pathway affecting the synthesis of ovarian androgens even when their serum levels of insulin are normal. It could also be possible that these medicines affect ovarian hormone production in ways that are separate from their effects on insulin.

What About Metformin in Women with Normal Androgen Levels?

Most of us who work with PCOS patients have seen women who don't ovulate regularly and who have irregular periods, weight gain and difficulty getting pregnant. But when we check their hormone levels, we find the androgens are in the normal range. Because of this, they don't fit the "classical" definition of PCOS and often get told they don't have PCOS and just to "eat less and exercise more." But these women tell me that as diligent as they are with diet and exercise, nothing works. So what's happening? Do these women have a variant of PCOS? Is it possible that metformin might help restore ovulatory cycles?

Drs. Carmina and Lobo addressed these issues in a study published in 2004 of 24 women with these characteristics. The study participants had serum androgen levels that didn't statistically differ from the control group with regular menstrual periods. They did have, however, higher fasting insulin levels than did the control group and were considered insulin resistant.

The women were randomized to take either placebo or metformin for three months, and the researchers found that women who took metformin had a higher frequency of ovulatory cycles than did the placebo group. 79% of the women met criteria for PCOS on pelvic ultrasound of the ovaries, even though they did not have high androgen levels.

This study suggests a couple of important points to keep in mind: (1) high androgen levels may not be as reliable a diagnostic feature of PCOS as we have thought, (2) loss of ovulation could be an effect of insulin resistance acting directly on the ovary or via the pituitary, and may be independent of androgen levels. This study suggests that metformin may be helpful for women who don't ovulate regularly, even if androgen levels are still normal.

I think what this means clinically for individual women is that there are still a lot of unanswered questions about PCOS, and we should not be too rigid in applying diagnostic criteria when our goal is to help women feel better, improve menstrual cycle function, and reduce long term health risks. This is particularly true with a medicine like metformin that generally has relatively few potential negative side effects.

Metformin in Pregnancy

Another encouraging study was published in 2002 in *Fertility and Sterility*. Researchers looked at all of the live births of women taking metformin during pregnancy and found gestational diabetes developed in 22 of 72 pregnancies (31%) in women who did not take metformin, but in only 1 of 33 pregnancies (3%) for women who took metformin. This is major improvement in risk by taking metformin.

Women who took metformin in this study had already had problems with gestational diabetes in 67% of their previous pregnancies, so they clearly were a group prone to developing diabetes again. It makes the reduction in risk with metformin even more remarkable. *There were no significant adverse effects on the fetus in any of the women taking metformin.*

But we still need more studies on the safety of these medications during pregnancy, so I think it is wise for women who want to use metformin during pregnancy to discuss this with their fertility specialist or obstetrician.

Tip: High androgen levels may not be as reliable a diagnostic feature of PCOS as we have thought

Good news! Researchers found a *10-fold* reduction in risk of gestational diabetes in women with PCOS who took metformin throughout pregnancy.

Metformin vs. Ovarian Surgery to Improve Fertility

Women with PCOS often have a dilemma when trying to explore the best ways to help achieve a pregnancy. Some doctors recommend clomiphene alone, some recommend insulin sensitizer medications like metformin, and other doctors recommend surgical procedures based on the earlier studies showing that removing part of the ovary could help restore ovulatory cycles in some women with PCOS.

Important Benefits: Women who took metformin had both a higher pregnancy rate and lower miscarriage rate.

To help clarify which approaches had the best chance of success, Dr. Palomba and colleagues conducted a well-designed, prospective, randomized double-blind, placebo controlled clinical trial. This type of study design is considered the "gold standard" in clinical research.

Their goal in the study was to determine whether metformin alone or ovarian surgery (using laparoscopic ovarian diathermy, or LOD) would be a better means to improve fertility in women who had not responded to clomiphene (brand name: Clomid) to trigger ovulation. There were sixty women in the study who were randomized into the following groups:

- Women who had the LOD surgery and then took a placebo for 6 months
- Women had a mock surgery and then took 1700 mg of metformin daily for 6 months

The researchers found that both treatments were equally effective in terms of the ovulatory rates achieved (55.1% and 54.8%, respectively). There was a striking difference, however, in the pregnancy and miscarriage rates between the two groups.

There was a remarkable 47% *decrease in miscarriage rate* in the women who took metformin after a mock surgery, compared to the women who had LOD surgery and took placebo. The decrease in miscarriages then meant that women who took metformin also had a higher live birth rate than women who had the surgery.

In my review of the literature, this is the first randomized clinical trial I have found that showed so clearly that women with PCOS who simply take metformin while trying to conceive can have *both* higher pregnancy rates *and* lower miscarriage rates. I think that is very good news for PCOS sufferers who have endured the heartbreak of recurrent pregnancy loss.

There are a number of ways that metformin could work to help women become pregnant, but at this time, researchers don't know all the reasons that metformin helps women with PCOS achieve pregnancy more easily. If these are issues that you have been struggling with, you may want to get a copy of this research paper and the editorial by Dr. John Nestler in the same issue (see Bibliography for complete reference), and discuss these with your physicians.

Metformin: Side Effects, Dosing and Monitoring

It is usually the annoying gastrointestinal side effects of metformin that bother people when they try it. These can include burping or dyspepsia, nausea, diarrhea, and less commonly, vomiting. These effects usually resolve quickly when the medicine is stopped or the dose decreased, so in that sense they are not medically serious.

I suggest that patients increase the dose very slowly over six to eight weeks, increasing the dose only every few weeks, based on how they tolerate it.

I find that if I starting with a lower than usual dose, and increase by only 250 mg at the time, it helps eliminate problems with diarrhea and gastrointestinal upset that can be very common if women are started on the usual 500 mg two or three times day.

Prior to starting patients on one of these medicines, I check measures of glucose and insulin, kidney and liver function, a fasting cholesterol profile with triglycerides in addition to the comprehensive hormone levels I feel are important.

Lactic acidosis is one reported side effect of metformin

Tip #1:
I find that we can usually avoid these side effects if I tell patients to start with just a half tablet, much lower than the usual dose.

Tip #2:
It may take longer to see the benefits of the medicine, but women are able to tolerate it if I go slowly with dose increases.

that can be very serious, even though it is quite rare. Most studies have found that this risk is not at all likely in those who have normal kidney function. Even in those with impaired kidney function, such as diabetics who have had damage to the kidney from their disease, lactic acidosis is still rare.

Current guidelines recommend that metformin *not be used* in people who have impaired kidney function, and that tests of kidney function (such as electrolytes) be done regularly while taking this medicine. If these guidelines are following, it is highly unlikely that am otherwise healthy person would develop complications from taking metformin.

About 7% of patients on metformin can develop low B12 levels, so I recommend that my patients take a B complex supplement when they are taking metformin to help avoid this problem.

Because it is fairly easy to prevent problems of low B12, I don't routinely check B12 levels unless a woman has been eating a vegetarian diet, or hasn't been taking any vitamins, or if she develops symptoms of low B 12. In these situations, it can be helpful to check a B12 blood level prior to starting treatment and recheck in 3-6 months after taking supplements to be sure any deficiency has been corrected.

I have used metformin successfully for many PCOS patients, and have found that it works well to reduce insulin resistance (and its complications) and facilitate weight loss in women who are not trying to become pregnant. Weight loss decreases risk for both diabetes and heart disease, and also helps reduce the insulin resistance in PCOS.

I really have not had very many patients who had so many side effects that they couldn't tolerate the medicine. I have seen many cases, however, of women having side effects and difficulty tolerating the generic metformin who did fine on the brand version Glucophage. Many times they were changed to the generic by a pharmacist

Tip:

Be alert to factors that cause side effects:

ॐ dose

ॐ generic vs brand

ॐ regular vs extended release

or an insurance plan, often without their knowledge. I have also seen a few patients who did better on the generic metformin but had bothersome side effects with the brand Glucophage. Some do better on the regular, some do better on the sustained-release form.

There is no way to predict ahead of time which form of the medicine may work better for you. If you try one version—brand or generic, regular or sustained release—and have bothersome side effects, then try another form and see if you do better. You can also try lowering the dose—sometimes women have diarrhea at 1500–2000 mg a day, but no problems at 750–1000 mg a day, and this is still enough to have a positive therapeutic effect for many women.

If side effects continue to be such a problem that you can't tolerate any form of metformin, then talk with your doctor about a trial of Actos or Avandia. These two insulin-sensitizing medicines don't tend to have the same side effects as metformin or each other, so having a problem with one doesn't mean you can't successfully take one of the others.

For women who don't respond fully to metformin alone, Actos or Avandia can also be *added* to the regimen. These medicines work in different ways to lower excess insulin, so the combination can give more benefits than seen with one medicine alone. Women taking these medications should have regular monitoring of electrolytes, liver function, fasting glucose, cholesterol and triglycerides.

Hormone Effects On Insulin Resistance

Estrogen and progesterone also play a role in insulin regulation, but each hormone has very different effects on insulin sensitivity. Although both hormones increase the pancreas' release of insulin after we eat foods high in carbohydrates, the similarity ends there.

Progesterone *decreases* insulin sensitivity, causing *resistance* to the glucose regulating effects of insulin.

Fact: Progesterone *decreases* insulin sensitivity. Estradiol *increases* insulin sensitivity.

Fact:

Progesterone dominance and low estradiol causes PMS, more sweet cravings, more water retention, more weight gain.

Progesterone's effect on insulin is quite rapid, and can be detected within ten minutes of taking the hormone. Researchers think it is a direct effect of progesterone on the pancreas itself. This is one of the reasons women often experience increased cravings for sweets when progesterone levels rise sharply in the second half of the menstrual cycle.

Estradiol, on the other hand, *increases* insulin sensitivity and improves glucose tolerance. Whether women are menstruating (pre-menopausal) or post-menopausal, estradiol improves glucose handling by the body, even in women who are diabetic.

Estradiol's beneficial effect on blood sugar is particularly noticeable if you are using the patch form of estradiol. Estradiol-triggered improvement in insulin sensitivity occurs at both fat cells (adipocytes) and skeletal muscle. The beneficial effect appears to occur by multiple pathways rather than just a direct effect on the pancreas.

In order to avoid making glucose control worse, mid-life and menopausal women who are getting fatter around the middle, or women of any age who have diabetes, need to *optimize* estradiol levels and take only the amount of progesterone that is necessary for preventing excess build-up of the uterine lining. Excess doses of progesterone can make insulin resistance and weight gain worse.

In a normal menstrual cycle with optimal hormone ratios, the opposing actions of estradiol and progesterone on insulin tend to offset each other, which suggests that the E:P *ratio* is more influential in determining the net metabolic effect. This has been one of the key factors in determining degree of symptoms in women whose hormone levels I have tested.

When premenstrual (luteal) phase hormone ratios are "progesterone dominant," and in women who have lower than optimal estradiol, the symptoms are classic: worse PMS, more intense sweet cravings, increased appetite, weight gain, bloating, fatigue, depressed mood, and more premenstrual water retention.

There is a lot of commercial marketing telling you to use over-the-counter progesterone creams. For women with PCOS, this can be a disaster. If you use progesterone supplements over a long time, and don't have the right balance of estradiol, you end up having *more* middle body fat gain, and more *insulin resistance*, and *more androgen production.*

All this means that you need to be very careful *which* hormones you take as a young woman with PCOS, or if you are beginning to have symptoms approaching menopause.

Warning: OTC progerterone creams can be a disaster if you have PCOS.

Oral forms of horse-derived estrogens like Premarin, or plant-derived estrone like Estratab and Cenestin, may make this insulin resistance-glucose intolerance pattern worse. Medical studies show that the "patch" form of estradiol delivery, improves glucose tolerance and lessens insulin resistance because it delivers estradiol through the skin, bypassing the first pass through the liver.

Approaches to Treat Mood Problems in PCOS

The hormone imbalances of PCOS have many mood-disrupting effects, and can even mimic bipolar disorder, dysthymic disorder, major depression, panic disorder, or generalized anxiety.

First, let's clarify some terms. Mood *symptom* usually refers to a brief period of mood change not severe enough or long-lasting enough to qualify for a formal diagnosis of mood *disorder.*

Mood *disorder* generally refers to a group of physical and emotional changes severe and sustained enough to meet certain diagnostic criteria for an illness that needs evaluation and treatment.

For example, about 90% of women in many different cultures experience *mood changes or symptoms* with their menstrual periods, post-partum and during perimenopause. Only about 5 to 10%, on average, experience symptoms severe enough to be considered a *disorder*, requiring more comprehensive treatment.

The same is true with anxiety, a widely used term, with many meanings. Some people use it to refer to a *mood*: "I'm feeling anxious." Others use it to describe a *characteristic or trait*— "She's always anxious and uptight." It can mean a brief *symptom*: "I had an anxiety attack over my bounced check." It can also mean a *sustained pattern* of physical and emotional changes called Generalized Anxiety Disorder, or Panic Disorder.

Warning: Low estradiol can also cause anxiety, depressed mood, fragmented sleep, and fatigue similar to major depression.

It is through a careful, detailed history, examination and labs tests that doctors can determine which type of problem you may have and what the most appropriate treatment may be.

All of the ovarian hormones have profound effects on the brain, as I have explained in more detail in my earlier books. That's why is it so crucial to check all of a woman's hormone levels as part of any psychiatric evaluation before assuming mood symptoms are caused by a psychiatric disorder alone.

Estradiol has multiple effects on serotonin, norepinephrine, dopamine and acetylcholine—*all* of our major mood regulating chemical messengers in the brain. It you take all its actions together, it has major antidepressant as well as sleep and pain-regulating effects that are like just about every class of antidepressants science has devised. It's not surprising that depressed mood can be a symptom of low estradiol, which is common in PCOS.

Estradiol helps our memory circuits function normally, and serves as a nerve growth promoter in the brain. This may help you understand why you feel "fuzzy" or "foggy" brain when it is too low. Falling estradiol also fires off the brain's alarm center and causes anxiety, racing heart beat, and palpitations that often get mistaken for an anxiety disorder.

Our brain makes it's own natural anxiety-relieving chemical, called *endozapine* which normally attaches to GABA receptors to help make us feel calm. If your brain doesn't make enough endozapine, you feel anxious. Prescription medicines like Valium or Xanax can help replace this brain chemical and thereby relieve anxiety symptoms. Taking benzodiazepine medicine to replace endozapine is similar in concept to replacing lost thyroid hormone with thyroid medicine. Several metabolic breakdown products of our ovarian hormone progesterone also attach to the brain's GABA receptors just like the anti-anxiety medicines to produce a calming, sleepy sensation. But for some women, this GABA effect of progesterone causes depressed mood, just as we see with the depressant effects of benzodiazepines, leading to low energy, blunted sex drive, and decreased memory and concentration.

Progesterone is more inhibitory than excitatory on the brain, so researchers describe its combined effects as *depressant*. Experiments show that it isn't just women who experience these sedative and depressant effects of progesterone; men given progesterone experience them too. Sometimes these sleep-inducing, anti-anxiety effects are beneficial, but if women have progesterone-producing ovarian cysts or are taking too much progesterone, it can cause significant depression and fatigue, as well as more weight gain, especially estradiol is too low.

Warning: High testosterone and DHEA can cause anxiety, agitation, irritability mood swings, and insomnia often mistaken for a bipolar disorder.

Testosterone and DHEA both have mood-lifting, energizing effects when the balance is in the optimal range for women. EEG studies confirm this, and show brain activation patterns very much like we see when people are given amphetmines.

At higher levels often occurring in PCOS, however, the androgens produce too much stimulation, much like the "manicky," irritable moods caused by too much amphetamine. This effect is intensified if estradiol levels are lower than they should be. Since fluctuating androgen levels can cause significant mood swings, it's easy to see how PCOS patients are often told they have "bipolar disorder."

Adding all the hormone effects on the brain together

with what I have described about the PCOS hormone imbalances, you can see how the hormone problems can cause serious mood symptoms. And if your psychiatrist is not checking hormone levels, you can also see how it may be easy to assume you have a primary psychiatric disorder, rather than the endocrine disorder of PCOS.

I think it is very important for you to have your hormones checked and the PCOS treated before concluding that you have a psychiatric disorder and need to take a load of "mood managing" medicines.

All of these medicines have the potential to have side effects, some that are minor and some that can be very debilitating. It's important to use them wisely, and after having a thorough evaluation for other causes of mood changes. Let's look at the various classes of "mood-managing" medicines available, and some pros and cons for each group.

Antidepressants

There are several classes of antidepressants available, and each class has different types of common side effects as well as different reasons for use. I will describe some highlights here, and also describe some potential pitfalls for women with PCOS.

Tip:
SSRIs differ, so if one doesn't work, try another one.

Selective Serotonin-Reuptake Inhibitors (SSRI)

These medications primarily act to boost serotonin activity in the brain and body by inhibiting the reuptake, or inactivation, of this chemical messenger by the nerve endings. There are several different ones, each with a slightly different side effect profile, length of action, and potency.

Generally, I find that the SSRI group of medicines give the best response in women with hormonally-triggered mood and sleep difficulties, and they have fewer side effects than the older tricyclic antidepressants. Although there can be many other side effects in some people, the common side effects of SSRI include nausea, diarrhea, anxiety or agitation, insomnia, decreased appetite and initially a small amount of weight loss, loss of sexual desire, and difficulty having an orgasm. Some of these problems resolve after you have been on the medicine for awhile, but some do not and may mean you need to try something else.

🐾 Important Cautions if you have PCOS

First, the longer you take SSRIs, the more likely they are to trigger increased desire for carbohydrate foods and weight *gain* rather than loss of weight. SSRIs can also cause weight gain by another pathway, since they may cause a rise in pituitary production of *prolactin*.

Second, sexual dysfunction occurs in 60–70% of women taking SSRIs, and tends to get worse the longer you take them. Sexual side effects are usually reversible once the medications are stopped.

Third, long-term use can lead to *serotonin excess syndrome* that is manifested by marked fatigue, lethargy, headaches, agitation, insomnia, and can even include worsening anxiety. Many times doctors don't recognize the problem of *excess serotonin* and continue to increase the antidepressant dose.

Estrogen acts to boost serotonin, so if you are taking an SSRI and then add estrogen, you may find you need to lower the dose of the SSRI to avoid serotonin excess symptoms.

SSRIs may also cause another strange side effect called *bruxism*, or clenching of the jaw and tooth-grinding that occurs usually during sleep. Nocturnal bruxism can lead to chronic daily headaches, neck and shoulder pain, cracked dental fillings, and wearing down of tooth enamel. This side effect of SSRIs is thought to be due to the fact that SSRIs cause a lowering of the chemical messenger, dopamine, that inhibits certain involuntary movements such as jaw-clenching.

Paxil and Luvox can have significant **withdrawal** syndromes if doses are skipped, missed, or decreased too

Warning: Many times doctors don't recognize the problem of excess serotonin and continue to increase the anti-depressant dose, creating a vicious cycle.

rapidly. Abruptly stopping one of these can cause severe anxiety, nausea and vomiting, diarrhea, muscle aches, muscle spasm/twitches, headaches and palpitations.

Do not stop these medicines abruptly—work with your physician to taper down gradually if you want to stop them. Longer acting SSRIs like Prozac, or lower potency ones like Zoloft, tend to be easier to stop, since their long half-life helps decrease the likelihood of withdrawal symptoms.

Tricyclic Antidepressants (TCAs)

This is an older class of antidepressant medicines, developed long before SSRIs were available. They have multiple effects on many different chemical messengers in the brain, which is one reason they have so many bothersome side effects.

Caution:
All TCAs can cause increased appetite and weight gain.

All of the TCAs tend to cause constipation, dry mouth, dry eyes, blurred vision, urinary retention, and difficulty having an orgasm. They may also cause high blood pressure, dizziness, and palpitations. Because of this, we don't use them as much anymore. Another drawback is that these medications can be lethal in an overdose, which generally is not the case with SSRIs.

For women with PCOS, the TCAs can be particularly bad choices because they all tend to cause increased appetite and weight gain. There are also many adverse cardiovascular side effects that can further aggravate heart problems caused by low estradiol and excess androgens in PCOS.

Mixed Serotonin-Norepinephrine Antidepressants—Effexor and Cymbalta

Both of these newer medicines are effective for depression and Effexor has also been used to treat hot flashes in menopausal women. They act differently from the SSRIs in stimulating norepinephrine as well as serotonin. Some women find that they feel more energy taking one of these medicines compared to an SSRI.

The mixed neurotransmitter action, however, gives these medicines additional side effects to watch out for, such as anxiety, agitation, insomnia, high blood pressure, nausea, dizziness and headaches.

Effexor and Cymbalta can have significant withdrawal syndromes if doses are skipped, missed, or decreased too rapidly. Do not stop these medicines abruptly—work with your physician to gradually decrease if you want to stop.

Caution: Withdrawal symptoms can be severe–taper down gradually!

Older Atypical Antidepressants—Desyrel (trazodone)and Wellbutrin (buproprion)

Desyrel (trazodone) is a much older antidepressant that has modest serotonin-boosting effects. It isn't used much for depression any longer because the doses that effective for depression (250–600 mg) are too sedating for most people to tolerate and we now have better options. It is effective in lower doses, 25–100 mg, to help sleep. It is not a brain depressant like sleeping pills are, so it is safer, does not cause dependency (addiction), doesn't disrupt the normal sleep stages, and it has fewer side effects than most sleeping pills. It also helps to decrease pain by enhancing the activity of serotonin and improving the serotonin–norepinephrine balance.

Wellbutrin (buproprion)

Wellbutrin is another older antidepressant that is being used more often now because of its low incidence of sexual side effects. In fact, it can actually help improve interest in sex. It has the added benefit for many women of decreasing appetite, which can help your diet and exercise efforts be more successful. For many patients who have found welcome relief of depression with SSRIs, but can't stand the sexual side effects of these medications, Wellbutrin has been helpful to allow normal sexual arousal and orgasm in both men and women.

Option: Wellbutrin has many helpful effects in women with PCOS.

One drawback to Wellbutrin, however, is that it may cause anxiety and insomnia if the dose is higher than you need. I usually start with low doses and work up gradually, which means better prospects for eliminating these side effects and still have the benefits. If you are taking Wellbutrin and feel too anxious or have problems sleeping, ask your doctor about whether it is possible to try a lower dose.

Monoamine Oxidase Inhibitors (MAOI)

This is a very old group of antidepressants that may be used in difficult-to-treat depressive disorders when other approaches have failed. These medicines are not often used today, because they have many very serious drug and food interactions that can be difficult to manage. I don't feel that these are very good options for mood problems in PCOS, because they are likely to cause more weight gain, high blood pressure, and headaches.

Anti-anxiety Medications (Anxiolytics):

The most common medicines in this group fall into two classes—benzodiazepines and others.

Good News!
I find that most of my patients don't need more medicine to control anxiety once the hormone balance is improved.

The benzodiazepines (Ativan, Klonopin, Librium, Serax, Transxene, Valium, and Xanax) act on the brain's GABA receptor sites to give multiple effects: anticonvulsant, sedative, muscle relaxant, and anxiolytic.

I find that these medications can be helpful for some patients, but they may also aggravate the dysphoric (or unpleasant) moods of PCOS, and cause daytime tiredness. They may also impair thinking, concentration, and memory in larger doses.

In addition, these medicines all act on the liver to speed up the metabolism of other medications, which can interfere with the effectiveness of birth control pills and other hormone products. The benzodiazepines produce a dependence syndrome requiring careful tapering off when being stopped. If stopped abruptly, they can cause a severe withdrawal syndrome. They are also drugs that tend to be frequently abused and have an additive adverse effect with alcohol. I don't recommend these very often.

If benzodiazepines are needed for management of anxiety symptoms in PCOS, I recommend they should be used in low doses and for as short a time as possible to keep symptoms controlled.

Of the benzodiazepines listed above, Xanax (alprazolam) is the only one that has been shown to have some mild antidepressant activity in addition to its anti-anxiety effects. This makes it a better choice to use when women are having problems with both anxiety and depression that haven't responded to other approaches.

Xanax is also the only benzodiazepine shown in double-blind, placebo-controlled studies to be effective in treating the mood changes of PMS. It can safely be taken just during the luteal phase when symptoms are present, and the taper off during your bleeding days. Used this way, in low dose, it usually does not cause any significant withdrawal symptoms.

Buspar (buspirone) is one of the "others" and belongs to a generation of anxiolytics that act primarily as a serotonin 1A receptor agonist (or booster) in the pre-synaptic nerve cells and a partial agonist in the post-synaptic nerve cells.

Buspirone is not an addictive or habit-forming drug, it usually does not produce withdrawal symptoms if stopped abruptly, and there is no known abuse potential. Buspirone is not a tranquilizer; it does not cause sedation or adverse effects on memory or coordination. Generally, it tends to cause relatively few side effects. It provides another option for you to discuss with your own physician.

Buspirone is not a medication to take "as needed" (or PRN). It takes at least seven days to effect a significant enough level in the brain to produce its beneficial effects and reduce anxiety.

It is crucial to check your hormones before adding anti-anxiety medication. The goal is to improve hormone balance and help you make lifestyle changes that will reduce anxiety symptoms in other ways.

Warning: It is crucial to check your hormones before adding anti-anxiety medication, since thyroid and ovarian hormone problems can cause symptoms that mimic an anxiety disorder.

Mood Stabilizers

Excess androgens and low estradiol in PCOS cause mood swings that can be mistaken for *bipolar* or *cyclothymic* disorders. This leads some physicians to recommend a "mood-stabilizer" medication. While there is certainly a role for these medications if you actually have a cycling mood disorder, I think it is unwise to over-use these medications **without** having checked first for hormone problems.

All of the medicines in this group have the potential to cause serious side effects. Many of these medications cause weight gain, already a problem in most women with PCOS. The medicines can also cause a rise in prolactin, which in turn can cause more weight gain, headaches, breast enlargement, and depressed mood.

Tip:

Make sure you really need these medicines. There are many potential side effects.

Depakote (valproic acid) is used more and more in young women as a mood stabilizer in bipolar disorders. It is also used for migraine headache management, and for chronic pain syndromes in addition to its use to prevent seizures. I do not recommend this medication for women with possible PCOS, since several studies have found it can actually *cause* an increase in ovarian cysts in 40–50% of female patients treated with it. It is not clear whether other anticonvulsants (Tegretol, Dilantin, Neurontin, Lamictal, etc.) have similar effects to trigger formation of ovarian cysts.

Remeron is often used as a "mood-stabilizer" in women even though it is well known to cause daytime drowsiness, weight gain and marked fatigue.

Neurontin, Tegretol, and possibly Lamictal, have potentially significant adverse drug interactions with oral forms of ovarian hormones, and may reduce hormone levels so that birth control pills are no longer effective for contraception, or no longer effectively suppress the ovaries when being used to treat PCOS.

Because of the risk of serious side effects or further adverse effects on ovarian function, I think it is crucial to have reliable testing of your ovarian hormone levels *prior to starting* one of these medications.

If your ovarian or thyroid hormones are out of balance, I feel it is important to restore those to optimal levels first. Then see how you do and whether you even still need one of the "mood stabilizers."

In Summary

Psychotropic medicines can be safe and effective when used appropriately after a thorough evaluation of non-psychiatric causes of mood and anxiety problems. If you suspect you have hormone problems, make sure you find someone to help you evaluate this possibility before you being an array of other medicines.

With any of the medicines in this category, a safe rule of thumb when starting psychotropics is to increase the dose slowly to avoid unwanted reactions and side effects. Then when it's time to stop, work with your physicians on making very small decreases in dose at one time, and come down very gradually to avoid withdrawal symptoms.

Tip: For best response, start low, go slowly, with any increases. Then taper down when stopping.

Medication Problems and Pitfalls to Avoid

Here's an example of what can go wrong with multiple medications being added by different physicians not taking drug interactions into account.

The first describes what happened to June, one of my patients, when another physician added Neurontin and Trazodone to the regimen I had her on. At her regular follow up appointment with me, she said:

> *"I know something is still awry with my hormones, and I knew something was happening three weeks before this ruptured cyst I had last week—I was cranky, irritable, my hair turned to hay, started feeling so fatigued, and I then had this bad lower back pain and pelvic pain. I believe that the cyst had already ruptured last Tuesday, but before it did, I was very bloated, I was crying all the time, I was very constipated, and then after the cyst ruptured, I started being able to go to the bathroom again."*

"I stopped the Ovcon for two days to have a period and it was a nightmare, the hot flashes were like waves, I was getting migraines everyday, and the symptoms were getting worse and worse, so I went back on the Ovcon. The past few days, I have been breaking out in sweats, and having more break-through bleeding as well as bleeding that's heavy like a period. I still have some pelvic pressure. I am feeling fatigued, my joints ache, I have leg pain at night and that had gotten better before this recent change. I am not sleeping well at all, feel like I am hypersensitive at night with the least little noise waking me up. All these were ways I had felt in the past, before you got me stabilized on the hormones and the Glucophage."

So Typical: June illustrates the problems that occur with over-medication when symptoms are treated one by one, and PCOS isn't diagnosed and treated as the metabolic-endocrine disorder it is.

I explained to June that her symptom pattern and physical body changes strongly suggest she had another abnormal ovarian cycle and a corpus luteum cyst producing excess progesterone. Adding Neurontin and trazodone, particularly since they were increased to high doses fairly quickly, can affect hepatic metabolism of birth control pills and reduce their effectiveness. This meant that her BCP was no longer effective in suppressing her ovarian cycles and cyst formation as had been the case before these medicines were added.

In addition, I told June that both trazodone and Neurontin can also cause significant daytime fatigue side effects, which may be aggravating her problems in feeling so tired and having trouble getting through the day. For this reason, and because of the hepatic interactions, I suggested she work with her other physicians to taper down both medicines as much as possible.

Over the next couple of months, these medicines were slowly tapered off, and her symptoms were once again controlled with just the birth control pill and metformin.

Another patient also illustrates this problem. When she first came in, Annette was 27 years old, severely obese, with painful acne. She was so self-conscious that she rarely looked up when talking. For several years, she had been ballooning up and frightened by a body out of control. Her acne was impossible to control no matter

DR. VLIET'S GUIDE TO
PSYCHOTROPIC MEDICATIONS

Antidpressants
- Selective Serotonin-Reuptake Inhibitors (SSRI):
- Celexa (citalopram)
- Lexapro (escitalopram)
- Luvox (fluvoxamine)
- Paxil (paroxetine)
- Prozac (fluoxetine)
- Zoloft (sertraline)

Mixed Serotonin-Norepinephrine Antidepressants
- Cymbalta (duloxetine)
- Effexor (venlafaxine)

Tricyclic Antidepressants
- Elavil (amitriptyline)
- Norpramin (desipramine)
- Pamelor (nortriptyline)
- And others

Older Atypical Antidepressants
- Desyrel (trazodone)
- Wellbutrin (buproprion)

Monoamine Oxidase Inhibitors (MAOI)
- Nardil (phenelzine)
- Parnate (trancylcypromine)

Antianxiety Medicines (also called anxiolytics)
- Ativan (lorazepam)
- Klonopin (clonazepam)
- Valium (diazepam)
- Xanax (alprazolam)
- And others

Mood-Stabilizers
Anticonvulsants:
- Depakote (valproic acid)
- Lamictal (lamotrigine)
- Neurontin (gabapentin)
- Tegretol (carbamazepine)

Others:
- Remeron (mirtazapine)
- Risperdal (risperidone)
- Zyprexa (olanzapine)
- Topamax (topiramate)

© 2005 Elizabeth Lee Vliet, M.D.

what she tried. She had other troubling symptoms for someone so young: hot flashes, insomnia, fibromyalgia-type muscle pain, anxiety that became worse with her periods, daily tension headaches, migraine episodes, severe fatigue, daytime sleepiness—especially after meals, inability to concentrate, and shortness of breath that made her fear a lung problem.

When I saw her, she was being treated by multiple specialists: a primary care physician, a neurologist for the migraines, a pain specialist for the daily headaches, a rheumatologist for the muscle pain, a psychiatrist for the anxiety, a pulmonary specialist to check for asthma, and her gynecologist who said her pelvic and Pap smears were normal, and she didn't have a hormone imbalance—she just needed to lose weight. No hormone levels were ever checked by anyone prior to her seeing me.

When I checked her ovarian, thyroid, adrenal and pituitary hormones, the results were staggering. Her estradiol was markedly low; all of the androgens were seriously elevated, especially the free testosterone. She had a high LH to FSH ratio and her adrenal hormone, cortisol, was quite elevated (another factor adding to her weight gain). She also had very high fasting insulin and glucose levels, and these were also high when measured two hours after eating. Prolactin was also elevated, adding to the depression, headaches and weight gain.

In short, she had all the classic indicators of PCOS. I felt sad that no one, out of all those doctors, had ever considered PCOS or checked her hormone levels, especially since her body shape and symptoms were such strong warning signals of PCOS, and she had such risk factors for diabetes.

By the time of her appointment with me, Annette took 13 medicines every day: a sleeping pill, two muscle relaxants, several pain meds, two mood-stabilizers, two antidepressants (one SSRI and one tricyclic), two anti-anxiety medicines, and a beta blocker.

Her medication costs were astronomical, but even more

frightening; many of the medicines were making her weight gain and hormone imbalances worse.

Tricyclics, added to use of SSRIs, can increase appetite, especially for carbs, which then increases insulin resistance and causes more weight gain. Tricyclics and SSRI can also elevate prolactin. Klonopin for anxiety and insomnia made her tired and sleepy during the day. The mood stabilizers added to her weight gain and tiredness during the day.

Beta-blockers make the insulin resistance worse as well, and can contribute to fatigue, depression, and shortness of breath due to effects on lungs and heart. Beta-blockers also interfere with normal thyroid function, further contributing to weight gain, low energy, and depressed mood. All of this pulled her further into the PCOS imbalances.

Turning this around would be a long struggle, because it could take a year or more to improve the hormonal balance and see which medicines could be gradually tapered off.

Sadly, so many other professionals kept telling her that her problems were not hormonal, she never had any support for trying to get off some of these medicines. These other doctors said she didn't have PCOS, and if she did, it "couldn't" cause such mood problems. With all this opposition from her other health professionals, I only saw her a few times and never got to help get the PCOS effectively treated so she could reduce her other meds.

My view has always been that ultimately it doesn't really matter who is "right" and who is "wrong" with a diagnostic label. Diagnoses are imperfect. What matters is whether the medicines make someone better, or whether they aggravate underlying problems and make people worse.

In her case, she *wasn't* getting better on all those medicines, and each had adverse effects that were well-documented in the medical literature, and were being overlooked as contributing to her problems. Her

Sad
It was a medication nightmare. She was trapped in the hormonal quicksand of PCOS and the quagmire of medication side effects.

headaches weren't controlled, she still had trouble sleeping, and she was still gaining weight and suffering from acne and excess facial hair.

So, if you see yourself in this picture, don't get hung up on diagnostic labels. Find out what's going on with your hormones, and find a physician who will listen to you and work with you on some of the approaches I have outlined to help you feel better.

Consensus on Antipsychotic–"Mood Stabilizer" Medications and Health Risks

Medication	Weight Gain	Increase in Diabetes	High Chol and TG
Clozapine	+++	+	+
Olanzapine	+++	+	+
Risperidone	++	?	?
Quetiapine	++	?	?
Aripiprazole	±	-	-
Ziprasidone	±	-	-

+ = increased effect
– = no effect
? = discrepancies in studies, no consistent results

Table adapted from: American Diabetes Association, American Psychiatric Association, American Association of Clinical Endocrinologists, North American Association for the Study of Obesity. Consensus development conference on antipsychotic drugs and obesity and diabetes. J Clin Psychiatry. 2004; 65:267-272.

Surgical Approaches Used in PCOS
Myomectomy

Myomectomy simply means removal of benign uterine tumors called myoma, which are more commonly referred to as fibroids.

Fibroids can interfere with a fertilized egg being able to implant normally in the uterus, leading to miscarriage or difficulty getting pregnant.

Fibroids can cause pain with sex, backaches, and pelvic pain. Erratic, heavy bleeding that is difficult to control is very common. Sometimes fibroids can be so large or positioned in such a way that they cause pressure on the uterus and/or bladder resulting in prolapse of these organs into the vagina and causing incontinence.

Fibroids often co-exist in women with PCOS. Myomectomy doesn't treat the metabolic problems of PCOS per se, but the procedure is often recommended when fibroids interfere with fertility, or fibroids are large enough to cause pain and/or bleeding that can't be controlled with medications.

In a myomectomy, the surgeon removes just the fibroids from inside the uterus, and leaves the uterus, cervix and ovaries intact. This is a more conservative surgery than hysterectomy since it does not remove the uterus, and leaves open the possibility for a future pregnancy.

Alert: Although fibroids are not cancerous tumors, they can cause a lot of bothersome problems.

Ovarian Wedge Resection and Laparoscopic Ovarian Drilling

Drs. Stein and Leventhal, the two physicians who first described in 1935 the cluster of problems we now call PCOS, also described a treatment approach called *wedge resection* of the ovary. This is a surgical procedure in which they removed half to three-quarters of an enlarged, cystic ovary in an effort to improve women's chance of ovulating and becoming pregnant.

After their initial reports of success in helping women conceive, more and more gynecologists used the wedge resection as a mainstay of treatment for PCOS. A medical article published in 1962 reviewed the outcomes of wedge resection in 1,097 women with PCOS. Pregnancy rates ranged from 13 to 89%, with an overall average of 63%.

This surgery was later discontinued in the 1960s and 1970s primarily because of the complications it caused. Any time the abdomen or pelvis is opened for surgery and the organs are moved around, there is a very high rate of scar tissue formation, called *adhesions*, resulting from manipulation of the tissues. Most of the time, adhesions don't cause major problems. But in women being treated for infertility, adhesions were a major culprit causing blockage or other malfunction of the Fallopian tubes.

Blockage of the tubes meant that women now had a mechanical cause of infertility added to the existing

Problem:
Wedge resection caused adhesions that often blocked fallopian tubes, causing infertility.

PCOS hormone imbalances causing infertility. In four early follow-up studies (see Appendix list of references), all women in the series (59 of 59, 16 of 16, and 7 of 7) or almost all (4 of 6) who had the surgery ended up having tubal adhesions. With such a bleak picture, you can see why doctors felt they had to give up this particular treatment approach.

Another development in the 1960s made ovarian wedge resection less needed. Medications to stimulate ovulation and treat infertility, such as *clomiphene citrate* (Clomid) and urinary or pituitary gonadotrophins, were developed. In the early years of its use, Clomid was reported to result in ovulation rates from 60% to 80% and pregnancy rates ranging from 33% to 60%. With medical approaches yielding such good results, and having fewer risks and complications than surgery, most doctors stopped using the ovarian wedge resection procedure.

But about 15% of women don't succeed in ovulating and becoming pregnant with clomiphene citrate alone. For these women, typically the next step is therapy with gonadotrophins. Again, results generally are good: overall, women with PCOS who had therapy with gonadotrophins had approximately a 70% ovulation rate and a 30% to 40% pregnancy rate, which further reduced the need for surgical intervention.

As time went on and more women were treated with gonadotrophin therapy, doctors began to discover that the ovaries in women with PCOS were more sensitive to stimulation with gonadotrophins. This meant they had a higher risk of having too many follicles develop at one time and then having to cancel that cycle of infertility treatment.

Women with PCOS also had a higher risk of developing ovarian hyperstimulation syndrome (OHSS) than other women undergoing gonadotrophin therapy. OHSS can cause serious medical complications, and also results in canceling the cycle of treatment.

Any time a cycle of fertility treatment has to be cancelled

early, regardless of the reason, it still means an enormous emotional and financial impact on the couple.

Gonadotrophin therapy also caused a higher incidence of multiple pregnancies—twins, triplets, quadruplets, and more—that meant increasing risks for the mother, particularly for women with PCOS who were already at higher risks of gestational diabetes than women who did not have PCOS. About two-thirds of triplet and greater numbers of fetuses in one pregnancy are caused by therapy with gonadotropins. In addition to the higher medical risks with multiple babies, couples also face the added financial and emotional stresses of taking care of several babies at once!

Some researchers think that high androgens and high levels of LH in women with PCOS is the primary reason that these women have a higher risk of too many follicles at one time, multiple pregnancy, and OHSS.

> **Important Difference:** Women with PCOS have a risk of multiple pregnancies with gonadotrophin therapy that is about 10%–15% greater than women who don't have PCOS.

Development of Laparoscopic Ovarian Surgery

So for women who don't respond to clomiphene, these additional risks led doctors to reconsider ovarian surgery as an option for treating infertility. At the same time doctors were seeing more complications from medical therapy with gonadotrophins, there were many less invasive surgical techniques being developed as a result of expanding use of the laparoscope.

Laparoscopic procedures allow use of very small incisions, and less manipulation of internal organs, so the complication rates tend to be much lower than surgeries in which the entire abdomen or pelvic is opened. In one series of 778 women between 1971 and 1987, Dr. Cohen (see reference in Appendix I) reported a pregnancy rate of 32% using laparascopic ovarian surgery. In another series from Sweden published in 1994, investigators reported a 92% ovulation rate and an 84% pregnancy rate in 252 women with PCOS who had undergone laparoscopic electrocauterization to remove part of the abnormal ovary.

Today's procedures are slightly different from the older wedge resection, in which a portion of the ovary was actually cut out and removed. Most surgeons today don't actually remove part of the ovary, but instead use lasers or electrocautery to punch multiple small holes in the ovary.

New Techniques: New techniques came into broader use in the 1970s, and meant doctors could accomplish benefits of older ovarian wedge resection with less risk of later adhesions.

As a result, the surgery is now often called *laparoscopic ovarian drilling.* Since there isn't the large cut surface of the ovary, or manipulation of the internal organs as with the earlier surgeries, there is much less likelihood of adhesions being formed later.

How Does Ovarian Surgery Work?

Studies show ovarian drilling also improves ovulation and subsequent pregnancy as was found with the earlier ovarian wedge resection. We don't fully understand all the ways it works, but doctors think that the both the older wedge resection and the newer ovarian drilling have similar effects on the ovaries to help restore more normal function in women with PCOS. There are several possible explanations how this occurs:

(1) In the early years using ovarian wedge resection, Drs. Stein and Leventhal thought that surgery to cut out the abnormally thickened capsule around the ovary actually removed a mechanical barrier. Follicles could then release properly from the surface of the ovary to become the egg produced with ovulation. Ovarian drilling likely has the same effect to open up the thickened tissue so that follicles can release properly for ovulation.

(2) Wedge resection and drilling both appear to also destroy, or ablate, some of the ovarian tissue, called the *stroma,* that produces excess androgens. This causes less androgens within the ovary, and less androgens circulating in the blood stream to disrupt pathways that regulate a normal menstrual cycle, follicle development, and ovulation.

Studies have found that androgen levels, particularly total and free testosterone, can decrease by 40–50% from the high levels seen before surgery. Researchers think that destruction of the stroma has both a direct effect to lower testosterone and other androgens, as well as an indirect effect to modulate the pituitary–ovarian axis that restores normal ovulatory cycles.

(3) Ovarian surgery also causes a decrease in production of LH from the pituitary. Most studies show that LH levels consistently fall a few weeks after these surgeries. LH is the major stimulator of excess androgen production in the ovarian stroma. When surgery causes a drop in LH, there is an added hormonal benefit to the mechanical destruction of stromal tissue to lower the excess testosterone and other androgens.

(4) Both types of ovarian surgery lead to decreases in sex hormone binding globulin (SHBG). This means that there is a higher level of free estradiol to feed back to the pituitary and help restore normal FSH: LH balance to oversee a normal progression of the menstrual cycle and development of follicles.

(5) Ovarian surgery also causes a rise in FSH, followed by restoration of its normal cyclical pattern that regulates ovulation.

Good News: Current studies have continued to show encouraging results on ovulation and pregnancy rates with newer surgical techniques.

How effective is ovarian surgery compared to using medications?

There have only been a few studies that directly compared the effects of using medications such as gonadotrophins instead of ovarian surgery to improve ovulation and pregnancy success. Dr. Gadir's group studied the responses of 88 women who had failed to ovulate with Clomid treatment. This non-randomized study, published in 1990, compared the women's responses to either ovarian surgery (electrocautery), or with medications, using either HMG or pure FSH.

The researchers found that ovulation rates among the three groups were fairly similar: 71.4% of the women who had electrocautery ovarian drilling ovulated, compared to a rate of 70.6% of the women treated with HMG and 66.7% of those treated with pure FSH stimulation.

In this study, women who became pregnant had a lower miscarriage rate (21.4%) with electrocautery compared to HMG (53.3%) and FSH stimulation (40%). The women treated with electrocautery also had a higher rate of live births (37.9%) compared to those treated with HMG (23.3%) or FHS (20.7%).

Since this 1990 study, there have been only four randomized controlled clinical studies (RCT) comparing laparoscopic ovarian surgery with ovulation induction using gonadotrophin medication. In all four studies, previous treatment with Clomid had been unsuccessful in stimulating ovulation for these women.

The success of pregnancy using the different methods differed according to length of follow up after the treatments: women followed for six months after ovarian surgery or after six cycles of treatment with gonadotrophins had higher pregnancy rates if they had received gonadotrophins instead of the surgery. Miscarriage rates were not significantly different between the women treated with surgery or gonadotrophins.

There are two common drawbacks of gonadotrophin treatment for infertility: increased risk of having twins or triplets or more babies in one pregnancy, and increased risk of ovarian hyperstimulation syndrome. In these four RCT, researchers did find a higher rate of multiple fetuses in pregnancies resulting from gonadotrophin compared to ovarian surgery.

It was encouraging, however, that there was no increased risk of ovarian hyperstimulation syndrome in the later two of these four studies. This suggests that newer medication protocols to reduce the risk of over-stimulation have been more successful than older approaches.

Two of these four RCT considered cost-effectiveness aspects of surgery versus medication treatment. Both found that for women who had not responded to Clomid to attempt pregnancy, it was about one-third lower in cost for each live birth to have laparoscopic ovarian surgery than to attempt ovulation induction with gonadotrophins. A study from the United Kingdom, published in 2000, also found that laparoscopic ovarian surgery was a more cost effective treatment for anovulatory infertility than using gonadrophins.

The studies so far indicate that women with higher LH levels, lower body mass index (BMI), and a shorter duration of infertility do better with ovarian surgery than women who do not have these characteristics.

Researchers have identified another potential advantage to laparoscopic ovarian surgery. It appears that women respond better to later use of medication approaches for inducing ovulation if they had the ovarian surgery first. Women who had ovarian surgery frequently required fewer and lower doses of gonadotrophins to stimulate successful ovulation.

What are the risks of ovarian surgery versus medications?

The primary problems that can occur with ovarian surgery are due to side effects of general anesthesia, or infection, or the formation of adhesions, and later on, the possibility of premature ovarian failure. Most of these complications are relatively rare with the new procedures used today, but women considering their options need to be aware that such problems can occur.

Adhesions are usually only a problem if they cause later pelvic pain, intestinal obstruction, or cause blockage of a Fallopian tube leading to mechanical interference with fertility. Pelvic infections are unusual complications now, because antibiotics are routinely given both before and after surgery. It is possible that ovarian surgery can lead to earlier decline in ovarian hormone production, but studies so for have not found this to be a significant problem.

Ovulation induction with gonadotrophins has two major risks that typically don't occur with ovarian surgery: the higher rate of multiple fetuses leads to increased risk for the pregnancy, and the higher rate of ovarian hyper-stimulation that can cause a medical crisis for the mother.

Note: Studies so far have not shown that either type of ovarian surgery has an effect on insulin production or insulin resistance as we see with some medications used to treat PCOS.

If you have already been through Clomid treatment and have not been successful in achieving ovulation, it is important to discuss these various options and risks with your fertility specialist in order to determine the best options for next steps in treatment. If you feel unsure about the information you are getting, then consider a second option with a different infertility specialist.

When Medications Fail: What About Hysterectomy?

Tip:

There are many options today to help infertility. Seek help from a qualified fertility specialist.

Hysterectomy. The word often conjures up images of horrible outcomes for women, and indeed, there are many books and websites that focus on the negatives of this surgery. I often see women with PCOS who have been told that they should have a hysterectomy and removal of the ovaries. Because of all the negative press about it, many of the patients I see are understandably scared and want to discuss their options before taking a permanent step like this.

Many women with PCOS have recurrent cysts that cause pain and disruptive hormonal swings, or they may have erratic bleeding, heavy or painful menstrual flow, fibroids, or difficulty tolerating side effects of medications. Some have had the recommendation to have hysterectomy and removal of the ovaries; others have been told hysterectomy doesn't help PCOS, so there's no reason to consider it.

Women in both groups are looking for options, and a way to make sense of conflicting recommendations. Whether to have a hysterectomy or not is a deeply personal decision in a woman's life. It is a decision that needs to be made on the basis of good information about options, and potential benefits as well as risks.

The complexities and nuances of how women can be affected take place at every level—physical, emotional, and spiritual—with the surgical removal of uterus and/or ovaries. I know from my clinical and personal experience that there are ways to restore optimal hormone levels and prevent women feeling robbed of their sexuality, their sense of womanhood, and their body-mind-spirit health.

I think there is a more balanced view about the surgery and there is also a systematic way you can go about making a decision whether this is an option for you.

As a nonsurgeon physician specializing in women's health for the last twenty years, and focusing my work on the incredible complexities of the myriad ways that our ovarian hormones are linked to the function of every cell and tissue of our bodies, I have personally treated several thousand women who have needed to find ways to restore optimal hormone health following pelvic surgeries such as hysterectomies.

Yes or No: Women need sound information on such an important decision.

Yet, I write this book not just as a physician and scientist. I write as a woman who has been there. A woman who has had this surgery herself. I know what it is like to go through the tumultuous feelings of grief and loss, even when accepting the medical reasons for having the surgery. I know what it is like to experience surgical complications, and have to go back into the hospital yet again. Then too, I know what it is like to struggle to find hormone balance again.

It isn't a simple matter. There is much to consider for women who are faced with whether or not to have a hysterectomy. The women's stories I hear daily in my practice have helped me understand just how profoundly hysterectomy can be a life-changing event—positive, negative, and all points in-between these opposites, no matter how needed the procedure.

Good News: Having a hysterectomy doesn't inevitably cause loss of one's quality of life or ability to be a fully sexual woman.

I have described many of these non-surgical options in this and earlier chapters.

But what about the woman who really has reached the end of non-surgical options available? What then? Hysterectomy is often thought to be the cause of depression, fragmented sleep, loss of energy, inability to function sexually, loss of bladder control, and a host of other problems, so many women don't want to consider having surgery.

The good news is that newer, carefully designed prospective studies do not support that removal of the uterus causes major depression or other psychologically damaging consequences in the majority of women.

In fact, *just the opposite has been found in a number of recent studies*: incidence of depression (as a mood state, not the illness), is about half the incidence found prior to surgery, with women showing improved psychological and physical well-being—including sexual enjoyment —after hysterectomy.

Hysterectomy today is usually done only when medical options have failed and there are very clear indications it is needed, such as severe endometriosis, excessive bleeding, extremely painful periods, severe fibroids that cause abdominal distension and pain with intercourse, and uterine or ovarian cancer.

Tip:

Most of these problems are due to low hormone levels, not the surgery itself.

I certainly see many patients who have low hormone levels and don't feel "back to normal" following a hysterectomy, but often these women are grateful the surgery took care of the bleeding or pain.

Why the discrepancy between the general perception of hysterectomy versus the positive outcomes from studies like these?

Let's look at some facts that often get overlooked

1. Surgeons rarely check hormone levels before surgery when women feel well to have a baseline for comparison later to determine whether the ovaries still produce optimal hormone levels. Doctors just assume the ovaries continue to work fine after a surgery that removes only the uterus. In many women, they don't.

Current studies show that 30–60% of women have menopausal levels of estradiol and testosterone as early as 2–3 years following removal of the uterus. Decline in ovarian hormone production wreaks havoc throughout our bodies, in every organ system, including the brain.

Most of these studies looking at hormone levels came from England, Germany, Italy and other European countries. In the United States, this issue has not been taken as seriously. It is not clear to me why doctors here don't think follow up checks of ovarian hormone levels are necessary.

Dr. John Studd, an internationally-known menopause researcher from London, is a strong advocate for follow-up tests of women's hormone levels after hysterectomy that leaves the ovaries. Dr. Studd says the majority of gynecologists and primary care physicians miss the diagnosis of premature hormonal decline after removal of only the uterus. He attributes the oversight in part to two factors: the loss of menstruation as a marker of the phases of the ovarian hormone cycle, and to doctors' assumptions that "vague" symptoms such as insomnia, anxiety, low libido, and depressed mood occur because of psychological reactions to losing the uterus, to feelings of lost femininity, or fear of aging.

This focus on assumed psychological issues completely overlooks the physical hormone effects on brain chemistry. There is laboratory confirmation of this endocrine connection in these symptoms: FSH is elevated to menopausal levels in about 30% of women who had removal of the uterus but still have ovaries. I certainly find these same objective confirmations—high FSH, low estradiol, and low testosterone, in my evaluations of patients.

How do women can become prematurely menopausal after a hysterectomy? The uterine artery has to be "tied off" (clamped) when the uterus is removed. Otherwise you would have uncontrollable bleeding. When this artery is tied off, it means a loss of over 50% of the blood flow to the ovary from the ovarian artery.

The ovary still gets some blood flow from another, smaller artery in the wall of the pelvis, but this does not make up for what is lost from the uterine artery. You can imagine how difficult it is for the ovary to make its hormones if it only has half it's normal blood supply.

2. Doctors tell women with one ovary removed, "Don't worry, the other ovary will take over and make enough hormones. You'll be fine." Try telling that to a man who

has lost one testicle. One ovary doesn't typically do the job of two. Women suffer symptoms of hormone loss.

3. Only about 25%–30% of women start hormone therapy even after complete removal of both ovaries and with the uterus causing instant menopause, with estrodiol levels plunging lower than a man's, and loss of about 90% of our testosterone.

Problem:
Even with both ovaries removed, only 1/4 of women take hormone therapy after a hysterectomy. Only about half of those women take it for longer than 5 years.

This means a huge number of women with no ovaries are going without any replacement of the very hormones needed for a myriad of body and brain systems. I don't believe it is the just loss of the uterus that causes so many health problems, including loss of sexual function. I think a bigger overlooked issue is the loss of our ovarian hormones.

4. Even if women do start hormone therapy after a hysterectomy, most still do not get "optimal" replacement of their ovarian hormones. The usual approach is to simply give estrogen, usually Premarin, a mixture of horse-derived estrogens foreign to our bodies. Premarin provides very little of the 17-beta estradiol our bodies have always made, and need. And hormone levels are rarely checked; there is typically no individualization of type, route or dose of estrogen.

Testosterone is rarely replaced after hysterectomy, particularly for women with PCOS who are often told they can never take testosterone because of their earlier problems with ovaries that produce excess androgens.

But what happens when your ovaries are removed? You have now lost the primary source of excess androgens. The longer you go without the ovaries to make more testosterone, the more likely you can reach a point of now not having enough of this crucial hormone. So, some women with PCOS may need replacement of testosterone after removal of both ovaries.

Testosterone enhances energy level, libido, sense of well-being and mood, bone and muscle formation and also (along with estradiol) improves the vaginal tissue to relieve dryness that causes pain during sex. Even though medical studies going back to the 1950s show the benefits, and safety, of testosterone replacement, the vast majority of women who have had a hysterectomy still are not offered testosterone therapy.

It doesn't have to be this way. I work hard to help my patients achieve optimal hormone replacement, and most are amazed at the degree of well-being that can return with the right type of hormone replacement, the right delivery approach and optimal levels.

5. Depression following hysterectomy is assumed to be a psychological reaction to losing the uterus. Dr. Studd's view, which is confirmed by my own clinical experience, is that "a more plausible cause of depression is the varying degree of ovarian hormone deficiency, which is often overlooked and untreated following hysterectomy."

Problem: Women don't usually get optimal balance restored after a hysterectomy

I certainly agree; clinical experience and a number of research studies show that depressed moods, low energy, sleep loss, anxiety, and loss of libido can be alleviated with good hormone management. But these problems are more likely labeled depression, chronic fatigue, anxiety or stress.

A long-term prospective study published in 1992 found no depression at 4 months after hysterectomy, but depression did develop after 24 months, which supports that depression is not likely just from an emotional reaction to hysterectomy but can occur as the ovarian hormones decline over time. Such a gradual decrease in estradiol and testosterone just may not produce noticeable symptoms for two or more years after the surgery.

What does this mean for you? If you are only 30 years old and have a hysterectomy, even if you keep both ovaries, you have a 30%–60% chance of having menopausal hormone levels within three years of the surgery though you are still in your 30s.

In fact, even when your ovaries work well for many years, studies show that you will become menopausal about 4 to 5 years earlier than average.

6. The hormone furor of 2002 and 2004, with major headlines screaming the dangers of "estrogen" based on studies (HERS, WHI, in particular) using only Premarin or Prempro, the horse-derived estrogen and synthetic progestin, has unnecessarily frightened many women into being afraid of taking "hormones" after hysterectomy.

Yet what is overlooked is that Premarin is not our natural estrogen, and Prempro contains a potent synthetic progestin that itself can have many negative effects.

Note:

If no one is checking your hormone levels with reliable blood tests, the hormone cause of symptoms is missed.

There is good news about the emerging research showing many benefits of estradiol—and testosterone—for many dimensions of women's well-being and health. Sadly, such positive findings often don't get reported in the media that seems to focus on sensationalizing the negative and promoting fear.

Clearly there has to be better efforts to educate doctors and women about the importance of hormone options, exercise, healthy diet and other medications to help overcome problems after hysterectomy and avoid the loss of sexual function and enjoyment, bladder problems or pain or sudden menopause that many women have experienced. You can feel good again after a hysterectomy, so don't discard this possible solution to pain or bleeding problems.

Summary

If you have spent years suffering, not feeling well, and going from doctor to doctor trying to find a way to relieve symptoms and to feel better, start your journey to regaining your well-being by insisting on having your hormone levels properly checked with today's "gold standard" blood tests. It is not difficult or overly expensive to do.

Then read about the many prescription options, lifestyle choices, and complementary approaches to help you regain hormone balance and health.

Take charge of this journey. There is hope, and help available.

Chapter 12

Lifestyle Strategies for Coping with PCOS

If you have PCOS, I suspect much of your focus has been on the "hormone problems." You may have viewed hormones with a negative connotation. I would like to turn that idea around and help you focus on the positive aspects that come with getting your hormones back in the right balance though healthy lifestyle choices added to the medication options I already discussed.

My integrated approach focuses on hormone balance together with the power that comes from a healthy diet, exercise and positive mental outlook. I call it **Your Hormone Power Life Plan**®. In this chapter, I have focused on the meal plans, vitamins and supplements and exercise to help you recapture your power and energy again! Then in Chapter 14, I will talk more about putting your *mind power* to work for you.

Good News: Hormone balance gives you the metabolic fuel, or power, for your body to function well and to feel good again.

Your Hormone Power Life Plan®:
Balancing Proteins, Fats and Carbohydrates to Restore Vitality... and Help Weight Loss

Most women with PCOS have been struggling to lose weight for many years by the time I see them. Most say they have tried every diet on the market. I have found, however, that with the insulin resistance and high cortisol that are so common in PCOS, women generally are able to lose weight more effectively with a lower carbohydrate intake than many diets recommend.

Pushing the carbohydrates too low as with the Atkins diet and some others like it, can interfere with optimal thyroid function and cause lower levels of the free, active form of T3 needed for a normal metabolic rate.

Diet Tip:

There are clearly many different approaches available, and no one approach is going to work for everyone.

Women's hormones play crucial roles in our metabolism in ways that are quite different from men's. It has seemed to me that most popular "diet" books are written by men, and don't seem to deal with women's hormones very well, or very accurately!

Over the years of working with patients, and working hard to deal with my own weight struggles, I have researched the "diet question" extensively to find a balance of proteins, fats, and carbohydrates that I think is more tailored to the needs of women.

I encourage you to read my book *Women, Weight and Hormones* for more background on these connections than I can include here. Here are the highlights of the meal plan balance that I have found works effectively for women with PCOS.

Your Meal Action Plan—The MAP for A Successful Journey to Weight Loss

Tip:

A balanced meal and snack also boost your metabolic rate more effectively, which helps you burn more fat all day long.

If you wanted to drive from the East Coast to the West Coast, you'd allow yourself plenty of time to make this long journey. You would also know that you needed a current map to show you the way so you didn't get lost. Old maps don't show new roads, or new ways to reach your destination.

Likewise, if you have tried many "diets" in the past and found that they didn't work for you, maybe you need a new food MAP for your weight loss journey… one that has the latest updates relevant to *women's* bodies, not one based on *men's* needs.

If you are going to be successful at losing excess body fat during the "hormonal challenges" of PCOS, then you will need a new food MAP that shows you how to turn all those fat-storing hormones into fat-burning ones.

That's what my Meal Action Plan, or MAP, is designed to do. Use this as a guide to help you plan your trip to a healthier body. You decide your pace for the journey.

My MAP features a higher protein intake than some current programs, but it is not the "high protein, high fat" diet similar to ones currently in fashion, such as Atkins. The key is to have enough carbohydrate intake that your thyroid works properly, and you avoid that "draggy" feeling that occurs with highly restricted carb intake, but without having so much carbohydrate that you overproduce insulin.

Give my MAP a chance and see if it helps your weight loss, especially if you combine it with getting the hormone balance you need, and a healthy exercise program, and your "mind power."

Learning How to Use Your MAP

To help you use my MAP with other programs you may be using, I have included the concept of "building blocks" or exchanges as used by the American Diabetes and Heart Associations. You can find a more detailed Exchange List in booklets from the American Diabetes Association.

Think of these building blocks, or exchanges, as ways you can *customize the meal plan for your tastes*, since you can exchange an apple for a pear or for an apricot, and you can swap your servings of meat for a protein equivalent of eggs or cheese.

The majority of the fat in my meal plan will come from your protein intake. I do not recommend adding many additional fat "building blocks," or exchanges, beyond what is included in the protein group.

In the sample meal plans, you will see that I have tended to use fruits that have a lower glycemic index to minimize insulin overshoot, and offer you more quantity and fiber for each fruit exchange.

Although my meal plan is lower in carbs than the ADA suggests, I still met the recommendations of the

A Guide: You can fill in my MAP with foods you like, just as you can choose the roads to travel on a car trip.

Healthy Swap: An **exchange** is simply a group of foods with similar nutritional value that you can swap, or exchange, for one another based on what you most like to eat.

Total Fat:
The total daily fat is comparable to that recommended in the American Diabetes Association (ADA) and American Heart Association (AHA) diets, about 27%–30% a day.

American Cancer Society for 5–6 servings of fruits and vegetables a day to give adequate fiber, vitamins and antioxidants.

Use shortcuts that help you incorporate this meal balance into your daily life. For example, you may take the basic meal ingredients and combine them into your favorite stew recipe that simmers in the crock pot while you are at work. Or buy bags of salad greens or frozen vegetables already washed and cut into pieces. The extra cost is still cheaper than a doctor's visit. The trick is to make these meals work for you and your family.

To make this MAP work, you need the right balance of protein, fat, and carbohydrate at EACH meal and EACH snack, not just for the day's total. I can't emphasize this enough.

If you eat only carbs, such as cereal or a bagel, for breakfast, your blood sugar falls an hour or so later. Then you are so hungry, you are likely to grab a donut or a soda when you walk into the office. Adding protein and fat for breakfast, and having a balanced snack mid-morning sustains blood sugar and energy until lunch. You avoid the drop in blood sugar that triggers cravings.

Diet Tip:
Focus on eating whole fruits instead of fruit juice in order to avoid excess insulin.

Balance Your Vitamins, Minerals and Supplements

Vitamins and minerals are essential to our survival. But many women are overdoing the vitamins and supplements today, especially those who are trying to lose weight. The plethora of weight loss products all with miraculous claims is mind boggling—and scary. Many of these are dangerous and may complicate underlying medical problems. This is especially true for women with PCOS.

You *need* a medically-sound, balanced approach to using vitamins and other supplements to avoid making the underlying PCOS issues worse. Most of us don't really eat a "balanced diet" these days. You can be overweight and actually malnourished.

Dr. Vliet's HORMONE POWER PLAN:
SAMPLE MEAL PLANS
Building Blocks for Each Meal

BREAKFAST:

	Protein gm	Fat gms	Carb gms	Calories
3 protein (low fat)	21	9	0	165
½ fat exchanges	0	2.5	0	22
1 bread	3	1	15	80
1 milk, skim	8	0	12	90
½ fruit	0	0	7.5	30
TOTAL PERCENTS	34 %	30%	36%	387

LUNCH

	Protein gm	Fat gms	Carb gms	Calories
5 protein (low fat)	35	15	0	275
½ fat	0	2.5	0	22
2 bread/starch	6	0	30	140
2 vegetable (non-starchy)	4	0	10	50
½ fruit	0	0	7.5	30
0 milk	–	–	--	--
TOTAL PERCENTS	33%	32%	35%	537

AFTERNOON SNACK

	Protein gm	Fat gms	Carb gms	Calories
1.5 protein (low-fat)	10.5	4.5	0	82
1 fruit	0	0	15	60
TOTAL PERCENTS	30%	28%	42%	142

This plan means that over 60% of daily calories are consumed prior to dinner, which helps prevent more fat being stored at night.

DINNER

	Protein gm	Fat gms	Carb gms	Calories
4 protein (low-fat)	28	12	0	220
½ fat	0	2.5	0	22
1 bread	3	1	15	80
2 vegetable (non-starchy)	4	0	10	50
1 fruit	0	0	15	60
½ milk	4	0	6	45
TOTAL PERCENTS	33%	29%	38%	477

BEDTIME SNACK

	Protein gm	Fat gms	Carb gms	Calories
1.5 protein (low-fat)	10.5	4.5	0	82
½ milk	4	0	6	45
TOTAL PERCENTS	46%	35%	19%	122

Dr. Vliet's Hormone Power Plan DAILY SUMMARY

I.   1600 CALORIE MEAL PLAN**

	Protein gm	Fat Gms	Carb gms	Calories
DAILY TOTALS:	141	56	149	1645
TOTAL PERCENTS:	35%	30%	35%	100%

II.   1800 CALORIE MEAL PLAN *

	Protein gm	Fat Gms	Carb gms	Calories
DAILY TOTALS:	154	61	164	1800
TOTAL PERCENTS:	35%	30%	35%	100%

HOW TO CHOOSE WHICH PLAN

*Women who weigh more than 190–200 lb. will need to eat more calories to provide adequate energy throughout the day, and avoid making your metabolism slow down even more. To increase from 1600 to 1800 calories per day, I suggest adding 1.5 protein exchanges and 1 bread exchange during the day, such as for a mid-morning snack. Or, you may add 1 bread/starch exchange to breakfast, and the 1½ meat exchanges to dinner.

** I really do not recommend decreasing daily caloric intake below 1600 calories for most women. Cutting calories too low simply makes your metabolism slow down even more and makes it harder for you to lose excess fat. Your body will hang on to all it has, because it thinks you are in a famine! Keeping your daily calories above the level of your resting metabolic rate will help jump-start your metabolism and rev up the metabolic rate if you are currently eating less than this amount.

EXCHANGES, OR BUILDING BLOCKS, FOR YOUR MEALS

I. PROTEINS = meats and meat-substitutes.

This group is divided into groups, based on fat content, which in turn affects the calories and fat grams, as shown in the chart.

	Protein gm	Fat gm	Calories*
Very lean meat, & meat substitutes7	0-1	35	
Lean Meat & meat substitutes	7	3	55
Medium-fat meat and substitutes	7	5	75
High-fat meat and meat substitutes	7	8	100

Protein Examples

*Calories based on serving size for one building block unit, or one exchange:

- 🐦 meat, chicken, fish: 1 ounce
- 🐦 hard cheeses: 1 ounce
- 🐦 soft cheeses (cottage, ricotta, farmers: ¼ cup
- 🐦 egg: 1 whole egg, or two egg whites (no yolk)
- 🐦 egg substitutes: ¼ cup
- 🐦 peanut butter: 2 tbsp (med-fat meat group)
- 🐦 soy milk: 1 cup
- 🐦 tempeh: ¼ cup
- 🐦 tofu: 4 oz. Or ½ cup
- 🐦 Beans, peas, lentils: ½ cup cooked, counts as one very lean meat AND one starch exchange

II. FATS: one building block, or exchange =

5 grams of fat
0 grams of carbohydrate or protein
45 calories

Sample foods:

all oils (vegetable and animal-derived), salad dressing, mayonnaise, butter, margarine, regular cream, sour cream, coconut, bacon, avocados, olives, nuts, seeds, tahini paste, shortening/lard/fatback/salt pork.

If you use a reduced fat version of butter, margarine, sour cream, mayonnaise or salad dressing this means you may increase the serving size as shown below to give the same total fat content.

Examples: One fat building block (exchange) =

- 🐦 1 tsp regular butter/margarine
- 🐦 OR 2 tsp whipped butter/margarine
- 🐦 OR 3 tsp (1 tbsp) reduced fat butter/margarine
- 🐦 OR 2 tbsp regular sour cream
- 🐦 OR 3 tbsp (1 tbsp) reduced fat sour cream
- 🐦 OR 1 tsp regular mayonnaise, salad dressing
- 🐦 OR 3 tsp (1 tbsp) reduced-fat mayo/salad dressing

TRY TO AVOID "TRANS" FATS

III. CARBOHYDRATES:

(A) BREAD/STARCH GROUP: one building block, or exchange,

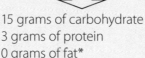

15 grams of carbohydrate
3 grams of protein
0 grams of fat*
80 calories

Sample foods: breads, cereals, grains, starchy vegetables (potatoes, beans, corn, green peas, yams, winter squash), crackers/snacks, beans, lentils, black-eyed or split peas.

*some starchy foods that are prepared with fat count as 1 starch exchange plus one fat exchange: biscuits, corn bread, crackers, croutons, granola, muffins, pancakes, bread stuffing, taco shells and waffles

(B) VEGETABLE GROUP: one building block, or exchange,

5 grams of carbohydrate
2 grams protein
0 grams fat
25 calories

Sample foods: artichokes, asparagus, green beans, beets, broccoli, brussels sprouts, cabbage, carrots, cauliflower, celery, cucumber, eggplant, green onions, dark greens (collard, kale, mustard, turnip, spinach), kohlrabi, mushrooms, okra, onions, pea pods, peppers, radishes, salad greens, sauerkraut, spinach, summer squash, tomatoes, turnips, water chestnuts, watercress, zuchini

(C) FRUIT GROUP: one building block, or exchange,

15 grams of carbohydrate
0 grams of protein or fat
60 calories

Sample foods: apples, apricots, bananas, blackberries, blueberries, cantaloupe, cherries, dates, figs, grapefruit, grapes, honeydew, kiwi, mandarin oranges, mango, nectarines, oranges, papaya, peaches, pears, pineapple, plums, prunes, raisins, raspberries, strawberries, tangerines, watermelon

IV. MILK GROUP:

Milk and milk products contain protein, carbohydrate, and fat "building blocks." The amount of fat a particular type of milk contains will determine both the fat grams and the total calories.

	Protein gm	Fat gm	Carb gm	Calories*
Fat-free (skim milk, Non-fat yogurt)	8	0	12	90
Low fat (1% milk, Low-fat yogurt)	8	3	12	100
Reduced fat (2% milk)	8	5	12	120
Whole milk	0	8	12	150

*Calories based on serving size for one building block unit, or one exchange:

milk (cow, goat, or kefir) = 1 cup   buttermilk = 1 cup

evaporated milk = ½ cup   yogurt = ¾ cup

fat-free dry milk = 1/3 cup powder

Note: rice milk is considered a starch exchange, and soy milk is considered a medium-fat meat (protein) exchange

© Elizabeth Lee Vliet, M.D. 1995-2005

Even if you do feel you eat a balanced diet, you still wouldn't get all the vitamins and minerals you need every day just from your food. One reason is that soils in which foods are grown today are often depleted of needed minerals. Another reason is that vitamins are frequently processed out of foods or lost in cooking.

Vitamins and minerals are called *micronutrients* because we need very small amounts each day, not because they are "micro" in importance. They are vital catalysts for all the chemical pathways our body uses to convert food into energy and for the body to make its critical hormones and chemical messengers.

Stress also increases the body's demands for the vital "micro" nutrients and antioxidants. Without them, stress causes chemical changes that lead to cellular damage throughout the body.

Most people today need a reasonable vitamin/mineral supplement daily to insure the right balance for optimal health.

Vitamin A

This fat soluble vitamin is important for many functions, and a rich food source is dark green, red, and yellow vegetables. Since it is stored in body fat, however, you can overdo by taking supplements that contain excess amounts of Vitamin A. Excess vitamin A can cause hair loss and pigment changes in the skin, increased risk of osteoporosis, as well as liver toxicity. Don't take any more than 5000 units daily in a supplement.

B Vitamins

Keep in mind
Taking supplements means learning the proper balance to make it work—too much of one vitamin may reduce the absorption and effectiveness of another.

B vitamins are involved as co-factors to make our hormones, as well as for carbohydrate metabolism, energy-generating, and fat-burning metabolic pathways. B vitamins are also critical co-factors in the brain pathways to make serotonin and other mood and metabolism-regulating neurotransmitters. Loss of B vitamins cause symptoms such as low energy, muscle fatigue, depression, insomnia, headaches, and anorexia.

Women taking birth control pills need higher intake of B vitamins, and the B vitamins are also rapidly depleted when you are under stress. This includes the physiological stress of dieting, as well as "life stress" every day.

The B vitamins include Thiamine (B1), Niacinamide (B3), Pantothenate (B5), Pyridoxine (B6), Cyancobalamin (B12) and folic acid.

B12 is only found in food of animal origin: meat/pork/poultry, eggs, cheese, milk, and fish. That's why women who follow a true vegan-type vegetarian diet are often deficient in B12.

Food sources for the other B vitamins and folic acid include enriched (or fortified) whole grain products such cereals, brewer's yeast, rice bran, wheat germ; legumes, nuts, meats, some vegetables, seeds, eggs, milk.

I recommend taking the complete B complex 25–50 mg formulated supplement rather than individual B vitamins because the B vitamins need to be present in the proper balance and ratio in order to work optimally. I suggest you avoid products derived from brewer's yeast, since many women are already having "yeast" problems.

The B vitamins are water soluble, so excess amounts are excreted in the urine rather than being stored in body fat. But you can still have problems from taking too much of the B vitamins in high dose supplements, since excess amounts cause saturation of the enzyme systems that depend on these vitamins. Then they can't function properly. For example, symptoms of excess B6 can be the same numbness and nerve tingling, called peripheral neuropathy, that occurs when there is a deficit of B6. So don't overdo it!

Wisdom:
Taking a B complex vitamin supplement is important for women with PCOS, for many reasons.

Vitamin D

Vitamin D deficiency may be more common than previously thought. Restoring vitamin D to optimal levels may reduce the risk of future fractures and may also help the healing of current hip fractures. If you already have bone loss, ask your doctor to check your blood level of Vitamin D to be sure that you aren't too low.

Make sure you are getting at least 400 IU of vitamin D daily. If you live in a climate that doesn't have many sunny days in winter, you will need to take a supplement.

As with Vitamin A, Vitamin D is a fat soluble vitamin and excessive amounts can cause damage. Stay within the recommended ranges, unless you have a medical reason for taking higher amounts and are under a doctor's supervision to prevent excessive buildup.

Tip:
You can get your vitamin D from about 20 minutes of exposure to sunshine daily

The Antioxidant Vitamins

All of the cells and tissues of your body are constantly subjected to highly reactive and unstable molecules termed *free radicals* that cause cell damage as they build up. These hostile free radical molecules are a normal by-product of life and chemical changes in the body. They also come from environmental sources (smoke, ionizing radiation, air pollution, toxic heavy metals and other chemicals. Free radicals also occur in oxidized (rancid) fats in our foods.

Anti-oxidants:
Antioxidants protect our tissues from oxidative damage by free radicals.

Free radicals by their very chemical nature promote a chain reaction of cell damage by forming more free radicals that in turn chemically alter important biological molecules your body needs to function. Eating food with plenty of natural antioxidants, and taking appropriate antioxidant supplements, helps prevent this type of cell damage.

Low intake of antioxidants is associated with higher risks of cancer, cardiovascular disease, arthritis, cataracts and many other degenerative diseases. Antioxidants also play a key role in the metabolic pathways for hormone production and weight regulation.

Make sure you get plenty of the following in your diet:

Beta-carotene

Caution!
Make certain you are not taking multiple supplements that give you excessive amounts when you add everything together.

Beta-carotene found in dark yellow vegetables such as carrots, pumpkin, winter squash, sweet potatoes; dark green vegetables such as collard greens, kale, spinach, Swiss chard, broccoli; fruits such as cantaloupe, mango, papaya, apricots. You need 10,000 to 25,000 IU daily. But don't overdo the supplements, try to get most of this from your food.

Vitamin C

Vitamin C is found in fruits such as oranges, grapefruit, cantaloupe, mango, kiwi, papaya, guava, strawberries; vegetables such as broccoli, bell peppers, Brussels sprouts, cabbage, tomatoes, spinach, kale, and potatoes. Daily intake should be anywhere in the range of 500 to 1000 mg. Higher intake also decreases risk of gallstones in women.

Vitamin E

Vitamin E plays a significant antioxidant role counteracting damaging free radical effects, including ones generated from excess glucose. Vitamin E reduces glucose levels and improves insulin sensitivity. It plays an important role in controlling platelet clotting and lowering platelet count.

Vitamin E is found in nuts such as walnuts, almonds, hazelnuts, peanuts, sunflower seeds; Oils such as wheat germ oil, vegetable oils; vegetables such as asparagus, broccoli, Brussels sprouts, corn, sweet potato, peas and beans (legumes); grains such as whole wheat, oats, whole grain cereals. Food sources are primarily the *gamma* form of Vitamin E, the most effective antioxidant.

Vitamin E
I suggest 100–200 IU daily instead of the higher amounts recommended in the past.

For Vitamin E supplements, use the *natural*, or "d" form (*d-alpha-tocopherol*), or one that says "*mixed natural tocopherols.*" *Synthetic* Vitamin E is identified with a 'dl' (*dl-alpha-tocopherol*) and it does not have the same benefits of the natural vitamin. The natural "d" form is more expensive, but it is worth spending the extra money.

Minerals

Selenium

This is an antioxidant mineral that is important in small amounts, up to about 100 mcg daily. Generally, there is enough selenium in a good multi-vitamin, so don't add extra as too much can be toxic. Selenium content of foods grown in soil varies a great deal due to the variability of the mineral in soil in different regions. It is found in vegetables such as broccoli, tomatoes, onions; or grains such as bran, wheat germ, whole grain products; fish, and poultry.

Boron

This is a trace mineral crucial for healthy bone, and it also helps reduce excretion of calcium and magnesium. It is found in a variety of vegetables such as green peppers and tomatoes. Check your multiple vitamin—it should contain boron. Too much boron is not good, so check your multivitamin. It should contain enough.

Iron

Women lose iron every month in their menstrual bleeding and most women today have decreased their intake of red meat, the primary food source of iron. Due to low dietary intake, and monthly loss of iron, many women have low iron stores, called *ferritin* (see also Chapter 8).

Tip
If your ferritin is lower than 60, take an iron supplement daily.

Low ferritin is associated with restless legs syndrome, insomnia, fatigue, muscle pain, poor exercise tolerance, thinning scalp hair and a variety of other problems. If you have these symptoms, taking a multivitamin with iron can help, *even if you don't have anemia.*

The concern about iron and heart disease is that *high* ferritin levels may increase risk of heart disease. I check ferritin on all my patients, and I have seen *high* ferritin levels in probably less than 1 out of 10 women. So don't stop taking multiple vitamins **with iron** unless you have your ferritin checked and find out it is actually high!

Magnesium

Magnesium is a critical mineral for hormone production, metabolic pathways, nerve cell conduction, muscle contraction, bone growth/formation, and it has an independent role in regulating blood pressure. It is an important factor in reducing migraine headaches and heart attacks because it helps prevent spasms of the blood vessels throughout the body, especially in the coronary (heart) arteries.

Ahhh...
A side benefit of optimal estradiol and optimal magnesium is improved bowel function, and... fewer chocolate cravings!

In the brain, magnesium is a cofactor in the production of mood-regulating chemical messengers such as dopamine that regulates appetite. It is also important in helping prevent, and possibly relieve, mood changes that occur with PMS and mild depression.

Several B vitamins require magnesium as a catalyst to make these vitamins biologically active in the body. Magnesium also is a cofactor for the chemical reactions to build protein for growth and repair of muscles and tissues. The pathways for the body to use carbohydrates are also dependent upon magnesium. Optimal magnesium decreases your risk of diabetes.

Optimal intake of magnesium and zinc (discussed next), as well as regular deep breathing, improves oxygen flow to the tissues, which helps your fat-burning and energy production pathways work more efficiently.

Magnesium is also important in preventing free radical damage to cells. When magnesium is low, we lose this protective effect. Low magnesium generates more free radicals leading to cell damage and aging effects. Women with PCOS need to be sure they are getting optimal magnesium intake, yet most American women are woefully deficient in magnesium.

Common problems that deplete magnesium:

- Drinking soft drinks daily—diet or regular—prevents absorption of magnesium and calcium since the phosphates (and phosphoric acid) in these beverages bind up magnesium and calcium and makes them insoluble
- Using foods and beverages with glutamate (MSG) and aspartate (Nutrasweet®) increase the body's need for magnesium
- High coffee consumption
- Excess catecholamine effects (e.g. from stimulant medications)
- Excess glucocorticoid effects (cortisone medications, and stress)
- Low estradiol decreases magnesium absorption from the gut and the uptake and use by the body's soft tissues and bone

Tip
Low Mg and low E2 add to high blood pressure, insulin resistance, weight gain, migraines, and risk of heart disease in PCOS

Caution: Taking estrogen, or birth control pills with estrogen in them, causes more of the magnesium to shift into the soft tissues and bone. This shift decreases magnesium in the blood, and causes imbalance in serum calcium and magnesium ratio, which then causes more muscle spasms and cramps. It also means you may be at higher risk to develop a blood clot because a shift in the calcium to magnesium ratio favors clotting (or coagulation). **If you are taking calcium and are on estrogen, it is critical that you also get enough magnesium each day.**

Tip:
The 2:1 ratio of calcium intake to magnesium intake is important for proper balance.

Getting Adequate Magnesium

The average American woman only gets about 100 to 200 mg a day of magnesium from her diet, and the RDA for magnesium is 400 to 600 mg daily. I recommend that my patients take 200 to 300 mg of magnesium supplement every morning and 200 to 300 mg every evening. Taking magnesium and calcium at least two times a day, generally AM and PM, provides better absorption and more even levels throughout the 24 hours.

I recommend magnesium capsules with easily absorbed magnesium powder, such as the Twin Lab brand. I've found absorption is poor with hard tablets and caplet forms. You may also find a liquid form is well absorbed and less irritating to the GI tract.

TIP
Adequate zinc is needed for healthy ovarian function and optimal insulin action

Magnesium's importance is often overlooked, and physicians often haven't paid enough attention to the importance of optimal magnesium intake to help relieve some of the symptons in muscle pain/spasms, fibromyalgia, PMS, headaches, high blood pressure, depressed mood, anxiety and a host of other woes.

Zinc

Zinc is as important as protein in the normal processes of growth and maintenance of body tissue, particularly the brain and nervous system. It plays an important role in DNA and protein synthesis, helps to regulate your blood sugar, aids in formation of healthy collagen (in skin and connective tissue), and plays a role in normal immune function. Zinc is also needed for optimal ovarian function. It is a helper for some 20 enzymes. It is involved in the action of insulin, the utilization of vitamin A, and the healing of wounds. It also helps decrease the spread of pain sensations.

Fact:
The recommended intake is 15 mg per day for the average adult.

Women have cut down on animal foods that are rich sources and often don't get enough zinc. Many plant sources, such as whole grains, now have reduced zinc content due to soil depletion from modern farming methods or from the refining and processing of foods.

Phytates in plant sources interfere with the absorption of several critical minerals (calcium, magnesium, iron), and particularly, zinc.

Animal foods and seafood are good sources of zinc. Plant sources include whole grains, and pumpkin seeds are a particularly rich source.

Vegetarians are more likely to have inadequate zinc intake, particularly if they eat a diet high in soy products as a main source of protein. Soybeans are more resistant than other beans and grains to the beneficial effects of long, slow cooking to reduce phytates that block absorption of key minerals. Only fermentation, such as involved in making miso and tempeh, will decrease the amount of phytates present in soybeans.

So if you rely on soy foods as your primary source of protein, you risk having significant deficiencies of zinc, iron, and B12 unless you take appropriate supplements.

Zinc supplements come in several forms, and I suggest *avoid piccolinate* and use either the arginate or citrate form. Be careful not to take too much zinc, since excess doses may interfere with copper absorption. Check your multivitamin to see that it contains 1.5 to 3 mg of copper, and take it at a different time of day relative to when you take the zinc. I suggest taking your multivitamin (with its copper) in the morning, and zinc at night.

Absorption of zinc depends on adequate dietary intake of tryptophan and B6. A deficiency of either will impair zinc absorption. Current studies have shown that 200-mcg of chromium once or twice a day is reasonable and has not shown any adverse effects. Higher doses can be toxic, so don't over do it. If you are overweight and have symptoms of glucose intolerance, adding chromium supplementation with zinc may be helpful.

Manganese

Manganese deficiencies are associated with osteoporosis, chronic depression, chronic pain, blood sugar problems, and allergies. Manganese is involved in a

Impairs Zinc absorption: Soybeans have the highest phytate (phytic acid) content of any grain or legume.

Warning: Recent studies in Germany found that the piccolinate form can cause liver damage

Tip: Supplementing with chromium can aid in zinc absorption and help keep blood glucose more stable throughout the day.

number of enzyme pathways needed for the utilization
of the B vitamins, vitamin E and vitamin C, as well as
the pathways of energy metabolism, glucose regulation,
and immune function.

In addition, manganese is a component of the antioxidant enzyme SOD, or superoxide dismutase, that controls superoxide free radicals formed in the body during cellular metabolism. SOD helps prevent the buildup of excess superoxide radicals that cause cell damage.

Dietary deficiencies of manganese are more common today due to several factors: soils depleted of manganese, diets high in simple sugars, high fiber diets that contain phytates, and soda beverages that contain phosphorus which impairs manganese absorption. Wheat milled to make white flour causes loss of manganese that is not added back even in flours marked "enriched."

Manganese is widely available in many plant foods. Examples include nuts, whole grains, raisins, spinach, carrots, broccoli, green peas, oranges, apples, tea leaves and wheat bran. You will get most of the manganese you need in a good multivitamin and a diet rich in the above foods. I don't think it is necessary to take additional manganese supplements.

Calcium

This is a mineral you hear a lot about for maintaining bone, but it is also critical in metabolism, mood and sleep regulating pathways, and for normal muscle function. The sad part is that even with so much emphasis on calcium, the average calcium intake for American women is still too low at only 450 milligrams a day. Low calcium also makes weight loss more difficult.

Many women cut back on dairy and milk and are drinking more diet beverages to lose weight, one reason for low calcium intake. They replace an important source of calcium, and phosphates in sodas prevent proper absorption of the calcium. Dairy products are still the richest dietary calcium sources. Vegetables contain much less calcium per serving, and the fiber in vegetables decreases calcium absorption.

I caution you to avoid calcium products made from oyster shell or dolomite. These have been found to be contaminated with toxic heavy metals such as lead, mercury, arsenic.

TUMS, pure calcium carbonate, is a simple and inexpensive option for getting extra calcium. Bioavailability studies of TUMS have shown it is readily absorbed, and well tolerated. TUMS contains no aluminum, so it is safe to take daily. It's easy to carry in your handbag, so there's no excuse for not taking your calcium. Calcium citrate is promoted as being better absorbed, but studies have not consistently confirmed this. Calcium citrate has less elemental calcium per tablet, so you have to take more tablets daily.

Calcium absorption can be checked by a 24-hour urine test of calcium excretion. This may be appropriate if you are not responding to bone rebuilding therapies (medication, exercise, hormones and supplements) or if you have greater bone loss than expected.

Two things I look at with this test: (1) very low urinary calcium tells me you're not absorbing calcium very well and may need additional calcium in the diet, or better estradiol level to help absorb calcium, or additional tests to find out why; and (2) very high urinary calcium tells me you are excreting more than you are absorbing, which typically occurs in women when estradiol levels are low.

One question my patients often ask me is "How do we get enough calcium without getting constipated?" I'll almost guarantee you that if you are getting enough magnesium, you won't have to worry about constipation from your calcium! Remember, Milk of Magnesia, is a laxative based on magnesium's ability to stimulate motility in the intestines. Too much magnesium quickly causes diarrhea, so you have a clear indication of getting too much, and when to cut back.

Warning: Avoid calcium products made from oyster shell or dolomite.

Tip If you don't eat dairy products, it really is important to supplement calcium every day.

Tip The recommended amount of calcium is 1000 to 1200 mg daily before menopause, and 1500 mg daily after menopause.

Mineral Summary

To review, the most important minerals for women experiencing hormonal problems are **magnesium, zinc, calcium, manganese, boron, and iron**. Focus on getting as much as possible from a healthy diet, and then supplement to reach the doses I have given as guidelines. You don't have to take the more expensive colloidal (fine particles suspended in a uniform medium) versions... regular capsules or tablets are readily absorbed by most people unless you have a disease affecting the gastrointestinal tract. In that case, you may consider a liquid form.

Enjoy
If you love chocolate, Viactiv is a chewy, chocolate calcium supplement.

Additional Supplements To Consider

Co-enzyme Q10

This is an antioxidant, vitamin-like compound that plays a critical role in the energy and oxygenation pathways throughout the body. It declines as we get older. It has effects similar to vitamin E, but is even more powerful. There is evidence that Co-Q 10 may help lower blood pressure, improve overall immune function, and improve cardiovascular response in people with congestive heart failure (CHF).

Sources:
Co-Q10 is found in oily, deep water fish such as salmon, sardines and mackerel, and in spinach and peanuts.

Statin medicines such as Lipitor and others to lower high cholesterol, can deplete Co-enzyme Q10. If you are taking one of these, talk with your doctor about whether to take Co-enzyme Q supplements.

There are many "CoQ10" products available now, but quality varies enormously and oral absorption is not always reliable. Since it is an oil-soluble compound, oral forms are better absorbed if taken with a meal containing oily or fatty foods, such as salmon or other cold water fish. Daryl Spence, R.Ph., recommends a compounded sublingual form, available with a physician's prescription.

Essential Fatty Acids

These are technically considered *macronutrients*, I discuss them briefly here since so many women take these as supplements.

The body needs a certain amount of the right kind of fat for critical life functions, such as to make hormone-like messengers called prostaglandins, to provide cholesterol as a building block for the steroid hormones (your three estrogens, testosterone, progesterone, and adrenal steroids such as DHEA and cortisol), to maintain normal nerve conduction and brain function, and for the essential processes of building new cells and repair of cellular damage.

Fatty acids are the building blocks the body uses to make necessary fats. There are two categories of EFAs:

> **EFAs**
> *Essential Fatty Acids* (EFAs) are ones the body cannot make, and must be supplied by the foods and/or supplements.

Omega-6-Fatty Acids

These include Linoleic acid (LA) and Gamma linolenic acid (GLA). GLA serves as a precursor for the body to form unsaturated fatty acids, which are important in making cell membrane structures, serving as cellular energy messengers, and to make *eicosanoids*, another group of important chemical messengers involved in pain, inflammation, immune control and other functions.

Omega-6-FA can be found in raw nuts, seeds, legumes, unsaturated vegetable oils (borage oil has the highest content), GLA is also found in evening primrose, grapeseed, and sesame oils.

> **Tip**
> Proper ratio of EFAs is crucial to keep the body from making more "bad" eicosanoids

Omega-3-Fatty Acids

These are alpha linolenic acid (ALA) and eicosapentaenoic acid (EPA). Good sources include fish oils—salmon, mackerel, and sardines contain the highest amounts per ounce; vegetable oils such as canola, flaxseeds and flaxseed oil, walnuts and walnut oil. I recommend you try to get your Essential Fatty Acids from the food you eat and the rich sources I have identified. **Avoid taking a very large amount of these supplements, which can lead to excess production of "bad" eicosanoids that can increase joint and muscle pain.**

If you take fish oil supplements, avoid ones that have been heat processed (destroys the EFAs), but do look

Tip:
The amount of EPA (omega 3) should be about 50 to 100 times the amount of GLA (omega 6) used.

for ones that have been distilled in a special process to remove contaminates.

However, if you are taking these supplements, balance is crucial. If you take GLA supplements, it is important that you also take EPA as well. Proper balance of omega 3 and omega 6 FAs is especially important for women with PCOS. To improve balance of the "good" eicosanoids, you should only need doses of GLA (omega-6 EFA) in the range of 1–10 mg accompanied by 50–500 mg of EPA (omega-3 EFA).

Supplements and Herbs—Pitfalls and Cautions for Women with PCOS

Caution:
Consumers in this country have no way to insure the quality and safety of what is in herbs and supplements.

As a result of the Dietary Supplements Health and Education Act of 1994, the Food and Drug Administration (FDA) is no longer allowed to oversee the supplement industry the way it watches over quality, safety, and effectiveness of prescription medications.

This is in contrast to Germany, where herbs and other types of supplements have been used as medicinal agents for years, and are overseen by the German Commission E, a government agency that checks the safety, purity, and effectiveness of herbs and other supplements that are marketed as having therapeutic benefits. Products have to meet the standards set by Commission E before they can be sold as medicinals in Germany.

Warning:
Reports on herbal products found contamination of lead, arsenic, pesticides and other adulterants. Many products didn't even contain what the label said.

How can you determine a product's safety and that it contains what it is supposed to? One resource is ConsumerLab, an organization that conducts detailed analyses of supplement products to help consumers know which brands actually provide what the label says they do, and are free of known contaminants. Another excellent, independent and unbiased resource is *The Comprehensive Database of Natural Medicines*, published by The Prescriber's Letter, also available on the web.

There are now thousands of vitamin and supplement products on the market that can vary enormously in quality and reliability as well as price. The most expensive is not necessarily the best, so shop carefully.

"Weight Loss" Supplements

The plethera of weight loss products all with miraculous claims is mind boggling—and scary. Many of these are dangerous and may complicate underlying medical problems. I think women with PCOS who are struggling with excess body weight are especially vulnerable to both the misleading advertising claims and to the damaging effects of many of these herbs and supplements.

Don't be misled by the word "natural" when looking for remedies for weight loss. Herbs may be "natural" plants, but many have toxic effects on the heart and liver as well as other side effects, just as some medications may have. This is the same reasoning I used in talking about the horse-derived estrogens, remember?

Many of the herbs are used in weight loss supplements or herbal remedies. **Do not use any products containing the following:**

St. John's Wort

St. John's Wort should not be taken with prescription antidepressants (may lead to serotonin excess syndrome), with birth control pills (leads to loss of contraceptive effectiveness), or prescription hormones (decreases effectiveness by 50% or more).

DHEA

I do not recommend over-the-counter DHEA. Most doses are more than women need, and women with PCOS already have problems from androgen excess that will be much worse if you take DHEA: weight gain, acne, facial hair, loss of scalp hair, irritability, restless sleep and sweet cravings.

Soy Isoflavones

Compounds in soy block conversion of your thyroid hormone T4 to the more active form T3 so taking soy and other isoflavone supplements can interfere with thyroid

Caution: Just because compounds are natural to plants does not necessarily mean they are natural for humans.

Potentially Dangerous ephedra (ma huang), OTC stimulants (phenylephrine, phenylpropanolamine), adrenal glandulars, thyroid glandulars, and ginseng

function. Soy and clover isoflavones also competitively inhibit estradiol binding at receptor sites. Studies in premenopausal women have found 20–50% reductions in production of both estradiol and progesterone, which clearly can cause major havoc in PCOS when your hormones are already out of balance and you may be dealing with infertility as well.

Warning:
With current concerns about prions causing Mad Cow disease, I don't recommend using ground-up, desiccated animal glands at all!

Ginseng

Often recommended as a "tonic" or energy-booster, ginseng is also marketed for weight loss and as an "immune-booster." I see many PCOS patients taking it for weight loss or in the belief that it will boost energy. But recent studies have found that it is no better than placebo and can cause serious problems, such as high blood pressure, which is often already a problem in PCOS.

Hormone Glandulars

I don't recommend the use of over-the-counter animal-derived "glandulars" (thyroid or adrenal) for weight loss. There is no regulatory oversight for these products, and no way for you to know the source of the animals, no matter what the marketing claims may say.

Caution:
Symptoms of low basal body temperature and fatigue are not reliable to diagnose adrenal or thyroid problems.

Taking adrenal glandulars is potentially dangerous in PCOS, since cortisol levels tend to be too high in PCOS, not low. The goal isn't to stimulate cortisol, as these products do, but to get it into the lower healthy range.

Whether you use over-the-counter glandulars or prescription thyroid medication, excess thyroid pushes your TSH too low, creating a hyperthyroid state. This causes heart arrhythmias and more rapid breakdown of bone and also causes the remaining bone to be more brittle. This is dangerous for women with PCOS who are also experiencing loss of estradiol that regulates bone metabolism and cardiovascular health.

There are now very effective and sensitive blood tests for measuring both adrenal and thyroid hormones, as well as tests for antibodies to the thyroid gland tissue and to your thyroid hormones. You don't need to take these supplements based on symptoms. Work with a knowledgeable physician to get properly tested, and when needed, use FDA-approved prescription products for thyroid or adrenal hormone replacement. See Chapter 8 for guidelines on testing.

HERBS TO AVOID

Known to cause acute liver injury, chronic hepatitis, cirrhosis and/or liver failure: chaparral, comfrey, coltsfoot, germander, margosa oil, mate tea, mistletoe and skullcap, Gordolobo yerba tea, pennyroyal (squawmint) oil, pyrrolizidine alkaloids, aflatoxins, Amanita phalloides, Jin Bu Huan (a Chinese herbal product), and others.

Known to increase heart rate, blood pressure (dangerous in people with heart disease): ephedra (Chinese name: mahuang), excessive amounts of caffeine (not generally shown on labels, but a common adulterant in "tonics"), and others.

Known to cause kidney damage (acute interstitial nephritis and/or renal failure): Tung Shueh pills found to be adulterated with an anti-inflammatory agent, mefanamic acid, not shown on the label; aristolochic acid; products adulterated with phenylbutazone.

Your Hormone Power Life Plan®:

Tapping Into the Power of Exercise

If you are struggling with PCOS, the last thing you want to be told by another doctor is "Just get out and exercise." Well, I am not saying 'just' exercise.

You cannot lose excess body fat without being more physically active, along with the right food balance and optimal hormone balance. I know. I have been there.

There are hundreds of studies to show that regular exercise improves energy, muscle mass, metabolic rate, and the production of fat-burning, mood-lifting, fatigue-fighting, pain-relieving brain chemical messengers.

To lose fat you have two options: reduce your caloric intake or increase your caloric expenditure. You cannot decrease your caloric intake much lower than 1400 to 1500 calories daily without slowing your metabolism

It's a fact:

I *am* saying
that physical
activity is
an *essential*
component
of an
integrated
treatment
program for
PCOS.
Period.

and getting fatter. So… you need to increase caloric expenditure… through more physical activity.

You can't do it all at once. You need guidance to begin at a level appropriate for you. You must start off slowly and increase your tolerance gradually as you build up stamina. This is crucial to prevent injuries and maintain your motivation.

Consult your physician before beginning any type of exercise activities, and ask for a referral to a physical therapist or exercise physiologist to help you get started on an appropriate program. Many hospitals now have fitness programs and are a good place to start. This is especially important if you are significantly overweight and haven't been exercising.

I find that many overweight women have joint and body pain and are reluctant to exercise, afraid it will cause more pain. After four spine surgeries over the years, I have found just the opposite: if I pace myself and gear my workout to what my body can do safely, then I actually have less pain than I have if I don't exercise at all.

Tips for Getting Started: It Doesn't Have To Be "All or Nothing"?

Good
medicine:

Physical
activity
improves the
function of
every single
part of your
mind and
body.

Generally, *anything* is better than *nothing*. This is especially true with physical activity.

Some people resist exercising because there is also a perception that they must run X amount of miles for X amount of time or there will be no benefits. This isn't true.

You simply need to be more active in your usual daily life. This is more realistic, more likely to be implemented, and more effective. Is this enough? To begin with, yes.

Over time, the amount of physical activity you need depends on your metabolism and how much excess fat you have to lose. Gradual increases in activity are very do-able, so let's look at some tips to get started.

TIP #1: WALK MORE

Walking helps stimulate your metabolism and helps your fat-burning pathways work more efficiently. You do not have to work up a sweat to benefit. Even if you only walk for 5–10 minutes at a time, it helps.

If you walk for 10 minutes three times a day, that adds up to several hours a week and puts a meaningful dent in your couch potato time.

Walk to lunch. Pack lunch and spend your lunch hour walking, not sitting in the office break room.

TIP #2: DON'T FALL INTO THE FOOD REWARD TRAP

Just because you have been "good" and increased your activity doesn't mean you can now eat anything you want. If you add activity and do not increase your food intake, you will see a steady loss of fat because you shifted to more calories out than calories in.

TIP #3: BOOST METABOLIC RATE WITH MORE MUSCLE

Increased activity levels help jump-start a sluggish metabolism. This occurs because more activity builds more muscles which in turn revs up your metabolism because muscles burn a lot more calories than fat.

Adding resistance or weight training to your workouts can greatly improve muscle mass over what you achieve with aerobic activity alone.

You burn more calories not only when exercising, but also when you are watching TV, driving a car, and even when you are sleeping.

TIP # 4: INCORPORATE MORE ACTIVITY INTO EACH DAY

- ❧ Walk up stairs instead of using elevators
- ❧ Avoid remote controls—get up and move to change the channel!
- ❧ Walk to do your errands when possible

Be creative!
After my cervical spine surgery, the physical therapist found ways for me to exercise even though I was in a neck brace and couldn't lift a water pitcher.

Just DO it!
No matter where, or how fast, just do it more.

ᘒ Park further away from entrances and walk more

ᘒ Stand more than you are sitting. You will burn more calories standing than sitting

ᘒ Walk for fitness at least a total of 30 minutes a day. Remember, you can break this into segments.

Tip:

Having more muscle means a higher metabolic rate over the whole day, every day.

TIP #5: INCORPORATE MORE STRENGTHENING ACTIVITIES INTO EACH DAY

The idea here is to look for the hard way to do things instead of the easiest.

ᘒ Sit down slowly using your muscles, rather than falling into the chair letting gravity do the work

ᘒ Rise from a chair without using your arms to help you get up

ᘒ Lift heavier objects with one arm instead of two

ᘒ Stand on one leg while waiting in line; then use the other leg. It's OK if you feel funny!

ᘒ Climb stairs without using hand rails to make your legs work harder

ᘒ Lift objects slowly to increase resistance rather than swinging them up using momentum to help

ᘒ Use your abdominal muscles to rise from a sitting position, instead of rocking to get up.

ᘒ Push down on floor with your toes while sitting, then lift your toes towards the ceiling and repeat these movements 10–15 times every hour

ᘒ Place hands, palms up, under your desk while you are sitting, and pull up against the desk several times a day.

ᘒ Push head back against high-backed seat, hold 10 seconds, release and repeat 20 times to help strengthen your neck

ᘒ Perform Kegel (pelvic floor) exercises any time, anywhere. No one will know why you are really smiling!

ᘒ Do abdominal tightening while riding in a car

Tip #5 is Adapted from

Exercise, Nutrition and the Older Woman Singh, (ed), CRC Press 2000

The "Lifestyle Approach" Grows Up and Becomes an Exercise Program

The "Lifestyle Approach" I outlined above is a good first step toward a more active life. An exercise program offers a more robust alternative. Once you've changed your habits, see progress, and feel better, you are ready for a more detailed plan designed to give greater results.

Let me set the record straight, however, on some common exercise misconceptions:

Misconception: "Exercise increases your appetite. I'll eat too much if I work out."

Fact: Exercise actually decreases your appetite if you are working out within your aerobic heart rate range. If your intensity is too high and you overshoot your aerobic range, you deplete muscle and liver glycogen stores, which makes you hungrier after a workout. If you stray, a slight increase in food intake is usually more than offset by two factors: (1) calories expended by the exercise itself, and (2) your increased metabolic rate for several hours after your workout is over.

Warning: Don't wear "sauna suits" or excess clothes to increase sweating.

Misconception: "The more you sweat, the faster you lose weight."

Fact: There is no benefit to excessive sweating, and it may be dangerous, particularly if you are on blood pressure medications or diuretics or are out-of-shape. Don't exercise in over-heated rooms either. You'll just get dizzy, faint and light-headed and only be losing water weight, not fat.

Misconception: "Women shouldn't exercise during their periods. Now that I hit perimenopause, I have a period every two weeks, and I don't feel like exercising, so I get out of the habit."

Fact: There is no medical reason for not exercising during your period. Physical activity actually helps the bloating and crampy feelings, and lifts low moods that hit at this time. If your energy is lower, or the bleeding heavy, just take it a little slower than usual, or maybe do a little shorter work out. If you are bleeding more often, it's time to ask your doctor about options to control the bleeding and better regulate your cycles.

Benefit:
Exercising at aerobic heart rate range three times a week for 20 minutes burns calories, stimulates your metabolism and leads to more fat loss.

Misconception: "In order for exercise to be effective, you have to work out every day, and I don't have time, so it won't do me any good."

Fact: You don't have to work out every day to see some positive changes. Simply increasing your physical movement throughout the day, every day, will help your body burn more calories. Can't you make 20 minutes, just three days a week, an important time commitment for YOU in the midst of all you do for others?

Misconception: "Exercise has to be strenuous to lose weight and I hurt too much to do anything strenuous enough to do me any good."

Fact: Exercise does not have to be strenuous to be effective. If you are overweight and out-of-shape, "really strenuous" exercise would probably put you above your aerobic range and would not be helping as much for losing fat. You will be surprised how quickly just simple walking will get your heart rate into the target range. This is all you need to do.

Good News:
Brisk walking for 30 minutes a day can burn up to 15 pounds a year. Not bad.

Misconception: "Aerobic exercise is no better than any other form of exercise for weight loss."

Fact: Getting your heart rate to the aerobic range will speed up your metabolism better, and also lasts 4 to 8 hours after you stop exercising, so additional calories will be burned off long after you finish working out. Non-aerobic exercise, like housework or gardening or weight-lifting, doesn't boost your metabolism to the same degree but they will improve muscle mass and strength, which has the benefits I listed above.

Finding Your Aerobic Range and "Target Heart Rate"

Aerobic heart rate is the number of heartbeats per minute that will increase the energy demands but still main-

CALCULATION OF TARGET HEART RATE RANGE

220 – age = PMHR X 0.6 = beats per minute for THR.

220 – age = PMHR X 0.85 = beats per minute for THR.

Divide the # of beats per minute by 6 to get beats per ten seconds

Then take your pulse for 10 seconds while you are exercising to see if you have reached the target range between 60% and 85% of predicted maximum heart rate (PMHR).

tain enough oxygen delivery to combine with glucose and "burn" to provide fuel. If you work too hard and increase your heart rate above this level, you force the body to use "anaerobic" (i.e. without oxygen) pathways.

If you exercise above your THR (anaerobic exercise), you will be burning muscle glycogen instead of fat, which accumulates more lactic acid in the muscles leading to stiff, sore muscles the next day. You will run out of "fuel" in the muscles, so you can't continue exercising very long.

Your maximum heart rate is based on age: the older you are, the lower the number of maximum beats per minute. To calculate your target heart rate range, use this formula (see chart) to determine your heart rate during exercise.

It's best to have your doctor give you a specific OK on these ranges since medications like beta blockers and some antidepressants may affect your target heart rate and make your target rate for exercise lower than what is calculated with the formula shown in the chart.

To make checking THR easier, I suggest purchasing a heart rate monitor to wear during exercise. These can be set to alert you when you drop below or go above your THR. There are many types, from basic ones to those that allow you to download exercise information into your computer or even wear while swimming.

If you exercise below the lower limit of your THR, you are not stimulating the heart enough to improve cardiovascular fitness or to promote significant fat burning.

THR:
Your target heart rate range (THR) is a heart rate between 60% to 85% of the heart's maximum beats per minute

Your Exercise Power Program: Aerobic Activities

When developing an exercise program you need to ask yourself "what activities do I like to do? If you don't like it, you won't keep it up. Then think about where you are going to exercise. If it isn't convenient, you won't keep it up. Consider working with an exercise physiologist or certified personal trainer who can set up a program for you and show you how to monitor your progress.

Monitor THR:

If you are not exercising in your proper target range, you won't see the benefits, and are less likely to keep up your program.

If you like to walk, is there a nearby walking path, school track, or shopping mall? If you hate walking and love the music and "energy" of aerobics classes, you may want to join a fitness center.

Do you like having the quiet time of exercising by yourself, or will you be more motivated to workout with a friend? Can you take your kids and the dog with you and make it a family outing? Are you a morning person, or do you feel better if you exercise at the end of the day?

Regardless of when you exercise, remember to do a 5–10 minute warm-up at the beginning of each session to gradually bring your heart rate up. Also remember to do 5–10 minutes of cool-down at the end, to gradually slow your heart back to normal.

I recommend aerobic activities that are low-impact to avoid injury to your joints. These include brisk walking (outside or on a treadmill indoors), swimming, water-walking, aqua-aerobics, bike riding or a stationary bike.

If you are overweight, it is especially helpful to do pool exercises because water helps support you and reduces strain on muscles and joints.

Your Exercise Power Program: Strengthening Activities

Aerobic activity improves cardiovascular fitness and increases the use of fat stores for fuel. Strengthening activities help to build more muscle mass and overall stronger bones and muscles. Strength, or weight, training, uses progressive resistance with machines or free weights.

You can do these at home with one of the excellent videotapes available for more intensive workouts, or you can work with a trainer at a health club. Both aerobic and strength-training components work together to help you lose excess body fat and feel better about yourself.

Your Exercise Power Program: Flexibility Activities

Flexibility, or the ease and degree to which a joint can move through a complete range of motion, helps prevent and reduce injury. Notice your cat or dog. They often stretch before they start moving. Stretching makes you more limber and helps improve circulation. I also highly recommend a book called "*Stretching*" by Bob Anderson. It describes ways to stretch all the muscle groups at many levels of difficulty and is well illustrated.

Examples to improve flexibility, balance and strength are TaiChi, Qi Gong, Yoga, Callenetics and Pilates. There are excellent videotapes available to help you start any one of these programs.

Do your stretching exercises as part of your final cooldown, after the aerobics and strength training. Stretching at the end of your workout when your muscles are warmed up helps prevent injuries. It also helps relax the muscles that are "tight" from your aerobic activity. Don't skimp on this area of your fitness program—your body will thank you!

Measuring Improvements

Remember that I said earlier you may not see loss of a lot of pounds on the scale, because you are replacing lightweight fat with heavier, denser muscle mass.

What you will see, though, is that your clothes fit better. You will notice that you are sleeping better, and awakening refreshed. Your resting pulse will start to decrease, another good sign of an improving fitness level.

Objective measures of your progress should be tracked in a chart that you keep in your health notebook. These include body measurements, BMI, body composition, Waist-to-Hip ratio, resting pulse, (and if you insist) your weight. But you only need to check these once a month.

As your fitness improves, you may need to increase the intensity of your aerobic training to stay in your THR range because you can do more work with less effort. This happens because your heart muscle has become stronger with exercise, it pumps more blood each time it beats, and your resting heart rate gets lower. This is a positive effect of exercise training and becoming more fit.

Adjust your workout routine to a higher intensity that will increase fat burning and maximize weight loss. You can do that very simply in several ways:

- Gradually increase your frequency of exercise
- Gradually increase your duration of exercise
- Increase the intensity of your exercise; for example, go from 60% to 75% of your predicted max heart rate (PMHR). For effective fat-burning, keep the intensity about in the middle of your predicted THR.

For example, if you are walking, now start swinging your arms more, or add some small hand weights, or try race walking, or find a hillier course. If you are doing your walking on a treadmill you can start gradually increasing the incline or the speed. Monitor your heart rate and stay in your THR range.

The Good News

Exercise and healthy eating need to become your cornerstones of managing PCOS. Neither is a quick fix that you stop when you lose a few pounds. They need to become your way of life, just like sleeping, breathing and drinking plenty of water.

The reason they are both so important is that they help you normalize body weight and lose excess fat. Loss of excess body fat is a specific way to improve PCOS.

For example, losing just 5–10% of your current body weight can achieve the following benefits:

- Decrease insulin resistance and excess insulin production
- Reduce excess androgens
- Reduce excess body hair
- Restore spontaneous ovulation
- Improve energy, mood and sleep

The good news is that once healthy eating and exercise become a habit, it will be easier to maintain your program than it was to start. When you start to get discouraged or bored or tired of exercising, or you want to overdo it with sweets, just remind yourself of how sluggish and lethargic you felt before you started your healthier program. If you have to miss for a day or so, don't take too long a break or you may not get back to it!

GO FOR IT! You deserve to feel better, and have a more fit body!

I know that if I do not do my pool exercises every day, or if I get too far off track with my healthy meal plans, I will pay for it in more neck and back pain, more stiffness, and feeling really sluggish. Since I don't like being in pain, I get in the pool every day and do my workout. I choose to exercise so I can continue feeling good, have the energy I want to do my work and enjoy activities I love!

Chapter 13

The Long Range—What About Menopause?

Does PCOS ever end?

PCOS has so many endocrine and metabolic effects that it isn't surprising that it can also have an enormous impact on the health risks women face with menopause and our later years. Untreated, PCOS doesn't just "go away" as we get older.

In fact, the health problems it causes—such as high blood pressure, high cholesterol, high triglycerides, insulin resistance, and others—usually get worse as we age.

Women *without* PCOS face a rising incidence of these problems after menopause, so you can imagine what the impact of PCOS can be when added to the changes that occur with age and menopause.

For women with PCOS, menopause is a time when you need to be even more aware of the potential health risks you face, and the benefits of appropriate hormone therapy, and balanced information about risks. You don't need the scare tactics and misinformation about hormones that is so rampant today.

My goal in this chapter is to give you straight talk about the benefits and risks based on the good science from international studies, and options to use to help you feel better now and improve your health for many years ahead.

> PCOS— affects more than just the ovaries. It is not something you outgrow when you reach menopause

Current research shows that there is a "window of opportunity" early in the menopause transition for hormone therapy to prevent damage to various tissues and organs.

PCOS is— a health problem you *manage* your whole life, not one that is *cured.*

Once this window of time is past, however, hormone therapy doesn't reverse damages that have occurred. We saw this clearly with results from the Women's Heath Initiative starting Premarin and Prempro 10–30 years after menopause in elderly women.

This chapter helps you understand that window of opportunity and how to better know when yours is at hand.

Understanding Hormone Headlines in the Aftermath of the Women's Health Initiative

The summer of 2002 brought a maelstrom of negative, frightening headlines about "hormones" and "hormone replacement therapy" (HRT). The headlines screamed that "estrogen" increased the risk of breast cancer. The newsmakers said HRT for menopause causes heart attacks and strokes, not prevents them.

The REAL Facts There are many well-studied, options for FDA-approved, bioidentical (or "natural") forms of hormones available, many FDA-approved, with fewer negative effects.

The headlines have made women feel terrified about hormones our bodies make naturally our entire reproductive life. Women are now fearful of all hormones, afraid to consider birth control pills, or menopausal hormone therapy. Why suddenly such intense negative focus on "hormones?"

An explosion of alarming reports from the Women's Health Initiative (WHI) and Heart and Estrogen/progestin Replacement Study (HERS) hit the media beginning in the summer of 2002. Each of these randomized clinical trials (RCT) used only one form of estrogen—Premarin—derived from the urine of pregnant horses, and a synthetic progestin—Provera—both hormones that are foreign to the human body, and not at all identical to anything we ever made naturally. This point is rarely mentioned in media coverage.

Why does damage found with one non-human horse hormone product get applied to all hormone preparations, even though they are chemically as different as night and day? We don't see that happening in any other field of medicine, or with any other class of medications. *But it did happen with women's hormones. And there's the tragedy that affects so many women now.*

The WHI was presented in the press as a study of "healthy" menopausal women. But these women in the study population *were not really healthy*—they just didn't have *symptoms* of menopause! Their average age was about 64 years, and almost 30% were over 70. This is 10–25 years *later* than most menopausal hormone therapies are started.

Healthy? Only in America would we call a group with these characteristics "healthy"—consider these statistics from the WHI study data:

- 35% of the women were already being treated for high blood pressure
- 35% were significantly overweight
- another 34% were obese *by the medical definition, making a total of 69% of the entire study group having an abnormal Body Mass Index, which affects all kinds of health risks from breast cancer to cardiovascular disease*
- 12.5% had high enough cholesterol to require medication
- 16% had a family history of breast cancer
- 4% had diabetes.
- *40% were former smokers, 10% continued to smoke cigarettes during the study*

These women were "typical" Americans, but certainly were not "healthy."

In the words of Professor A. R. Genazzani, a world-renown physician researcher and the President of the International Society of Gynecological Endocrinology, "We would never choose that kind of combination

The REAL Facts
These women, like the older women in the HERS study, already had evidence of heart disease, high cholesterol and high blood pressure.

REAL Risk
A woman's risk of hip fracture is equal to her combined risk of breast, uterine and ovarian cancer.

(Prempro) for our elderly patients with those clinical characteristics."

The position paper of the *International Menopause Society*, published in September, 2002, concludes: "The WHI results, and particularly the data on cardiovascular disease risk, should only be related to the continuous combined treatment of 0.625 mg CEE (conjugated equine estrogens) together with 2.5 mg MPA (medroxy-progesterone acetate), prescribed to elderly, obese women with characteristics similar to those depicted in the WHI study." [parentheses explanations of terms mine—not in original quote] Full reference in Appendix.

The REAL Facts

The WHI authors indicated that the average risk in an individual woman is 0.1% per year for breast cancer or heart attacks. You probably never saw that number either. Your risk of having a car accident is far greater than your risk of getting breast cancer. Have you stopped driving your car?

In fact, the above comments and WHI findings, validate concerns I have been raising about Premarin and Prempro in my previous books and medical articles for more than a decade.

The press shouted there was a 26% increase in risk of breast cancer. What they didn't say was that the statistical increase was minute: of 10,000 women taking Prempro, *only 8 more would develop breast cancer than women not taking Prempro.*

Most women, and even most doctors, still don't know that the WHI data re-analysis showed no statistical difference between breast cancer rates in the Prempro group and the placebo group. I think that is a disgrace professionally, and a national tragedy for women who need reliable information to make informed health care choices.

The alarmist headlines made it appear that more women *died* taking hormones. *This was not so.* Articles neglected to say that the *death rate* from breast cancer or heart disease was not increased in the WHI Prempro group. They also neglected to say that in the estrogen-only group of the WHI, there were *fewer* breast cancers than in the placebo group.

Why don't you get a full picture of the studies? Why

are the negative results trumpeted and crucial positive findings downplayed or ignored? The focus on fear of breast cancer appears to sell newspapers and magazines. That same fear is also used to sell everything from herbs and soy supplements to new and expensive "designer estrogen" prescription products.

Instead of balanced information, we are bombarded with poorly researched and hastily presented stories with a biased focus on breast cancer to the exclusion of other serious disorders—osteoporosis, diabetes, and cardiovascular disease are prime examples—that kill many times more women every year.

Fact Check:

- 90,000 women per year die of diabetes-related complications, twice the number who die of breast cancer
- 450,000 women per year die of cardiovascular disease, more than TEN times the number who die of breast cancer
- Women suffer 1.5 million osteoporotic-related fractures per year, about 7.5 times the number of women who are diagnosed with breast cancer per year.

All you hear about is the slight increase in risk of breast cancer that may occur with some—not all—types of estrogen–progestin therapy after menopause. There are other links to breast cancer that are far more ominous such as obesity, alcohol and tobacco use, exposure to pesticides.

Researchers in Finland found that women with the highest lindane residues were 10 times more likely to have breast cancer than women with lower levels. An analysis of Connecticut women in 1992 showed levels of PCB, DDE and DDT in the breast tissue of breast cancer patients were 50–60% higher than in women without cancer.

And the ultimate irony— When all the cancer cases were checked by independent experts, (*adjudication*) they found that the differences in breast cancers between the hormone group and the placebo group were no longer statistically significant. **This point never made it to the lay press.**

You need sound facts about other factors in this hormone–breast cancer link before you "throw the baby out with the bath water" on prescription hormones.

My Philosophy and Recommendations

I use a science-based focus and the international research studies to form the basis for my clinical work and to strip away the myths and misconceptions surrounding hormones and hormone therapy for you to consider.

Common misconceptions include the following myths:

- hormones cause cancer
- all estrogens are the same
- all progestins are the same
- how you take them doesn't matter
- hot flashes and vaginal dryness are the only "true" symptoms of menopause (said by a male expert, of course!)
- The "cookie-cutter" approach works for all. One form of estrogen derived from pregnant horse's urine has been used in the United States for over 50 years for about 85% of all HRT prescriptions—in spite of prescription hormones bioidentical to those made by the ovaries approved in the US by the FDA since 1976. You wouldn't see 85% of men with heart disease given the same drug, and same dose.

Women are individuals, with individual body chemistries. Women vary in response to hormones just as they do with all other classes of medicines (and herbs) we use. Women desire, and must have, hormone options individually tailored to their needs for optimal response.

Bioidentical human forms of hormone products need to be used instead of "one-size-fits-all" horse-derived or synthetic progestins that have very different—and often negative—effects in the human body.

How do we determine the appropriate dose for you? We can measure hormone response with objective tests. The "gold standard" serum (blood) tests for hormone levels are reliable for management of infertility in younger women. We must apply these same reliable objective tests for management of midlife and menopausal hormone issues. Saliva tests and hair analysis simply are not reliable or adequate to make dosing decisions for the complexity of women's hormones.

One size does not fit all–dose matters! Doses need to be adjusted to the individual woman, not the insurance company, manufacturer or FDA "accepted" dose for all.

Some women may find that health measures check out fine and they don't need hormones at all. In that case, I suggest that you re-evaluate your picture in a year or two, and keep track of how your body is changing. The key is to intervene with positive action (hormones, other medication, etc.) *before more serious disease develops.*

Current recommendations are that hormones may be started when:

(1) symptoms appear and quality of life is diminished (regardless of age),

(2) when disease risks are identified,

(3) actual disease, such as osteopenia or osteoporosis, is present, or

(4) a combination of these issues.

Hormone Therapy: Options and Choices To Individualize Your Program

Different Estrogens, Different Effects

Our medical establishment and the media present "estrogen" and "Premarin" as the only option but it's not true. Premarin is only one brand of estrogen among many brands available. It is made from the urine of pregnant mares and contains a mixture of estrogens that the horse makes, but most are never found in a human female body!

Warning! All estrogens are not the same, and Premarin is not the only estrogen product available.

Sadly, most women in the United States do not know that we have had an FDA-approved bioidentical form of 17-beta estradiol available on the market, and covered by most health plans, since 1975.

Fact: Premarin only provides a small amount of the 17-beta estradiol that your body made before menopause

Fact:
Premarin is natural for the horse, but is *not* "natural" for your body.

That's right—a bioidentical estradiol for women available in the U.S. for more than 30 years! The brand is Estrace.

If you have PCOS, Premarin (and the Provera prescribed with it) often aggravates the weight problems and heart disease risks of PCOS, for a variety of reasons that I explain later, and as found in the WHI.

What are the Natural Human Estrogens?

Estradiol, Estrone, and Estriol as I defined these in Chapter 3. Here's a quick refresher:

17-beta Estradiol (E2), or just estradiol: our primary, biologically active, premenopausal estrogen that is the optimal "key" to activate our estrogen receptors and provide all the benefits we associate with "estrogen therapy."

Estrone (E1): made in the ovary and fat tissue; after menopause, the estrogen that is still made in fat tissue from the androgen, androstenedione; it is the one that is associated with higher risks of breast and uterine cancers. It is metabolically less active than E2, and is often already too high in women with PCOS.

Estriol (E3): the weakest estrogen, made in the placenta during pregnancy, not normally found in high levels in a non-pregnant woman. Many studies have shown it does not preserve bone, heart or brain benefits seen with E2. There really is little reason to use this for menopause hormone therapy, and newer research suggests it may actually be one of the estrogens that *increases* breast cancer risk rather than being protective as John Lee and others claimed.

Product Options for Estradiol (E2)

There are several brands of 17 beta-estradiol commercially available in this country, and all of these brands use a form of estradiol that is derived from soybean or wild yam building block molecules and purified in the laboratory to make *the identical molecule made by our ovary* before menopause.

Comparative studies that have been done show that the bioidentical human form of 17-beta estradiol is more easily tolerated, with fewer side effects and better positive effects on glucose regulation, insulin sensitivity, muscle and connective tissue, brain function, pain regulation, and bone markers.

Keep in mind that 17-beta estradiol is what your ovary made before menopause, and what keeps your body's cellular machinery working at optimal effectiveness. When you think about hormone replenishment for the optimal metabolism, energy and well-being, think about restoring the "key" that your body always had.

FDA-approved 17-beta estradiol brands in the United States:

These are bio-identical options—

- Estrace tablets and vaginal cream (FDA approved in 1975),
- Gynodiol tablets and generic estradiol tablets
- Climara, Vivelle, Vivelle DOT, Estraderm, and generic transdermal patches (all come in multiple strengths)
- Estrasorb transdermal lotion
- Estrogel transdermal gel
- Femring (vaginal ring for systemic estradiol)
- Estring (vaginal ring for topical vaginal estradiol)
- Vagifem vaginal tablets

Not true! Some claim "bio-identical" hormones are only available from compounding pharmacies. Not so!

FDA-approved combination products (17-beta estradiol with a progestin):

- Activella tablets
- Angelique tablets
- Climara PRO patch
- Combi-patch
- Ortho Prefest tablets

In addition to these FDA-approved branded products,

estradiol USP is available for various generic products. Not all are as reliable as the brands, however, so be aware of this problem. Estradiol USP is also used by compounding pharmacists in making tablets, creams, gels, and injections in other dose strengths than are available in the FDA-approved products. Compounded hormones are not FDA-approved.

Attention!
What do obesity, alcohol and Premarin have in common related to breast cancer? They all cause higher than normal levels of estrone.

Products Delivering Primarily Estrone (E1): Caution!

There are a number of commercial products that deliver mainly estrone. I do not recommend these if you have PCOS and/or have gained a lot of weight. Overweight women already have higher estrone relative to estradiol, so using an estrone product just makes this imbalance worse and makes your metabolism even more sluggish.

I think women with PCOS should avoid the estrogen products that give high levels of estrone and relatively little of the 17-beta estradiol such as:

- Premarin, PremPro and PremPhase (combined horse estrogens with synthetic progestin)
- Estratab
- Estratest (estrone and others with <u>methyl</u> testosterone
- Cenestin
- Menest, Ogen, Ortho-Est

Estriol (E3) The Pregnancy Estrogen:

Estriol has been studied extensively in Europe over several decades. It really isn't the "forgotten estrogen" as some books claim; it just isn't used much because many well-done studies from a variety of countries have clearly shown that it doesn't provide the degree of protective effects on bone, heart, brain, and nerves as does 17-beta estradiol. Consequently, there are no FDA-approved estriol products in the United States.

Since menopause is not a time you are planning to be pregnant, taking estriol doesn't make much sense, and could be harmful.

Some authors claim estriol prevents breast cancer, but no protective effect of E3 has been found in reputable medical studies, other than the known effect of full-term pregnancy prior to age 30 in reducing breast cancer risk. Whatever role estriol plays in reducing breast cancer risk does not appear to be an independent effect of estriol, but seems to occur along with other breast changes that occur with a full-term pregnancy before age 30.

Many studies have demonstrated that estriol does not improve sleep, in contrast to what has been shown with 17-beta estradiol. Estriol also does not have significant beneficial effects for improving pain, memory, mood, and the "brain fog" symptoms that are so common in mid-life and are clearly helped by estradiol. I have treated a lot of women who had been put on estriol and suffered from "brain crash" when it didn't work as well as estradiol on these crucial brain pathways. Women who use estriol have it made by compounding pharmacists. For some women, estriol relieves milder symptoms (vaginal dryness, mild hot flashes, for example).

Fact

If someone tells you that your estriol level is low, that's a normal finding if you are not pregnant.

Don't be misled by "Natural hormone" practitioners who use estriol and tell you it is "safer." Studies from England over the past 20 years showed that higher doses of estriol needed to give symptom relief will also stimulate the endometrium of the uterus to thicken just as other estrogens do. Thus, if you take enough estriol to really help your symptoms, you have to still watch for endometrial thickening, heavy bleeding and hyperplasia just as you would if you took any of the estradiol products.

New research has also found that estriol is one of the estrogens on the "bad" metabolic pathway that increases risk of breast cancer. This is another reason not to depend on estriol for hormone benefits after menopause.

Plant Estrogens (Phytoestrogens):

These are estrogenic compounds found in several hundred different plants, including soybeans, red clover, grains, and many others. The phytoestrogens are biologically weaker than the native human estrogens and don't have the same effects at the human estrogen receptors as our own estradiol.

Fact:
Taking phyto-estrogen supplements does not provide the critically necessary 17-beta estradiol.

Some of the phytoestrogens are "activators" (agonists) and some are "blockers" (antagonists), and some have mixed agonist–antagonist effects. These different actions are dose- and concentration-related, and occur due to small chemical changes in molecular arrangements.

All of the phytoestrogen precursors require chemical conversion in the laboratory to make the bioidentical human form of 17-beta estradiol because the human body does not have the enzymes needed for these changes.

Fact Check:
Ginseng is recommended as a "natural" estrogen. Ginseng gives little estrogenic effect, and can cause high blood pressure, insomnia, anxiety, and agitation if taken in large amounts.

These differences help explain an apparent discrepancy: in China and Japan, where diets are high in phytoestrogens, women do not typically describe hot flashes, but they do continue to have bone loss and cognitive decline after menopause. Japanese researchers report a serious problem with osteoporosis in Japan; and their studies show that phytoestrogens alone do not provide enough estrogen effect to protect against osteoporosis.

Phytoestrogens are less potent than 17-beta estradiol, but because the blood concentrations are so much higher when today's isoflavone supplements are used, it is quite easy to "overwhelm" the tiny concentration of estradiol. By competing with your body estradiol at cellular receptors, these high concentrations of iso-flavone phytoestrogens can interfere with action or production of your own body estradiol, progesterone and testosterone.

Synthetic Estrogens—Chemically Different Options

All of these estrogens have slightly different chemical structures and are more potent than ovarian estrogens. As a result, they have somewhat different beneficial effects as well as side effects.

Ethinyl Estradiol (EE): The most common form of estrogen found in the birth control pills that are widely used to help relieve the symptoms of PCOS and in perimenopausal women who may need better control of irregular cycles, symptoms, and erratic bleeding.

BCP are not widely used in the U.S. for postmenopausal HRT because they provide more estrogen effect than is generally needed after a woman reaches menopause. But, EE is found in a new menopause product, Femhrt, in a much lower dose than in birth control pills.

The problem with Femhrt is that it has as much progestin as many birth control pills (1 mg norethindrone), but so little estrogen that women in our practice who tried it didn't like the way they felt. Plus, they gained more weight because the high progestin content made them so hungry!

Estradiol valerate: a chemically different estrogen, more potent than 17-beta estradiol, and rarely used in the U.S. for hormone therapy. It is used commonly overseas for postmenopausal ERT in oral and intramuscular injectable forms.

Ogen (piperazine estrone sulfate): a synthetic estrone that is chemically similar to, but not exactly the same as, human estrone. If you have PCOS, using a product with more estrone simply doesn't make sense to me when what you need is estradiol.

Women using Ogen often tell me they have some residual symptoms. This is due to the lower amount of estradiol and the piperazine chemical ring part of the molecule. I have found that this chemical difference makes Ogen more likely to aggravate muscle and bladder pain in menopausal women.

Non-Human, Mixed Estrogens: More Chemical Differences

Cenestin: a plant-derived estrogen product formulated to have the same mixed estrogens found in Premarin;

> **Proven:** Double-blind, placebo-controlled, prospective studies have found that phyto-estrogens were no more effective than placebo for controlling hot flashes.

Fact:
Methyl testosterone was banned by the German Endocrine Society in the 1980s as too dangerous to use for hormone therapy in men.

In an ironic twist,
Methyl testosterone is still used for women's menopause therapy in the United States, while the FDA denied approval for a safer bioidentical form of testosterone in a patch delivery system.

delivers predominately estrone but has many other estrogenic components *not normally found in human females.* I find women don't get very good sympton relief with Cenestin.

Premarin: conjugated equine estrogens derived from pregnant mares urine; *delivers high levels of estrogens not found in the human body,* plus higher levels of estrone and very little 17-beta estradiol. Prem-Pro and PremPhase contain the horse estrogens plus synthetic MPA, or medroxyprogesterone acetate (also called Provera).

Estratab: esterified estrogens, similar to Premarin, plant-derived; delivers primarily estrone. **Estratest:** esterified estrogens plus methyl testosterone, a very potent synthetic testosterone. **Methyl testosterone** has been found to cause liver damage and increased risk of liver cancer due to the added methyl group.

Why *Horse* Estrogens?

In the past, we did not have a way to give estrogen orally, because it would be broken down and lost in the digestive process before getting into the bloodstream. About 65 years ago, scientists developed a way to extract estrogens from the urine of pregnant mares, purify the extract containing "conjugated equine estrogens" (CEE), and then coat the estrogens in a matrix of binders (called enteric coating) that allowed the tablet to survive digestion in the stomach, reach the small intestine, be absorbed into the bloodstream, and then produce an estrogenic effect on the body organs.

This product, Premarin (PREgnant MARes urINe), has been the primary type of estrogen used in the United States ever since, accounting for about 85 to 90 percent of the prescriptions written for estrogen in the United States.

An oral dose of Premarin produces low blood levels of the two primary estrogens also found in humans, estradiol and estrone, but it also produces high blood levels of equine estrogens native to horses, also called equilin estrogens.

A typical oral dose of 0.625 mg Premarin produces most of the total circulating estrogens as equilin compounds or estrones; only about 0.5% of the total estrogen present is the estradiol found in humans according to published data from the manufacturer.

Three decades ago (late 1970s, early 1980s), two leading British menopause researchers, Drs. Whitehead and Campbell, did studies of the potencies of the different types of estrogens and the effects of the various estrogens on different organs in the body. Their work raised some serious issues about adverse effects of horse-derived estrogens for women, but most of their questions and concerns have been ignored in the United States. What are the concerns they and others have raised?

(1) Conjugated equine estrogens in Premarin are about three times more potent in stimulating the liver production of renin substrate, which is used to make angiotensin in the body, a factor that causes increased blood pressure. Estrace and Ogen, two other estrogens used in Campbell and Whitehead's work study, did not show this elevation of renin substrate, and didn't have the tendency to cause high blood pressure that was seen with Premarin. If you have PCOS and already have high blood pressure, this is an important difference.

(2) Premarin was more likely to lead to elevated triglycerides than the human estradiol, particularly when estradiol was used in patch form and bypassed the liver "first-pass" metabolism. This is also important for women with PCOS who tend to already have high triglycerides.

(3) Other important differences, particularly relevant for overweight women, emerged from the Nurses Health Study. This study reported an increased risk of breast cancer in women on long duration estrogen. But what the news articles failed to tell you was that these women were primarily taking Premarin, and *the Premarin users who also drank alcohol regularly were the ones who had the increase in breast cancer risk.*

Disadvantages of Horse-derived Estrogens

We know several important things about the horse-derived estrogens:

(1) equine estrogens stay in the human body much longer than our natural estradiol, anywhere from 8–14 weeks after the last dose;

(2) equine estrogens have stronger "attachment strength" (affinity) for our estradiol receptors (especially the breasts, where estrogens may concentrate in the fat tissue), and

(3) equine estrogens give much higher total blood level of estrogens following an oral dose of Premarin than is seen with a comparable dose of Estrace. All of these problems are made worse when women have high estrone due to excess body fat.

(4) The WHI found that oral Premarin and PremPro increased risks of blood clots and stroke. This is the opposite of studies showing *no such increased risk with non-oral estradiol.*

Development of Bioidentical Estradiol

In 1976, the FDA approved a new product (brand: Estrace) as a form of native human estrogen, *micronized 17-beta-estradiol* derived from soybeans.

Micronization means making the molecule particles small enough that they can be rapidly absorbed into the bloodstream before being broken down by digestive acids and the liver. Many recent studies have shown that the smaller the particle size, the better the absorption and the more reliable the blood levels obtained. Micronization is used to make many therapeutic medications and has been particularly helpful in developing native human forms of estradiol (estrogen), progesterone, and testosterone because these hormones typically were inactivated or destroyed by digestion when taken orally.

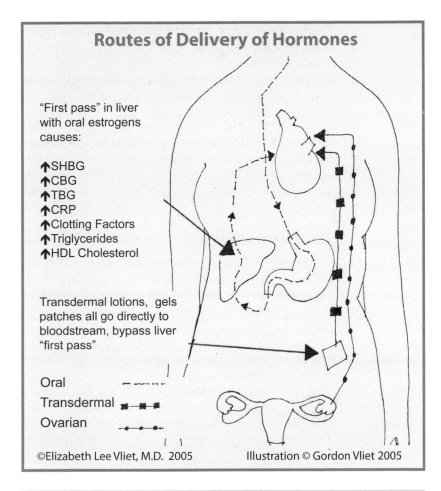

Routes of Delivery of Hormones

"First pass" in liver with oral estrogens causes:

↑SHBG
↑CBG
↑TBG
↑CRP
↑Clotting Factors
↑Triglycerides
↑HDL Cholesterol

Transdermal lotions, gels patches all go directly to bloodstream, bypass liver "first pass"

Oral
Transdermal
Ovarian

©Elizabeth Lee Vliet, M.D. 2005   Illustration © Gordon Vliet 2005

Advantages and Disadvantages of Various Delivery Systems

Oral Estrogens

Various 17-beta estradiol products deliver the identical estrogen made in our body. Oral delivery has some pluses and some minuses. If you have a very low level of HDL, you may want the boost of having the oral estrogen stimulate the liver to make more HDL. This is a pharmacologic, or drug-like, effect of estrogen first going through the liver. For women who have high total cholesterol and low HDL, however, an oral form of estradiol provides more decrease in total cholesterol and a more significant increase in HDL.

Patches, creams and gels give you the beneficial physiological (natural) effect of estradiol to maintain the normal level of HDL cholesterol, they just don't give you that rapid, extra liver stimulation to make more HDL. The patch may be all that is needed for women who have a normal cholesterol profile.

Oral estrogens in some women may lead to higher blood pressure, higher triglycerides, higher estrone and more likelihood of gallstones *if you have a predisposition to those problems*. Otherwise, which form you use—pills or patches—becomes a matter of personal preference.

Get Balanced
About 24% of hip fracture patients over age 50 die in the year following their fracture.

Transdermal Estradiol: Patches, Lotion, Gel Options

Transdermal estradiol patches deliver the human 17-beta estradiol in a way that is the most "natural" of all. The estradiol is absorbed through the skin, directly into the bloodstream, similar to the ovarian process before menopause. Direct delivery to the bloodstream bypasses the "first pass" metabolism in the liver that breaks down estradiol and increases the unwanted estrone.

The estradiol patches stick to the skin and stay in place for several days for the hormones to be slowly absorbed. Each brand of patch lasts for a slightly different period of time. Women metabolize the hormones at different rates, so it may take a little experimenting to find the patch change schedule that is right for you.

Advantages of the Patch, especially if you have PCOS:

1) patches keep blood levels of estradiol fairly steady, similar to the hormone production by the ovary (helpful for women with blood pressure or "hormonal" headache problems);

2) estradiol by patch gives better improvement in glucose control and insulin sensitivity than oral estrogens

3) patches do not lead to further elevation of estrone (as seen with oral forms) since the estradiol bypasses the liver "first pass";

4) estradiol in a patch is less likely to be adversely affected by other medications, since the estradiol is not metabolized first in the liver

5) transdermal delivery of estradiol does not elevate triglycerides as occurs in some women taking oral estrogens

6) estradiol by patch is less likely to cause gallstones

7) patches maintain benefits of estradiol on HDL to LDL cholesterol even though this form of estradiol delivery doesn't raise HDL as rapidly or quite as high as oral estrogens.

8) transdermal estradiol does not increase renin, CRP, TBG, CBG, SHBG, or some clotting factors such as oral estrogens can.

There really are only two drawbacks to this form of estradiol:

1) the skin irritation from the adhesive may bother some women, although adhesives vary by manufacturer, so experiment with different brands;

2) some women don't like the cosmetic appearance of having a patch on their body.

Creams, Gels, Injections and Implants (Pellets)

All of these delivery methods bypass the liver "first-pass," so they will have similar results and benefits as I outlined for the patch. Their main drawback, as a group, is that the stability in estradiol level is not as good as with the pills and patches. Creams and gels may rise too fast and wear off too quickly for some women, leading to more symptoms from the fluctuations in estradiol blood levels. Other than that problem, these can be good options.

Injections and implants, in the usual way they are used, tend to cause excessively high levels at the outset and then wear off unpredictably, leaving you again feeling like you are on a roller coaster ride. While I have used all of these approaches, they are a little more tricky to stabilize and keep estradiol even and consistent each day. Sometimes, what I find works best is a combination of the above options. The key is finding what gives the best results for each individual women and not being locked in to any one approach.

PROGESTERONE and PROGESTINS

There are several terms that many women find confusing.

Attention:

If you don't have a uterus any longer, progesterone's metabolic effects aren't needed after menopause when you are not trying to be pregnant.

Progestogen is the broad term used to describe any substance that has chemical effects to prepare the body for sustaining a pregnancy, called "progestational" activity.

Progesterone is a biologically natural "progestogen" produced by the corpus luteum (egg released from the ovary) before menopause, by the placenta during pregnancy, and to a much smaller extent, by the adrenal gland. Progesterone acts to help prepare the mother's body to sustain a pregnancy by overseeing a number of metabolic effects in the mother's body that will help her carry the baby full-term.

If you have a uterus after menopause, you need progesterone opposing estrogen effects on the uterine lining to prevent hyperplasia and possible development of cancer of the uterine lining.

Progestin is the term that generally refers to chemical compounds made in the laboratory that have properties similar to progesterone, but they have a different molecular structure and are more potent than natural progesterone.

Progestins are members of the larger group of progestogens because they do have progestational ("pro-pregnancy") activity, but they are not compounds normally found in the human body. Technically, progesterone itself is a "natural" progestin, but we don't usually mean "natural progesterone" when we use the term progestin.

Progestins may be made in the laboratory using the natural hormones progesterone or testosterone as the basic building block. Each of the chemically different progestins has slightly different properties, depending on whether progesterone itself or testosterone is used as a starting point, and depending on what chemical modifications are made. Therefore, each type of progestin has slightly different benefits and side effects.

Since all of the synthetic progestins are significantly more potent than progesterone itself, they are used in much lower doses than are needed for progesterone. As a result of their potency and their chemical differences, progestins can produce desirable effects that are beneficial, or they can cause bothersome side effects.

Why even use the synthetic progestins if they tend to cause so many side effects? There are some medical situations, such as suppression of fibroids or endometriosis or ovarian cysts, when the more potent synthetic progestins are needed. And, some women actually feel better on the synthetic ones!

Development of Bio-Identical Progesterone

Progesterone USP is the form of natural progesterone made in a laboratory from "building block" molecules (disogenin, diascorea and others) found in wild yams and soybeans. These plant precursors are chemically different from progesterone.

The yam and soy "building block" chemicals have to be changed in the laboratory in a series of steps to make the bioidentical molecule of progesterone that can be biologically active in the body. Our bodies do not have the enzymes to make progesterone from simply consuming yams and soybeans or using creams with these precursors in them.

This synthesized progesterone is then purified to meet FDA standards, and is now called USP (or pharmaceutical grade) progesterone.

USP progesterone is used by pharmaceutical companies

to make the FDA-approved commercial products: tablets (Prometrium), and vaginal gel (Crinone and Prochieve) used in menopausal hormone therapy and for infertility patients. USP progesterone is also used by compounding pharmacists to make individual prescriptions of tablets, suppositories and creams for patients.

USP progesterone is the active form of the hormone that is commonly added to "wild yam" creams. When given in the correct dose and schedule for hormone therapy regimens, progesterone generally has fewer unpleasant side effects than a synthetic progestin like Provera.

For many years, Progesterone in oil was available in the U.S. in injectable form made by Upjohn, the company that also makes Provera and Depo-Provera. The injectable form of progesterone USP in oil has been widely used by gynecologists for years to treat bleeding problems, and I was taught to use it more than 25 years ago while in medical school. So natural progesterone really isn't an overlooked hormone or a new idea, but since most women don't want to get an injection on a regular basis, this form of progesterone has not been widely used for menopause therapy.

Progesterone wasn't well-enough absorbed orally to be a reliable way to use it for uterine cancer prevention until the process of micronization (ability to make the hormone particles smaller) was developed in the 1970s. This made it possible to make oral forms more reliable.

Progesterone as individually made prescriptions tended to cost a lot more than the commercial products. In addition, each compounding pharmacy has its own formula, making it difficult for doctors to trust the reliability of compounded products.

Now that we have FDA-approved commercial products that are standardized in the manufacturing process, have reliable quality control, and are covered by most insurance plans, more and more physicians are now using these progesterone products for menopause regimens.

I have used natural micronized progesterone in my

women's health practice with a great deal of success. I have learned a lot over the years about the nuances of dose, side effect changes based on how it is given (tablets, suppositories, prescription creams, injectable) and ways of working with progesterone to create individualized regimens and fewer side effects for my patients with all kinds of hormone problems.

This 53-year-old woman had been having very bothersome side effects of depression, weight gain, lethargy, and "all that PMS feeling again" with the Provera phase of her HRT, until I changed her to natural progesterone with the Estrace:

> "I'm feeling great! I am so pleased with the changes and this combination. I'm floored by all of this. I can't believe the difference in how I feel taking the natural progesterone, it's nothing like what I felt on the Provera. I don't feel so depressed and slowed down like I did. I used to hate those 14 days on Provera, and sometimes I didn't even take it. I didn't want to tell my doctor, but I just didn't like how I felt on the Provera. I'm thrilled, the natural progesterone worked like clockwork, and my period started within 24 hours of stopping the progesterone. It was like a normal period, no pain or any problems."

If the dose or type of oil base (peanut) or dyes in Prometrium cause problems for some women, then we still have the option of micronized progesterone obtained from independent pharmacists who compound the prescription individually for patients based on the physician's prescribed amount.

Even with natural progesterone, there are still some women who simply aren't able to tolerate any progestogen, synthetic or natural. Women who are markedly sensitive to progesterone or progestins may experience intolerable degrees of depression, loss of libido, pain flares, headaches, lethargy, bloating, breast tenderness and weight gain. Changing from an oral form to a vaginal form can help reduce such side effects.

Why Take Progesterone or a Progestin?

The primary reason any progestin (synthetic or natural) is added to a menopausal hormone regimen is to oppose estrogen effects on the lining of the uterus and reduce the risk of endometrial cancer in women who have a uterus.

Adding a progestogen (synthetic progestin or natural progesterone) stops the endometrium from growing and allows it to be shed as a "withdrawal bleeding" when the progestogen is stopped. Shedding the uterine lining at regular intervals, whether monthly or every couple of months, protects against the buildup of endometrium that can later lead to malignant changes.

Since all progestins, including natural progesterone, reduce the benefits of estrogen, increase the risk of breast cancer over that of estrogen alone, and also have their own side effects, most physicians who understand the metabolic effects of progesterone/progestins don't recommend their routine use if you no longer have a uterus.

Take Note
If you have had a hysterectomy, you no longer have a uterine lining to become cancerous and you don't need a progestin or natural progesterone added to hormone therapy.

Types of Progestins

Provera (generic name: medroxyprogesterone acetate, or MPA) is the most commonly used synthetic progestin in the U.S. for menopause therapy, although it was never actually approved by the F.D.A. for that purpose. Other brand names for MPA include Cyrin, and Amen. MPA was originally approved by the FDA in the 1960s for contraceptive use under the brand name Depo-Provera and has since been used to treat abnormal uterine bleeding and some types of amenorrhea.

In more recent years, MPA and other progestins have been used for protection of the uterine lining in menopausal regimens. MPA is derived from progesterone, and is more progestational and less androgenic than progestins derived from testosterone.

In the past, the dose of Provera has typically been 10 mg. I find that is too much for most women, and produces an unacceptable degree of unpleasant bloating, breast tenderness, feelings of lethargy and depressed mood; or as some women tell me, "I feel like all that awful PMS has come back again."

The more common recommendation today is 5 mg of Provera or equivalent amount of another progestin or natural progesterone. At the International Menopause Society conferences for the past few years, more and more menopause specialists are recognizing the problems with the higher doses of the synthetic progestins and are urging physicians to use lower amounts or change to natural progesterone.

Another group of progestins, such as norethindrone (brand names: Aygestin, Micronor, Nor-QD, Norlutate,) are derived from the male hormone 19-nor-testosterone, and as a result they have more androgenic effects similar to testosterone in addition to their progestational activity. This group of progestins is often used when women are experiencing a loss of libido since they have less libido-robbing effects than Provera or other progestational progestins.

My patients tell me that the androgenic progestins typically cause less bloating, breast tenderness, weight gain and depression than Provera and other brands of MPA. The more androgenic progestins may not be the best choice for women with high cholesterol and low HDL, particularly in the high doses that have been used in the past. But the more androgenic progestins tend to have fewer depression-causing side effects than Provera-type progestins.

Another new combination product that has worked well for many of my patients is Activella, which contains 1 mg 17-beta estradiol and 0.5 mg norethindrone. This estrogen–progestin ratio is better than most of the other combination products on the market, and it is the natural human form of estradiol. We have seen *less bleeding* and spotting with this product compared to PremPro, Combi-patch, and Femhrt. Women also

Notice
All of the progestins and natural progesterone can cause unwanted side effects, particularly if doses are too high relative to estradiol. The trick is to find the type and dose that works best for you.

tell us that they don't have as much bloating, breast tenderness and weight gain with Activella as they do with the other combination products.

Side Effects to consider

Synthetic progestins, whether in birth control pills or given in postmenopause, are the most common cause of unpleasant side effects associated with "hormone therapy": increased ("ravenous") appetite, weight gain, fluid retention, irritable mood, depressed mood, headaches, decreased energy, bloating, breast tenderness, loss of libido, among others.

Important Fact: There is evidence from the WHI that estrogen alone is safer than estrogen plus progestin for breast cancer risk. If you do not have a uterus, there are many reasons to avoid taking progesterone /progestins.

To minimize the negative effects, it is important to consider:

1) the relative balance of progestational and androgenic activity,

2) the balance of progestin relative to estrogen in the preparation

3) the route of delivery

If you have PCOS and a weight problem, and have had a hysterectomy, then I would strongly urge you NOT to add progesterone (pills, patches, creams or gels—either prescription or over-the-counter) to your therapy.

Why complicate the problems of PCOS if you no longer need to protect the uterine lining from developing hyperplasia or cancer?

Route of Delivery

How you take progestin is another factor that will influence side effects. Oral progestins or progesterone are more likely to cause depression, fatigue, headaches and increased appetite because of the compounds that are made by the liver in the "first-pass" metabolism.

If you take progesterone or progestins vaginally or as a patch, you avoid this first-pass through the liver, and don't have these depressant compounds made the same way. Side effects tend to be much less when you use a

---

FDA-approved Products for Progesterone and Progestin—Used for HRT in Menopause

- ❧ Micronized progesterone: Prometrium, Crinone or Prochieve
- ❧ Androgenic progestins: Norethindrone: Micronor, Aygestin; Levonorgestrel: Mirena IUD
- ❧ Anti-androgen progestin: Drospirenone: Angelique
- ❧ Progestational progestins: Medroxyprogesterone acetate: Provera, Cycrin, Amen, DepoProvera
- ❧ Combination products (estrogen and progestin): Activella, Combi-patch, Climara PRO, Ortho Prefest, Femhrt

©Elizabeth Lee Vliet, MD 2001-2005

---

reliable, non-oral form. You may have to try different products to see what works for you.

A progestin-containing IUD is another option to explore if you have gained a lot of weight and have trouble with increased appetite when you take the progestin or progesterone. The IUD with progestin releases a small amount of progestin daily directly to the lining of the uterus, and there is very little progestin absorbed into the total body circulation.

The dose of progestin is smaller because it is delivered directly to the uterine lining. These two reasons are why it does not have the usual unwanted side effects of progestin or progesterone taken orally or transdermally.

Mirena and Progestasert are two intrauterine progestin-delivery systems approved in the U.S. for contraception. But this option is widely used overseas for perimenopausal women to reduce bleeding and cramping, and for a low dose progestin option for menopause.

A number of studies have shown that these products deliver enough progestin to effectively suppress the build-up of the uterine lining. If you have a uterus and want to continue estrogen but nothing else has worked to give you a progestin you could take, you may want to ask your doctor about Mirena or Progestasert.

To Bleed or Not to Bleed with Progestins

If you are on a cyclic progesterone or progestin regimen, when you stop the progestin each month, you will have some degree of menstrual-type "withdrawal" bleeding. This is what you want to have happen in order to reduce the endometrial cancer risk by getting rid of the lining of the uterus. Current research has shown that it is sufficient to reduce endometrial cancer risk if you cycle the progesterone or progestin every other month or even every third month.

On the other hand, if you don't like having menstrual-type flow after menopause, you may choose to take a progestin every day. Daily use suppresses the lining and stops bleeding in about 80 percent of women after about six months of continuous progestin use. The other 20% of women taking progestin daily tend to continue to have annoying, erratic bleeding and spotting. If you fall in this last group, you may want to talk with your doctor about going back to a cycling regimen so that you have more predictable bleeding patterns.

The longer you are on hormone therapy, what characteristically happens is that the uterine lining does not build up as much as it did earlier in your life so the actual flow is shorter and lighter.

Taking estrogen and progestin every day can work well, unless you are a woman with significant heart disease, diabetes or elevated blood pressure or triglycerides, or a history of headaches or fibromyalgia or depression. The daily progestins tend to make these conditions worse.

We still have a lot of unanswered questions about the continuous–combined regimen, including potential negative effects on heart disease risk, more problems with weight gain, interference with optimal estrogen effects on the brain, and others. This regimen still needs further evaluation for its long-term safety.

Taking the progestin (or even natural progesterone)

Recent research has shown Whether the progestogen is given monthly or every two or three months, it is the duration that is needed to protect the endometrium from hyperplasia.

every day also tends to cause more weight gain and more side effects in women who are sensitive to the depression-causing effects of the progestin. For women with a family history of heart disease, the progestin every day may negate some of the benefits of the estrogen on the heart and the lipid profile. Daily use of the progestin may also contribute to difficulties regulating blood sugar in women with diabetes or insulin resistance.

If you are considering this option you may want to review these pros and cons with your physician. Just keep in mind that this option is one for which we don't have as many studies on long term effects.

Whether the progestin is given cyclically or daily, the goal is to use the least possible dose that protects the endometrium in order to reduce the likelihood of unpleasant side effects and to decrease the amount of progestin or progesterone effects on the breast.

Caution!
Be aware that many of these products have significant progesterone effects, even though they are sold as "natural" and/ or as "wild yam extract."

Duration of Progestin/ Progesterone Cycles

One study of 398 women found that in those who took the progestogen for only 7 days, 3.5 percent (14 women) developed cystic hyperplasia after several years. When the duration of progestogen was increased to 10 days or more, not a single woman developed cystic hyperplasia.

If you are supposed to be taking a progestogen, make certain you take it for the full time your physician has recommended, even if you should start bleeding earlier, before you have finished your progestin/progesterone cycle. If you continue to start bleeding early each time, talk with your doctor about changing the dose or type of progestin.

Be aware:
Many of the OTC progesterone creams deliver amounts far in excess of progesterone in FDA-approved Prochieve 4% cream.

What about Wild Yam and Progesterone Over-the-Counter Creams?

Disogenin (and others) is a plant precursor molecule found in wild yams, soybeans and a variety of other foods, which has some very mild effects similar to both progesterone and estrogen. This is used in many OTC nonprescription creams. These phytosterols (phytoestrogens, phytoprogestins, etc.) can be synthesized into progesterone or estradiol in a laboratory, **but not in your body.**

These plant precursors are not the same chemical molecule as either progesterone or estradiol, and do not have the exact same effects in the body—even though the marketing claims try to make you think they do.

Caution

If you are using an OTC progesterone product, let your doctor know. Read the label carefully to see if it says "progesterone" in addition to wild yam extract.

OTC progesterone or wild yam creams will not prevent endometrial cancer, so you can't depend on these for this purpose.

A lot of women have been misled about these OTC creams sold in health food stores, on the internet and in health catalogs. Women are treating themselves using these products in the mistaken idea that they are "safe," have "no side effects" and can even help weight loss. These claims are not substantiated by reputable medical research. In fact, as I have explained, *progesterone promotes fat storage.*

Many have very high doses of USP progesterone added to them, sometimes shown on the label and sometimes not. The standardized FDA-approved prescription progesterone vaginal cream Prochieve 4%, delivers 40 mg per application, and the recommended amount is one applicator every other night for only 6 doses a month.

Using Prochieve 4% cream would deliver an average of 20 mg a day over 12 days. This is the non-oral amount that research to date has shown is sufficient for preventing endometrial hyperplasia.

Excess progesterone in OTC creams can account for side effects such as weight gain, bloating, breast tenderness, headaches, low libido, acne, sweet cravings, depressed mood, lack of energy, fatigue, back aches and other effects of high levels of progesterone.

Just think about the last trimester of pregnancy when

progesterone is highest. This is when women have increased risk of gestational diabetes, fatigue, swollen ankles, back aches and low energy. That should give you have an idea of how progesterone in skin creams can affect you.

If you have been having any of the symptoms I mentioned above since starting one of these products, I suggest you stop the product and observe how you feel off it.

Women, and many doctors, tend to focus only on bleeding problems that occur when there is excess estrogen relative to progesterone. Too much progesterone relative to estrogen can be another cause of heavy bleeding and painful cramps. Many women don't know this, and the makers of these creams don't tell you.

Natural vs. Surgical (Induced) Menopause

Many patients ask about the difference between natural menopause and a surgical menopause: hysterectomy with removal of the ovaries is what is generally meant by "surgical menopause," although some people use the term to refer to removal of the uterus alone.

If you have had a hysterectomy without removal of the ovaries, you will still have ovarian cycles and will be producing your own estrogen, progesterone, and testosterone. Correctly speaking, you are not in the endocrine state of menopause, although you will no longer have menstrual periods because the uterus is removed.

Women who have had a hysterectomy without removal of the ovaries do typically, however, have an earlier menopause. This is believed to be due to interruption of the blood flow to the ovaries during surgery. Dr. Phillip Sarrel from Yale Menopause Center published a study in the 1990s showing that 25 percent of women will have loss of ovarian function within three months of having a hysterectomy even though only the uterus is removed. He also found that by three years after

Fact: If your ovaries are present, you may still have PCOS problems because it is related to ovarian hormone cycling, not to the presence of the uterus.

removal of the uterus, about 60 percent of women will have menopausal levels of ovarian hormones, and show a marked decline in estradiol.

It is crucial for YOU to know this, because most doctors don't know it. It is still a common belief that women who have their ovaries after hysterectomy do not become menopausal until about age 50.

Vital Info:

If you've had a hysterectomy *with removal of the ovaries,* then it is even more crucial that you have adequate hormone replacement.

Many women today have had a hysterectomy in their early- to mid-30s, and even though they still have their ovaries, may have markedly low estradiol and testosterone levels within two or three years of their surgery. This means they begin suffering from the many problems associated with loss of these key metabolic hormones: worsening PMS, severe fatigue, weight gain, headaches, muscle and joint pain, fibromyalgia, disturbed sleep, memory and concentration problems, loss of libido, incontinence, vulvodynia/interstitial cystitis, and many others.

Checking Hormone Levels After Hysterectomy

If you begin to have symptoms of menopause following hysterectomy, no matter what your age, I think it is important to check your hormonal levels to see whether the ovaries have declined in hormone production to the point that you may be endocrinologically menopausal.

But if you don't have a uterus, checking remaining ovarian hormonal function becomes a little more difficult because you don't have the external marker of the bleeding days to know when to draw the blood tests.

I usually ask the woman to let me know when she has any body changes like she had the week before her period (breast tenderness, mood swings, etc.). I draw hormone levels at that time, and again about a week or so later to get a picture of the most likely low point of the ovarian cycle (the time that you would have been bleeding, if you still had your uterus).

This helps determine the relative pattern of residual ovarian hormone cycles and actual levels that correspond with various symptom patterns. It takes a little more "detective work" but the effort is worth it to get the answers we need in order to decide about helpful approaches to relieve symptoms.

I also encourage a woman in this situation to have a bone density test along with the urinary marker, NTx, of bone break-down. Women who have had hysterectomies at a relatively early age, even if their ovaries are remaining, are still at higher risk of bone loss than women who have a gradual, natural decline in hormone production.

The younger you are when you have the uterus and ovaries removed, the more important it is to be sure you are on the proper replacement hormone amount. The sudden loss of estrogen and testosterone can have a profound impact on all of the health concerns I have been describing. In this situation, it truly is replacement therapy, because your own ovaries were *prematurely removed*, and the body needs the ovarian hormones to function properly.

Warning: If you are a smoker, you will metabolize the estradiol faster, and may need to change a patch sooner.

Many times a woman who may have a complete hysterectomy with removal of the ovaries at 38 or 40 may be given just the lowest dose of estrogen. That often is not enough for a younger woman. Her needs are different and the amount really has to be adjusted to what her body needs.

Many women who have had a surgical menopause are also going to need testosterone. This can even be true for women with PCOS who had higher levels of testosterone when they had ovaries producing it.

I listen to the patient, and I take my clues from what she describes. A patient may tell me, "I've had a hysterectomy, my ovaries were removed and I'm on 0.625 mg of estrogen, but I don't have any energy. I don't have any libido. I'm still having hot flashes. I'm not sleeping well. And I just don't feel quite right." Her description tells me that she's probably not on the right type of estrogen or an adequate amount for her, and that she may need testosterone as well. And yet over and over women are told, "Well you couldn't possibly be having symptoms because you're on 0.625 milligrams of Premarin."

Important:
The key is not what dose you are taking, but what level of estradiol is produced in your body from what you are taking.

Optimal estradiol levels to help you feel your best are typically the levels produced for most of the time in a healthy menstrual cycle, i.e., somewhere in the range of 90–150 pg/ml.

Even though you may be taking estrogen, if you have not yet had an optimal response, because you are not getting enough of the bioidentical form of 17-beta estradiol that your ovaries made before surgery or before a natural menopause. I would encourage you to talk with your physician about trying one of the many types of FDA-approved 17-beta estradiol options available.

Keep in mind with the estradiol patches all contain the same type of 17-beta estradiol. The difference among the patch brands is primarily in the type of adhesives they use, and how long the patch is designed to last. If one causes skin irritation or won't stay on your body well, try another brand.

And be ready to ask your doctor to write your prescription so you can change the patch sooner than the manufacturer says if you find your "estrogen-loss" symptoms coming back before you are scheduled to change your patch. This can happen if you exercise a lot. "Brain fog," loss of word recall, hot flashes, restless sleep, night sweats and/or headaches are some of the common "brain" clues that the patch is wearing off sooner than it is supposed to.

Taking steroids (as for arthritis or asthma) or antibiotics will also increase the metabolism of your ovarian hormones and affect how often you need to change your patch or take the estrogen tablets.

These are some of the many issues we deal with every day in my practice trying to help women find the right type and amount of hormone to use. Keep in mind that there is a lot of fine tuning that can be done in order to come up with an optimal approach that works well for you.

Potential Pitfalls and Problems with Hormone Therapy

As new data emerges, there have become fewer and fewer reasons not to consider taking hormones after menopause. The primary remaining concerns, or potential "risks," have to do with breast cancer, uterine cancer (addressed earlier in this chapter), headaches, high blood pressure, stroke or blood clots, and risk of gallstones.

I have discussed extensively in *Screaming to Be Heard* the hormone–breast cancer issues, and have tried to give you a balanced view of the data on this complex topic.

Headaches can occur with various forms of hormone therapy if the dose or type isn't right, but I find that most of my headache patients actually see reduction in headache frequency on hormone therapy, once we have found the right type and dose, especially with progestins.

Hormone therapy, particularly oral estrogens, has also been implicated in causing gallstones in some women. This potential "pitfall" can be avoided by using transdermal estradiol that allows bypassing of the liver "first pass" and, therefore, eliminates most of the unwanted effects on the biliary (gallbladder) system.

Another question that comes up frequently is "what about blood clots and the possibility of stroke?" The newest research from European centers, published since 1990 in the international menopause medical journals, has shown that non-oral estradiol used for menopause therapy does not cause adverse effects on clotting factors. Transdermal forms of estradiol bypass the liver "first pass" metabolism and do not therefore stimulate liver production of clotting factors.

The PEPI trials in the U.S. further supported the lack of adverse effects of estrogen on clotting factors, and also that women on ERT or HRT had lower levels of fibrinogen (one of the clotting-forming factors) than women not taking hormones.

In addition, the type of estrogen makes an enormous difference in your risk of thrombophlebitis. Dr. Malcolm Whitehead in England published in 1982 his studies showing that the conjugated equine estrogen (Premarin) was more likely to adversely affect clotting factors than is the native human 17-beta estradiol. This is thought to be due to the higher potency and stronger receptor binding of the equilin group of estrogens in Premarin. The same problem is likely to be found with the other "mixed-estrogen" products, Estratab and Cenestin.

Crucial finding: Recent studies using the patch form of 17-beta estradiol have shown that estradiol decreases fibrinogen.

I definitely would not prescribe the conjugated estrogens, whether derived from plants or horses, to women who have a history of a blood clot or a strong family history of clotting problems. This is especially the case after the WHI results.

Transdermal 17-beta estradiol is much safer in such situations, and there is a significant amount of data now showing there is no increase in clot formation in women using the estradiol patches.

In fact, restoring the estradiol levels to optimal amounts has a number of important effects to reduce the likelihood of clots being formed to cause strokes and phlebitis.

There is encouraging news from current research that many diseases of the blood vessels, which can lead to stroke, hypertension, ischemia, and heart attacks, are decreased by estrogen therapy, *if it is begun at meno-pause instead of after the disease has developed.*

You and your doctor need to work together to find a solution that works for you, rather you just stopping on your own. She or he cannot do the best job for you if you don't speak up about your needs and communicate about things you may be doing on your own.

If you stop taking a medication of any kind and you don't tell your physician, he or she may not know to see that you get monitored properly for possible consequences. It's so important to your health and well-being for the long run for you to work in an active partnership with the physician you choose.

Taking a Look at The Big Picture: Symptoms and Health Risks

So often, I hear women saying "I'm confused. There doesn't seem to be an answer. Every book I read says something different. Everybody I talk to is doing something different. Or, Everybody I talk to is on the same thing. Why? What about herbs for hot flashes? What about progesterone cream for osteoporosis? What's the difference with all the estrogens? How do I make sense of all this?"

Keep in mind these *two critical points* when reading any book on menopause or thinking about hormone therapy:

POINT 1. The real issue is not an "either-or" approach: "If I am having symptoms of menopause, do I take hormones or not?" I'm not having symptoms, so I don't need hormones, do I?" Your key question here, and any decision about taking hormones, should not just be focused on whether or not you have symptoms.

You need to look at the big picture of your health and ask questions specific to YOU: "What are my health risks? Which of my health risks will be helped by hormones? Which of my health risks could be made worse by the type of hormones I use? Which type of hormone therapy, and route of taking hormones, is best suited to my individual needs? What options do I have?"

In my opinion, when women ask whether to take hormones just based on symptoms, they are missing the most important point. Hormones are not the only way to manage symptoms. There are many other ways to minimize symptoms...from acupuncture to herbs to non-hormonal medications to zen meditation.

No RX swap! Just because you enjoy trading kitchen recipes does not mean that it's a good idea to trade hormone recipes or swap prescriptions when you run out.

The crucial issue is whether you may be missing silent, subtle changes that may significantly affect your future health, like bone loss, brain effects, glucose intolerance or cholesterol changes.

For example, both acupuncture and some herbs may reduce hot flashes, but don't provide protection against bone loss that you may not identify for another ten years. How will you feel down the road when you have lost two inches in height from vertebral bone loss, you have daily back pain from vertebral fractures and your doctor says that you could have prevented this bone loss with good hormone therapy or anti-resorptive medication taken earlier?

Self-Test
If you found out you had osteopenia, or osteoporosis would you be upset with yourself for not taking more aggressive steps than just herbs in order to prevent bone loss? If the answer is "Yes," then pay attention and check into your options more thoroughly.

You simply can't assume that all is well inside your body if you don't have any symptoms that you notice. You need the reliable, objective tests at an early stage so that you have this critical information to guide your decision-making for now and the years ahead.

POINT 2. Every woman's body is different. Any hormone options must be designed to provide what you need for your body. The amount and type of hormones you take is not likely to be the same as what your friend takes *if it is truly individualized to your needs.*

We cannot continue this crazy "cookbook," "one-prescription-fits-all" approach to women's hormone needs that has been the standard approach in most gynecology settings in the United States for decades.

The emphasis has to be on individualizing the prescriptions, and using the many new FDA-approved natural bioidentical hormone products available.

Your body. Your genes. Your metabolism. Your health. Your diet. Your exercise. Your stress level. *All of these factors, and more,* will determine what type of hormone and what amount you need at any given time.

Women also have different preferences. Some women "hate" the patch; other women "hate" taking pills. Vive le difference! *Your preference counts!*

Each of us reaches a time when we need to make our own decision for our own health. How do you do this in an educated, informed way?

First, do I think all postmenopausal women need estrogen? No. Many women are healthy and have no symptoms without adding hormones, and they are blessed with good genes and lifestyle habits that give them great bone density, a normal cholesterol profile and great memory as they grow older.

But the problem is, how do you determine who does and who doesn't have reasons to use hormones? I have often referred to osteoporosis, heart disease, and dementia as the "silent thieves" of later life and health because they are ones that typically do not announce themselves with many early symptoms. You really need objective information to determine the best answer for you.

I was an example of someone who had no disease like bone loss and no heart disease risk but I was experiencing a great number of really disruptive symptoms beginning about age 38: fragmented sleep, waking up many times at night and then feeling exhausted the next morning; and what must have been hot flashes but they didn't feel exactly like what I thought hot flashes were like. Also, because I was only 38, neither my gynecologist nor I recognized these symptoms as the beginning of ovarian decline.

I started to have frequent ovarian cysts. Premenstrual mood changes suddenly became noticeable and bothersome. These were all perimenopausal symptoms. When I was checked, my bone mineral density was above average, my cholesterol was 130, and I had an HDL of 70. My doctor said he had never seen a cholesterol/HDL ratio that low. I have been exercising most of my adult life, and I also have a heavier body build that helped prevent bone loss.

Since I did have a lot of symptoms that were interfering with my quality of life, I elected to start a low dose of supplemental 17-beta estradiol, using the estradiol

Fact: Some women have marked symptoms and little disease risk; others have no symptoms and major disease risk.

patch. Within a couple of weeks, it made a world of difference in my sleep and my energy level; even my clarity of thinking and word recall improved. I had not realized how much I was having these subtle changes until I tried the estradiol patch.

At the time, it definitely was not the standard practice to start premenopausal women on even a low dose of additional estrogen. My doctor and I were later vindicated in the validity of our decision as more data became available. Even before that, however, I felt validated by the rightness of my decision, for me, based on my significantly enhanced sense of feeling well and feeling back to my normal self.

A woman I treated illustrates the same point. She was in her 40s, has PCOS, and was now struggling with fibromyalgia, and bad insomnia. Our testing revealed low estradiol, as well as low thyroid function. I started her on a 17-beta estradiol, low-dose thyroid, cyclic natural progesterone (Prometrium), and tapered off her amitriptyline that was causing weight gain and other side effects. I received this letter four months later, after having only two appointments with her:

"I also want to tell you how good I am feeling. I have a life back. In fact, it is so noticeable that within the past 24 hours, I have been asked by 3 different women about what I have done. One has my book written by Dr. Vliet, one has borrowed a copy and one is looking in the book store for a copy. There is a common thread to their conversations with me. They all have health problems and have all been told by their doctors that it could be hormonal but no tests are offered or a way of addressing that situation. Their doctors have even said that there is not a test for hormones, and all have been given antidepressants, like I was, and told to try to cope. I was not doing well at all on the PremPro. I am so grateful to be feeling so much better and be able to get around, free of pain, and do things again."

Chapter 14

Putting It All Together—Living and Thriving Despite PCOS

By now, you've seen what PCOS can do to your health, and that this overlooked disorder is a major health problem for young women. The earlier PCOS is recognized and treated, the better your chance of avoiding serious disease or permanent complications.

Unfortunately, PCOS is the overlooked culprit for about 80–90% of women who have irregular periods, increased body and face hair, acne, and abnormal weight gain. These symptoms are often minimized by physicians, hormone levels aren't checked, and PCOS rarely gets diagnosed as early as it should.

The good news is that PCOS is a *manageable* health problem if recognized and treated early with an integrated approach. Women assume that treatment should wait until research is complete…but it never is! Research always needs to be ongoing. Don't wait.

You need effective treatment *now*, based on the best available information available. This is what I have tried to provide.

Another patient with a message is Marge, a 34-year-old woman with PCOS, who also had an unusual autoimmune dermatitis whenever she ovulated and her progesterone rose. She had been on chronic corticosteroid medications for many years trying to control the dermatitis, and had many adverse side effects from these medicines. She had noticed the connection with her menstrual cycle, but as often happens, doctors dismissed her ideas and said it couldn't be related.

She came for a consult, and I identifed several hormone imbalances that caused her symptoms, and recommended that she take a steady dose birth control pill to reduce the excess androgens and stop the cyclic rise in progesterone that triggered her skin reactions.

A year later at her third follow-up appointment, she had the following to say:

> "I feel great now. I am doing so well... I couldn't ask for a better treatment...I feel so even-keel. You have really changed my life, my skin has cleared up, the self esteem effects of that are great, I sleep well, it's such a positive effect. It is truly remarkable...I used to feel so out of synch every morning and now I feel so in-synch and even. The Yasmin is a wonderful pill, and the great thing is I don't have to have a period all the time. And my skin is finally so much better now. I don't have the acne, I don't have all that itching and breakouts on my arms either. I am just thrilled! We spent thousands of dollars and saw so many doctors and you were the one that figured it out and gave me some help."

There is a hopeful message for you as you go forward from here with more information about PCOS. Remember Suki, from Chapter 2? Let's review what she said about her treatment and how she feels now:

Suki talks about *managing* her PCOS, not about being cured or being *free* from PCOS.

> "...I know that while I do have PCOS, it is manageable. Before it seemed like something that was going to destroy any attempts of normalcy...
>
> I do have to maintain a healthy diet and get a lot of exercise, which in the long run is beneficial to anybody, but it is such a relief to know that I don't have to spend the majority of my day trying to remember what medicine to take next.
>
> In the short period of time that my PCOS has been managed properly, I have noticed an incredible difference in my overall well-being. I don't have the horrible mood swings I used to go through; the exercise has helped not only in managing my PCOS, but is a great stress reliever and is tons of fun: especially, when you take dance-aerobics with a great instructor. I no longer have irregular

periods or acne, which is a great relief!

*All the frustration that I went through in high school;
taking care of the PCOS symptoms as well as the social
aspect of it have finally disappeared. But mainly the most
important thing that can be shown from my experience is
that PCOS doesn't have to be limited to a certain group
of people. It can happen to someone as young as fourteen
or even younger. And being thin does not eliminate the
chance of your having PCOS. But, that doesn't mean
that having PCOS is the end of the world and since it
is manageable PCOS doesn't have to dictate how one
lives one's life."*

Suki has adopted a proactive, positive attitude that
is essential to her continued success in managing her
PCOS.

I understand that it may be easier to have this positive
attitude once you are feeling better physically. Even
when you aren't feeling well, however, it can help for
you to focus on the positive things you *can accomplish*
with the right combination of medications and lifestyle
changes.

During the summer of 2005, Suki's mother wrote me a
letter describing the changes in her daughter over the
past year of integrated treatment for the PCOS:

> *"On the happy side, Suki's PCOS is markedly im-
> proved. This summer, she went to India and my brother
> (who happens to be her favorite uncle) remarked at
> how changed she was. The silent, sullen moodiness was
> replaced with a happy smile and humor. She enjoyed
> all her social contacts and participated in all the family
> events. Her uncle was so astounded at the change in her
> behavior; he asked me, 'What happened and how did
> she become so different?'*
>
> *"My answer is correct medical management and
> balancing of her hormones by you coupled with prayers
> of her spiritual mentor and love of her family has saved
> her from a diagnosis of bipolar disorder. My advice to all
> young women in Suki's situation is do not be fooled by
> your psychiatrist's diagnosis. He was certain that such*

Insight: Suki recognizes that PCOS will be part of her life, but it doesn't have to *be* her life or *ruin* her life.

'mild' disturbance in her hormones couldn't cause such major mood problems. The truth is that it (hormone imbalance) does. It can cause moodiness and mood swings severe enough to mimic a mood disorder. It can make family members who see it feel hopeless and despair for their child who goes from a happy, vibrant daughter to a moody, irritable, distant one."

"Suki's illness was not 'neglected' medically. She had seen an ob/gyn in our home town, her family physician, an ob/gyn at UCLA, a psychologist, and a psychiatrist, an endocrinologist. No one hit the correct diagnosis. Her endocrinologist thought she was just insulin resistant, the psychiatrist thought she had a mood disorder, and the ob/gyn didn't even test her for a hormone imbalance. I can't thank the almighty enough that I found you and Suki went under your excellent management."

Keep in mind: Medications alone are not likely to be successful in managing PCOS.

PCOS is a complicated problem that affects many aspects of your health. You are going to need *all the approaches* I have outlined in Chapter 12 on lifestyle strategies.

And, you are going to need a healthy positive mental outlook too. I call this part of *Your Hormone Power Life Plan®* tapping into your *mind power* for healing. This chapter will focus on strategies to help you develop an optimistic outlook and attitude about PCOS. I want to help you learn to focus on what is possible to achieve in managing PCOS over the long term.

Your Hormone Power Life Plan® Strategy #1: Overcoming Stress Traps

All of us live with stress, all of the time. Not all stress is bad. Without some stress, we wouldn't get out of bed in the morning. Yet, too much stress can make you not *want* to get out of bed.

Stress sets off a series of hormonal changes that are more profound for women than for men, especially for women with the metabolic imbalances in PCOS. The abnormal hormone production of PCOS triggers the outpouring of additional stress hormones that further aggravate the metabolic imbalances of PCOS, add to more body fat storage and cause more mood problems and fatigue.

Stress also saps our mental ability to focus on constructive solutions and explore new strategies for success. Stress keeps us stuck in our comfortable, and often unhealthy, patterns.

Too much **stress** is what affects your hormones and can have adverse effects on your health.

What are some simple, effective ways to break out of the vicious cycle of stress that may be sabotaging your efforts to cope with PCOS?

1: Look for ways of reducing *avoidable* negative stresses, and look for ways of minimizing the adverse effects of unavoidable stresses.

2: If stresses in your life can't be changed or eliminated, try physically working out the negative effects. For example:

> ❧ Use deep breathing,
>
> ❧ Go out for a power walk,
>
> ❧ Hit tennis balls against a backboard,
>
> ❧ Use a plastic bat and beat on a bed
>
> ❧ Find another physical release form you like... just make sure it's socially acceptable!

3: Learn the "relaxation response," used for hundreds of years in many cultures. You can use a variety of techniques: visualization, progressive muscle relaxation, self-hypnosis, autogenic conditioning, meditation and others. There are many good books and tapes available to guide you in using these approaches.

4: Get a massage. This is an incredibly effective stress management technique, especially during the premenstrual week when you feel bloated and out of sorts. Massages improve relaxation, boost your endorphins, improve circulation, and decrease muscle tension, headaches, and back pain. Look for a registered AAMT certified therapeutic massage therapist in your phone book. If you feel guilty about doing this for yourself, get your doctor to write a prescription for massage therapy for stress or pain management.

5: Try a personal coach or professional counselor to help you find more effective ways to deal with stress. It is amazing how much those outside, objective eyes can see things we miss when we are "up to our ass in alligators," as the saying goes.

There are often a variety of counseling options through your health plan or through your work place employee assistance program. Getting an outside perspective on what you can do helps you feel more in control, which then decreases the body's "fight or flight" outpouring in response to stress that adds more fat to your middle.

Tip:
If the "blues and blahs" become a major depressive episode, you may need professional intervention and possibly medication treatment.

6: Don't overlook major depression that can sap your mental and physical energy and robs your spirit. Nearly everyone has occasional down, moody times or bouts of sadness and discouragement that may last for a short time. If a severe depressed mood settles in and remains for more than a few weeks and starts to sap your energy, affect your appetite, make you lose interest in life and activities you usually enjoy, and disrupts your sleep, you may be clinically depressed and need to see a professional for evaluation and consideration of antidepressant medication. This is especially true if you feel so overwhelmed or sad that you are thinking about taking your life.

Clinical, or biological, depression is a medical illness that is caused by chemical imbalances in the neurotransmitter or "messenger" molecules in the brain. It is two to three times more common in women, with the gender differences beginning in puberty and ending after menopause. These rates are even higher in women who have PCOS and are obese, due to the many metabolic and hormonal factors I have been describing. By restoring hormone balance, however, you may not even need an anti-depressant.

Lack of proper treatment causes not only untold suffering, lost productivity, diminished quality of life, but is also a major risk factor in suicide. This is a tragic loss when we consider that treatment of depression is successful for 80%–90% of sufferers, with proper diagnosis and careful use of medication.

This physical, or biological, form of depression is not likely to be cured by "talk" therapies alone. Proper medical evaluation can identify this form of depression, rule out medical causes for the symptoms, and prescribe medication to reestablish the normal chemical balance. Don't let yourself go without professional help if you have any of the symptoms I have described.

Fact: The lifetime risk of death from suicide in major depressive illness is greater than the lifetime risk of death from breast cancer.

Your Hormone Power Life Plan® Strategy #2: Tapping Your Mind Power

I have profound belief in, and respect for, the power of the mind and spirit in all aspects of health, disease, and the healing process. Indeed, these dimensions may be the most critical of all as we seek the "wellness of being" that is at the core of our human quest, instead of our cultural emphasis on *doing* and *achieving*. I know from a deep personal level and from my professional experience that, in its fullest sense, healing must include attention to our battered spirits, as well as our damaged bodies.

The body feels the pain of our soul and spirit, which your mind may block out of consciousness. Your mind and your thoughts affect your body in many ways, both chemically in the physical sense, and psychologically in how you see yourself. Our cells know and communicate things about us that are invisible to our eyes and ears. If our mind is permeated with negative thoughts, it is like sludge blocking the free flow of water in a creek.

Tip: For women, one of the biggest saboteurs is a negative self image.

Feeling dissatisfied with, and even angry at, your body because you don't like how you look tends to rob you of the energy you need to move forward. Instead of struggling with the burden of your perceived inadequacies, use these thoughts as a foundation for change. Experience these feelings as a way out of the depths of pain from being overweight and unhappy with your body.

Mind Power

Tapping into your mind power means getting in there and "mucking out the stables" of all the negative thoughts that sabotage your efforts to reach your goals.

Think of this process of regaining your healthy body as one of moving from creating beauty in the cosmetic sense to creating the beautiful person of YOU:

- One who has known struggle and come out of it.
- One who has faced uncertainty, and found her strength.
- One who accepts that none of us have a "perfect" body, and yet we are all beautiful in some way to those who care about us.

Your Hormone Power Life Plan® Strategy #3: Face Your Fears, Accept Change

For many women, being told you have a medical problem of any kind, but especially something like PCOS that affects so many areas of your health, can be a time of uncertainty and even fear. Or, it can be empowering, now that you have answers and a plan to move forward. How you view change and challenge determines in large part what the health impact will be.

You!

Celebrate what is right, good and wonderful about you as a person, and your body, no matter its current form.

Do you feel overwhelmed by challenges and changes in your life, or are they exciting to you? Do you see them as threats, or crises, or opportunities? Even positive changes create a stress response in our bodies as we adapt. The degree of impact on our health is dramatically intensified when we perceive changes as negative.

One woman, facing a major change, even though a positive one, described her feelings: "I feel a sense of petrified excitement!" Her words really hit me. In those two words "petrified excitement," she captured the essence of the mixture of emotions that often hits us when we have significant changes in our lives.

If you feel overwhelmed, seek professional help to guide you. Having a sense of control over, and acceptance of, changes that come in our lives will enhance our inner strength, and also facilitate a healthier view of self.

Your Hormone Power Life Plan® Strategy #4: Know Yourself

If you are going to better understand who you are and what you want out of life, it will take time *being with your self and your thoughts and feelings*. This seems so obvious, and yet how often do you take the time to do it? In addition to the demands of work, you are likely giving to others day in and day out—as a 24-hour a day mother, an attentive wife, a dutiful daughter, a dedicated community volunteer, a caretaker for ill family members or friends, a teacher for your children, as well as other roles.

Women are constantly "switching hats," as multiple roles require that we dip into diverse areas of skills, insights, and wisdom when new demands emerge. A man may have one primary career focus for his entire life. Women have many.

Instead of investing everything in *doing* for others, this is a time to invest in *being* with yourself, getting to know the inner you, and what is important for your sense of soul purpose. This investment in you will nourish you for the years ahead.

Do you really know who YOU are and what you want out of life? Are you trying to meet someone else's ideal for you, or are you living the life YOU want to live? Finding out you have PCOS can be a blow to your sense of self-esteem, your sense of self confidence, and even your sense of who you are.

Your sense of self-worth and feeling of direction in your life can be greatly enhanced by setting aside time to explore what's meaningful to you, either or your own in quiet moments of reflection and journaling...or with a professional counselor.

Remember

If you focus on daydreaming about the person you would like to be, you end up wasting the time to enjoy being the person you are now.

Take time right now to write down the first six things that come immediately to mind as you read these statements:

- ❧ I want to be healthy because:
- ❧ Three things I really like about myself are:
- ❧ Three things I would like to change about myself are:
- ❧ If I knew I only had six months to live, I would want to accomplish/finish:

Now, meld these answers in a way that fits for you. Use your imagination. Look at your lists. Are you doing things for yourself or for others? Do you see regaining your health as a way to help you accomplish the items on your fourth list?

Take your own personal "sabbatical" to look a little deeper into your life and the aspects that you might want to change, improve, expand.

Take control
Take a step outside any self-imposed limits.

Embrace solitude, take "me" time, meet a physical or intellectual challenge that is meaningful to you, go out and be in nature, whatever works for you.

"You have to leave the city of your comfort,
and go into the wilderness of your intuition...
What you'll discover will be wonderful.
What you'll discover will be yourself!"

—Alan Alda

Your Hormone Power Life Plan® Strategy #5: Touching Your Spiritual Self

In the 6ᵗʰ Century B.C., Pythagoras wrote:

"The physician's task is to teach men and women the physical and spiritual laws of life, and to live in accordance with God's purpose for them."

From ancient times, the healing arts of all cultures have traditionally focused on the whole person, addressing spiritual needs as well as physical and emotional needs. As the "science" of medicine evolved, in the last hundred years or so, the care of patients has become very compartmentalized and more focused on the physical body, with medical and surgical specialists to take care of its needs. Other specialists—Psychiatrists or psychologists—attend to the needs of the mind. Our soul or spirit pain is turned over to ministers, rabbis or priests for "treatment."

Often, these different specialists aren't talking to each other to develop an integrated approach to the whole person. Ultimately, splitting mind, body, and spirit leads to artificial divisions that don't lead to true healing and wellness.

Saboteur
Anger, bottled up inside, saps physical and spiritual energy.

Just as our bodies and minds change, our spiritual needs grow in different directions as we travel on our life journey. Being faced with an illness like PCOS at a young age causes a major upheaval in our lives that affects us physically as well as psychologically and also spiritually.

Do you find you feel angry at the Universe for being dealt this hand? Do you feel angry at doctors that didn't diagnose it earlier? Do you want children and haven't been able to get pregnant?

Do you need to take some time to focus on developing new skills and insights to help you deal with these challenges and changes? How are you going to weave them into new ways of understanding about your life? Do you need people with whom you can share these innermost struggles? Make time for this dimension of your life.

Listen
Your survival, spiritually and physically, may well depend on your listening to your soul and heeding its needs.

Even with my emphasis on the importance of hormone connections in this book, I believe that we all yearn for a sense of purpose in life and a belief in something greater than ourselves as a foundation for our life. On this base of faith and purpose, we can build a wellness lifestyle, and add medical approaches (hormones, medications, surgery) when needed.

I know firsthand how important all of these are in achieving optimal health. I have sunk to the depths of despair during my own health crises, and have been forced to heed the call of my spirit to attend to that dimension in my healing journey.

Be still…and listen to the unspoken messages of your body, as it calls you to pay attention to its needs and those of your battered spirit…you'll be guided on the steps to take toward healing and wholeness.

Your Hormone Power Life Plan® Strategy #6: Getting the medical help you need—Finding a good doctor

PCOS and Syndrome X desperately need careful attention by you and your physicians. If you have body changes like I have described, or suspect an imbalance in any of these hormone systems, get evaluated properly.

Seek out a physician who is experienced in these problems and who will help you get answers. You do not have to put up with feeling lousy and missing out on your life.

Many women depend on their gynecologist for primary care as well as annual pelvic exams. Women with PCOS are often seeing gynecologists, and this is both appropriate and reasonable.

But you may find, as have many of my patients, that family medicine or internal medicine physicians are more open to the idea of checking hormone levels than are many gynecologists. I think this is related to the fact that medical specialists are more accustomed to using laboratory tests both to evaluate health problems and to monitor response to medications.

You may also find that internists and family physicians are likely to be responsive to your written summary of the patterns you notice in relation to your menstrual cycle, so keep track of these observations and share them with your physicians.

If you are not satisfied with your physician's evaluation, don't hesitate to get a second opinion. Addressing these hormonal imbalances in young women prevents many of the chronic weight and health problems commonly seen today.

You may also find the PCOS Support Association (www.pcosupport.org) helpful in finding a local doctor that treats PCOS. You can access their list of physicians at their website.

Becoming The Savvy Woman: Living and Thriving with PCOS

As you utilize the combined strategies of *Your Hormone Power Life Plan®*, remember balance can be achieved in different ways, with different techniques, for different individuals. The key is to weave and blend my suggested therapeutic approaches into your own tapestry.

Women like you have done it.

Now it is your turn.

Pay careful attention to healthy food, optimal hormonal balance, exercise, optimal vitamin and mineral supplements, and moving the body.

Pump up your positive attitude. Find pleasure in your life.

Use meditation and prayer. Find what works for you and what support systems you need to put in place to help you.

Now that you know what is going on and what to do, it is a matter of assembling all the pieces and putting them together in the way that works best for you and your needs.

There *are* answers and help available.

There is no need to wait another 10 or 15 years to address the situation, as Noel, a 28-year-old patient with PCOS and insulin resistance happily found out. With a change in her birth control pill and the addition of Glucophage, spironolactone and a higher protein meal plan, she said at her recent follow up appointment,

Possible

Yes! It *is* possible to find a way out of the hormonal haze and middle spread of PCOS. Don't be afraid to ask for help.

"I didn't realize how messed up I was until I got better. I had adapted to all those symptoms and didn't realize how bad it was. I am eating better, I don't crave carbohydrates like I did, my body is reshaping, I am less heavy on top, I see my waist coming back, my headaches are almost gone, and I am not as depressed and foggy-brained as I was. I feel so encouraged, Finally I have hope for a healthier future."

This book is not just about PCOS. It is about *health*. Your health. Your zest. Your energy. Your life.

Taking steps to lose weight, to exercise, to develop a positive mental outlook is not just about how to deal with PCOS. It is about creating a healthy body and mind to carry you with strength into the years ahead.

You can have PCOS and still have your power to be as healthy as possible. Your power comes when your body, mind and spirit are whole and balanced again. You control achieving that balance.

Remember Suki's words, profound insights from someone so young:

Claim it. You can reclaim *your* power over *your* life.

"In the short period of time that my PCOS has been managed properly, I have noticed an incredible difference in my overall well-being. I don't have the horrible mood swings I used to go through; the exercise has helped not only in managing my PCOS, but is a great stress reliever and is tons of fun...

...having PCOS is not the end of the world and since it is manageable PCOS doesn't have to dictate how one lives one's life."

Remember the words of a great First Lady:

"You gain strength, courage and confidence by every experience in which you really stop to look fear in the face...You must DO the thing you think you cannot do."

—*Eleanor Roosevelt*

Keep in mind the following benefits that can be achieved in PCOS:

PCOS is highly treatable and manageable with proper combined treatment approaches:

- There are effective ways to lose weight safely with diet, exercise and the right medications to help
- Excess body hair can be decreased
- Acne can be cleared up
- Hair on your head can grow back
- Bleeding problems and irregular cycles can be controlled
- Fertility is achievable for many
- Mood "swings" can be evened out and depression relieved
- Risk of diabetes, uterine cancer and heart disease can be significantly decreased
- You CAN feel good again.

©Elizabeth Lee Vliet, MD 2001-2005

And heed this poignant warning, said by a woman who didn't listen to her own words….and died early of a drug overdose:

"DON'T COMPROMISE YOURSELF. YOU are all you've got."
—Janis Joplin

Appendix I

Bibliography References

It is not possible to list the hundreds of medical and scientific peer-reviewed articles from reputable medical journals that I have read and studied for my clinical work and this book. This is a list of selected historical and current articles that may be of interest for those of you who want a reference for your physician, or for your own reading of the medical literature. I have included older articles to illustrate how long this information has been available and how our current understandings have evolved from this historical foundation. Many of the concepts I described in this book have been described in the medical literature, but ignored, for many years. The current research articles help you see the depth and breadth of our existing science explaining PCOS. Each article provides additional references if you wish to pursue a topic in more depth.

For this book, I have focused on medical research articles published in the major, peer-reviewed national and international medical journals.

For additional information about PCOS and other important hormone connections in women's health, and more resources, you may find it helpful to read my other four books:

The Savvy Woman's Guide to Testosterone, HER Place Press, 2005; *It's My Ovaries, Stupid!*, Scribner, New York, 2003; *Women, Weight and Hormones*, M. Evans, New York, 2001, and *Screaming to Be Heard: Hormone Connections Women Suspect and Doctors Still Ignore*, Revised Edition, M. Evans, New York, 2001.

Abbot DH, Dumesic DA, Franks S. Developmental origin of polycystic ovary syndrome–a hypothesis. *J Endocrinol* 2002;174:1-5

Abraham GE. Ovarian and adrenal contributions to peripheral androgens during the menstrual cycle. *J Clin Endocrinol Metab* 1974;39:340-6

Acbay O, Gundogdu S. Can metformin reduce insulin resistance in polycystic ovary syndrome? *Fertil Steril* 1996 May; 65(5):946-9

Adashi EY, Resnick CE, D'Ercole AJ, et al. Insuline-like growth factors as intraovarian regulators of granulose cell growth and function. *Endocrin Rev*. 1985;6:400-20

Agrawal R, Sharma S, Bekir J, Conway G, Bailey J, Balen AH, Prelevic G. Prevalence of polycystic ovaries and polycystic ovary syndrome in lesbian women compared with heterosexual women. *Fertil Steril* 2004; 82:1352-7

Alexander CM, Landsman PB, Teutsch SM, Haffner SM. NCEP-defined metabolic syndrome, *Diabetes*, and prevalence of coronary heart disease among NHANES III participants age 50 years and older. *Diabetes*. 2003;52:1210-1214.

Amato P, Simpson JL. The genetics of polycystic ovary syndrome. *Best Pract Res Clin Obstet Gynaecol* 2004;18: 707-18

Anderson KE, Sellers TA, Chen PL, et al. Association of Stein-Leventhal syndrome with the incidence of postmenopausal breast carcinoma in a large prospective study of women in Iowa. *Cancer* 1997;79:494-99

Archer JS, Chang RJ. Hirsutism and acne in polycystic ovary syndrome. *Best Pract Res Clin Obstet Gynaecol* 2004;18: 737-54

Archer C, Thiers J. Le virilisme Pilaire et son association a L'insuffisance glycolytique. *Bull Acad Natl Med*. 1921;85:51

Arner P. Effects of testosterone on fat cell lipolysis. Species differences and possible role in polycystic ovarian syndrome. *Biochimie*. 2005 Jan; 87(1):39-43

Aruna J, Mittal S, Kumar S, Misra R, Dadhwal V, Vimala N. Metformin therapy in women with polycystic ovary syndrome. *Int J Gynaecol Obstet* 2004; 87:237-241

Azziz R, Ehrmann D, Legro RS, et al. PCOS/Troglitazone Study Group. Troglitazone improves ovulation and hirsutism in the polycystic ovary syndrome: a multicenter, double blind, placebo-controlled trial. *J Clin Endoc Metab* 2001 Apr; 86(4):1626-32

Bahceci M, Tuzcu A, Canoruc N, Tuzun Y, Kidir V, Aslan C. Serum C-Reactive Protein (CRP) Levels and Insulin Resistance in Non-Obese Women with Polycystic Ovarian Syndrome, and Effect of Bicalutamide on Hirsutism, CRP Levels and Insulin. *Horm Res*. 2004; 62: 283-7

Baillargeon JP, Jakubowicz DJ, Iuorno MJ, Jakubowicz S, Nestler JF. Effects of metformin and rosiglitazone, alone and in combination, in nonobese women with polycystic ovary syndrome and normal indices of insulin sensitivity. *Fertil Steril* 2004; 82:893-902

Baillargeon JP, Jakubowica DJ, Iuomo MJ, et al. Effects of metformin and rosiglitazone, alone and in combination in nonobese women with polycystic ovary syndrome and normal indices of insulin sensitivity. *Obstet Gynecol Surv*. 2005 Mar;60(3):l78-9

Balen A. The pathophysiology of polycystic ovary syndrome: trying to understand PCOS and its *Endocrinology*. *Best Pract Res Clin Obstet Gynaecol* 2004; 18: 685-706

Barbieri RL, Makris A, Ryan KJ. Insulin stimulates androgen accumulation in incubations of human ovarian stroma and etheca. *Obstet Gynecol*. 1984;64:73S

Barbieri RL, Makris A, Ryan KJ. Insulin stimulates androgen accumulation in incubations of ovarian stroma from women with hyperandrogenism. *J Endocrin Metab*. 1986; 62:904

Bartnik M, Malmberg K, Hamsten A, et al. Abnormal glucose tolerance–a common risk factor in patients with acute myocardial infarction in comparison with population-based controls. *J Intern Med*. 2004;256:288-297.

Battaglia C, Mancini F, Persico N, et al. Ultrasound evaluation of PCO, PCOS and OHSS. *Reprod Biomed Online*.2004 Dec;9(6):614-9

Bayram F, Unluhizarci K, Kelestimur F. Potential utility of insulin sensitizers in the treatment of patients with polysystic ovary syndrome. *Treat Endocrinol* 2002; 1(1):45-53

Beigi A, Sobhi A, Zarrinkoub F. Finasteride versus cyproterone acetate-estrogen regimens in the treatment of hirsutism. *Int J Gynaecol Obstet*. 2004; 87: 29-33

Bergamaschi R, Livieri C, Candeloro E, Uggetti C, Franciotta D, Cosi V. Congenital adrenal hyperplasia and multiple sclerosis: is there an increased risk of multiple sclerosis in individual with congenital adrenal hyperplasia. *Arch Neurol* 2004; 61: 1953-5

Bhathena RK. Drospirenone and PCOS. J. Fam Plan Reprod Health Care. 2005 Jan;31(1):81

Bickerton AS, Clark N, Meeding D, et al. Cardiovascular risk in women with polycystic ovarian syndrome (PCOS). *J. Clin Pathol*. 2005 Feb; 58(2):151-4

Blogg, W. Waist circumference linked to blood pressure, insulin sensitivity. *Reuters Health*

Info 2005. Re article in Hypertension (Mar, 2005), research by Poirer P, et al Laval Hospital Research Ctr, Sainte-Foy Quebec, Canada

Brown AJ. Depression and insulin resistance: applications to polycystic ovary syndrome. Clin *Obstet Gynecol* 2004; 47: 592-6

Bruns CM, Baum ST, Colman RJ, Eisner JR, Kemnitz JW, Weindruch R, Abbott DH. Insulin resistance and impaired insulin secretion in prenatally androgenized male rhesus monkeys. *J Clin Endocrinol Metab* 2004; 89: 6218-23

Buster JE,Casson PR.Where androgens come from, what controls them, and whether to replace them. In: Lobo RA (Ed).Treatment of the PostmenopausalWoman, *Lippincott-Raven*,1999, Philadelphia, PA

Buttram VC, Vaquwero C. Post-ovarian wedge resection adhesive disease. *Fertility and Sterility* 1975;26:874-876

Carmina E, Longo RA, Rini GB, et al. Phenotypic variation in hyperandrogenic women influences the findings of abnormal metabolic and cardiovascular risk parameters. *J Clin Endocrinol Metab.* 2005 Feb 22; Epub

Carmina E, Lobo RA. Does metformin induce ovulation in normoandrogenic anovulatory women? Am J *Obstet Gynecol* 2004; 191:1580-4

Carmina E, Orio F, Palomba S, et al. Evidence for altered adipocyte function in polycystic ovary syndrome. *Eur J Endo*, 2005 Mar;152(3):389-94

Carmina E, Lobo RA. Polycystic ovary syndrome (PCOS): arguably the most common endocrinopathy is associated with significant morbidity in women. *J Clin Endocrinol Metab* 1999;16:1897-9.

Castelli WP. Cholesterol and lipids in the risk of coronary artery disease--the Framingham Heart Study. *Can J Cardiol.* 1988;4(suppl A):5A-10A.

Cattrall FR, Healy DL. Long-term metabolic, cardiovascular and neoplastic risks with polycystic ovary syndrome. *Best Pract Res Clin Obstet Gynaecol* 2004; 18:803-12

Ceriello A. Postprandial hyperglycemia and *Diabetes* complications: is it time to treat? *Diabetes.* 2005;54:1-7.

Chang RJ, et al. Diagnosis of polycystic ovary syndrome. *Endocrinol Metab Clin North Am.* 28(2):397-408, vii.1999.

Chang RJ, Mandel FP, Lu JK, Judd HLCharmandari E, Brook CG, Hindmarsh PC. Classic congenital adrenal hyperplasia and puberty. *Eur J Endocrinol.* 2004; 151 (Suppl 3): U77-82

Cheatham B, Kahn CR. Insulin action and the insulin signaling network. *Endocrin Rev.* 1995; 16:117.

Chekir C, Nakatsuka M, Kamada Y, et al. Impaired uterine perfusion associated with metabolic disorders in women with polycystic ovary syndrome. Acta *Obstet Gynecol* Scand. 2005 Feb;84(2):l89-95

Chen EC, Brzyski RG. Exercise and reproductive dysfunction. *Fertil Steril* 1999; 71(1):1-6

Chhabra S, McCartney CR, Yoo RY, et al. Progesterone inhibition of the hypothalamic GnRH pulse generator: evidence for varied effects in hyperandrogenemic adolescent girls. *J. Clin Endocrinol Metab.* 2005 Feb 22 (Epub)

Chiasson JL, Josse RG, Gomis R, et al. Acarbose treatment and the risk of cardiovascular disease and hypertension in patients with impaired glucose tolerance: the STOP NIDDM trial. JAMA. 2003;290:486-494.

Chobanian AV, Bakris GL, Black HR, et al. The seventh report of the joint national committee on prevention, detection and treatment of high blood pressure. The JNC 7 report. JAMA. 2003;289:2560-2572.

Ciraldi TP, El-Roeiy A, Madar Z, et al. Cellular mechanism of insulin resistance in PCO. *J Clin Endocrin Metab* 1992; 41:1257-66.

Cook DG, Mendall MA, Whincup PH, et al. C-reactive protein concentration in children: relationship to adiposity and other cardiovascular risk factors. *Artherosclerosis* 2000; 149:139-150

Cook S, Weitzman M, Auinger P, et al. Prevalence of a metabolic syndrome phenotype in adolescents: findings from the Third National Health and *Nutrition* Examination Survey 1998-1994. *Arch Pediatr Adol Med* 2003;157:821-827

Cook S, Weitzman M, Auinger P, Nguyen M, Dietz WH: Prevalence of a metabolic syndrome phenotype in adolescents: findings from the Third National Health and Nutrition Examination Survey, 1988-1994. *Arch Pediatr Adolesc Med* 157:821-827, 2003

Cooper HE, Spellacy WN, Prem KA, Cohen WD. Hereditary factors in the Stein-Leventhal syndrome. *Amer J Obstetrics and Gynecology* 1968; 100:371-387.

Cooper RI, Kavlock RJ. Endocrine disruptors and reproductive development: a weight-of-evidence review. *Journal of Endocrinology* 1997; 152:159-166.

Creighton S, Kives S. Early versus late intervention of congenital adrenal hyperplasia. *J Pediatr Adolesc Gynecol* 2004; 17:411

Cullberg J. Mood changes and menstrual symptoms with different gestagen/estrogen combinations. *Acta Psychiatr Scand* (suppl) 236: 1, 1972.

Cussons, AJ, Stuckey B, Walsh, J et al. Polycystic Ovarian Syndrome: marked differences between endocrinologists and gynaecologists in diagnosis and management. *Clin Endocrinol* (Oxf). 2005; 62 (3): 289-295

D'Ercole AJ, Underwood LE, Grokle J. Leprechaunism: Studies on he relaionship among hyperinsulinemia, insulin resistance and growth retardation. *J Clin Endocrin Metab* 1996; 81:302-9

Danesh J, Wheeler JG, Hirschfield GM, Eda S, Eiriksdottir G, Rumley A, Lowe GD, Pepys MB, Gudnason V: C-reactive protein and other circulating markers of inflammation in the prediction of coronary heart disease. *N Engl J Med* 350:1387-1397, 2004

Dansinger ML, Gleason JA, Griffith JL, et al. Comparison of the Atkins, Ornish, Weight Watchers and Zone Diets for weight loss and heart disease risk reduction. JAMA. 2005;293:43-53, 96-97.

Davoren JB, Kasson BG, Li Ch, et al. Specific insulin-like growth factor (IGF-l and II) binding sites on rat granulose cells. *Endocrinology* 1986;119:2155.

de Zegher F. *Endocrinology* of small for gestational age children: recent advances. *Horm Res* 2004; 62 (Suppl.3): 141-2

De Vries MJ, Dekker GA, Schoemaker J. Higher risk of pre-eclampsia in the polycystic ovary syndrome. A case control study. Eur J *Obstet Gynecol* Reprod Biol 1998;76:91-5

De Lignieres B, Dennerstein L, Backstrom T. Influence of route of administration on progesterone *Metabolism. Maturitas* 21, 251-257, 1995

Diamanti-Kandarakis E, Alexandraki K, Bergiele A, et al. Presence of metabolic risk factors in non-obese PCOS sisters; evidence of heritabilityof insulin resistance. *J Endo Invest.* 2004-Nov; 27(10):\931-6

Diamanti-Kandarakis E, KouliC, Tsianateli T, et al. Therapeutic effects of metformin on IR and hyperandrogenism in PCOS. *Eur J Endocrin* 1998; 138:269-74

Dickey, RP. Managing Contraceptive Pill Patients. Eleventh Edition, 2002. Available from: Essential Medical Information Systems, Inc., P.O. Box 820062, Dallas, TX 75382 or website: www.emispub.com

Dimitrakakis C, Zhou J, Bondy CA. Androgens and mammary growth and neoplasia. *Fertil Steril* 2002;77:S26-S33

Doldi N, Gessi A, Destefani A, et al. Polycystic ovary syndrome: anomalies in progesterone production. *Hum Reprod* 1998; 13:290-3.

Douchi T, Oki T, Yamasaki H, Nakal M, Imabayashi A, Nagata Y. Body fat patterning in polycystic ovary syndrome women as a predictor of the response to clomiphene. Acta *Obstet Gynecol Scand* 2004; 83: 838-41

Dreno B, Bettoli V, Ochsendorf F, Layton A, Mobacken H, Degreef H. European recommendations on the use of oral antibiotics for acne. *Eur J Dermatol.* 2004;14:391-399

Dreno B. Acne: Physical treatment. *Clin Dermatol.* 2004; 22: 429-33

Duggirala MK, Mundell WC. Low carbohydrate diets as compared with low fat diets. *N Engl J Med.* 2003;349:1000-1002.

Dumesic DA, Schramm RD, Abbott DH. Early origins of polycystic ovary syndrome. *Reprod Fertil Dev.* 2005;17(3):349-60

Dunaif A, Segal KR, Futterweit W, Dobrjansky A. Profound insuin resistance, independent of obesity, in polycystic ovary syndrome. *Diabetes* 1989; 38; 1165-1174.

Dunaif A, Segal KR, Shelley DR, et al. Evidence for distinctive and intrinsic defects in insulin action in PCO. *Diabetes* 1992; 41:1257-66.

Dunaif A. Insulin resistance and the polycystic ovary syndrome: mechanism and implications for pathogenesis. *Endocr Rev* 1997;18:774-800

Dunaif A, Xia J, Book CB, et al. Excesive insulin receptor serine autophosphorylation in cultured fibroblasts and in skeletal muscle: a potential mechanism for insulin resistance in the PCO. *J Clin Invest* 1995;96:801-10

Ehrmann DA, Cavaghna M, Imoperial J, et al. Effects of metformin on insulin secretion, insulin resistance and ovarian steroidogenesis in women with PCOS. *J Clin Endocrin Metab* 1997 82:524-30

Ehrmann DA, Barnes RB, Rosenfield RL, et al. Prevalence of impaired glucose tolerance and Diabetes in women with polycystic ovary syndrome, *Diabetes Care* 1999; 22:141-146.

Ehrmann DA, Barnes RB, Rosenfield RL. Polycystic ovary syndrome as a form of functional ovarian hyperandrogenism due to dysregulaion of androgen secretion. *Endocr Rev* 1995;16:322-53.

Ehrmann DA, Schneider DJ, Sobel BE, et al. Troglitazone improves defects in insulin action, insulin secretion, ovarian steroidogenesis, and fibrinolysis in women with polycystic ovary syndrome. *J Clin Endocrinol Metab* 1997 Jul; 82 (7):2108-16

Enhanced disparity of gonadotropin secretion by estrone in women with polycystic ovarian disease, *Journal of Clinical Endocrinology & Metabolism*, Vol 54, 490-494, Copyright © 1982 by Endocrine Society

Erturk E, Kuru N, Savci V, Tuncel E, Ersoy C, Imamoglu S. Serum leptin levels correlate with obesity parameters but not with hyperinsulinism in women with polycystic ovary syndrome. *Fertil Steril* 2004; 82: 1364-8

Escobar-Morreale HF. Macroprolactinemia in women presentino with hyperandrogenic symptoms: implications for the management of polycystic ovary sindrome. *Fertil Steril* 2004; 82:1697-9

Fabregues F, Penarrubia J, Vidal E, Casals G, Vanrell JA, Balasci J. Oocyte quality in patients with severe ovarian hyperstimulation syndrome: a self-controlled clinical study. *Fertil Steril* 2004; 82: 827-33

Farquhar CM. The role of ovarian surgery in polycystic ovary syndrome. *Best Pract Res Clin Obstet Gynaecol* 2004;18: 789-802

Ferraroni Am, Dearli A, Franceschi S and La Vecchia C. Alcohol consumption and risk of breast Cancer: a multicentre Italian case-control study. *European J of Cancer* 1998; 34:1403-1409.

Ferriman D, Gallwey JD. Clinical assessment of body hair growth in women with hyperandrogenism. *Endocrinol Metab* 1961;21:1440-47

Festa A, D'Agostino R Jr., Howard G, et al. Chronic subclinical inflammation as part of the insulin resistance syndrome: the Insulin Resistance Atherosclerosis Study (IRAS). *Circulation* 2000;102:42-47

Festa A, D'Agostino R, Howard G et al. Chronic subclinical inflammation as part of the insulin resistance syndrome. The Insulin Resistance Atherosclerosis Study. *Circulation*. 2000;102:42-47.

Fleming R, Harborne L., MacLaughlin DT, et al. Metformin reduces serum mullerian-inhibiting substance levels in women with polycystic ovary syndrome after protracted treatment. *Fertil Steril*. 2005 Jan;83(1):130-6

Floter A, Nathorst-Boos J, Carlstrom BK, et al. Androgen status and sexual life in perimenopausal women. *Menopause* 1997;4:95-100

Fontbonne A, Eschwege E, Cambien F, et al. Hypertriglyceridaemia as a risk factor of coronary heart disease mortality in subjects with impaired glucose tolerance or *Diabetes*. Results from the 11-year follow-up of the Paris Prospective Study. *Diabetologica*. 1989;32:300-304.

Forest MG. Recent advances in the diagnosis and management of congenital adrenal hyperplasia due to 21-hydroxylase deficiency. *Hum Reprod Update*. 2004;10: 469-85

Franks S. Polycystic ovary syndrome: N Eng J Med 1995; 333:853-61

Fraser IS, Kovacs G. Current recommendations for the diagnostic evaluation and followup of patients presenting with symptomatic polycystic ovary syndrome. *Best Pract Res Clin Obstet Gynaecol* 2004;18: 813-23

Frohlich M, Imhof A, Berg G, et al. Association between C-reactive protein and features of the metabolic syndrome: a population-based study. *Diabetes Care* 2000; 23:1835-1839

Gambacciani M, Genazzani AR. Hormone therapy: the benefits in tailoring the regimen and dose. *Maturitas* 2001; 40:195-201.

Gambacciani M, Genazzani AR. The Missing R. (editorial). *Gynecol.Endocrinol* 2003; 17:91-94.

Garg A, Grundy SM. Nicotinic acid as therapy for dyslipidemia in non-insulin dependent Diabetes mellitus. *JAMA.* 1990;264:723-726.

Gatelais F, Berthelot J, Beringue F, Descamps P, Bonneau D, Limal JM, Coutant R. Effect of single and multiple courses of prenatal corticosteroids on 17-hydroxyprogesterone levels : implication for neonatal screening of congenital adrenal hyperplasia. *Pediatr Res.* 2004; 56: 701-5

Gelfand M. Estrogen-androgen hormone replacement therapy. *European Menopause Journal* 2:22-26, 1995.

Genazzani AR, Gambacciani, M. A personal initiative for women's health: to challenge the Women's Health Initiative, *Gynecol Endocrinol* 16:255-257, August, 2002.

Genazzani AR, Bernardi F, Spinetti A, et al. The brain as target and source for sex steroid hormones. Third International Symposium Women's Health and Menopause. June, 1998.

Genazzani AR, Gadducci A, Gambacciani M. Controversial issues in *Climacteric* medicine II: Hormone replacement therapy and *Cancer.* International *Menopause* Society Expert Position Paper. *Gynecol Endocrinol* 2001; 15:453-465.

Genazzani, AR (President of the International *Menopause* Society). HRT and breast *Cancer*: is there any news? A clinician's perspective (editorial). *Climacteric: The Journal of the International Menopause Society*, 2000:3:13-16

Gerli S, Casini ML, Unfer V, Costabile L, Mignosa M, Di Renzo GC. Ovulation induction with urinary FSH or recombinant FSH in polycysatic ovary sindrome patients: a prospective randomized analysis of cost-effectiveness. *Reprod Biomed Online* 2004; 9:494-9

Giordano MG, Oliveira CA. Immunohistochemical analysis of IGF-1 and IGF-2 receptors in ovaries of patients with polycystic ovary syndrome. *Int J Gynaecol Obstet* 2004; 87: 256-7

Girard J. Mechanisms of action of thiazolidinediones. *Diabetes Metab* 2001Apr;27(2-C2):271-8

Glintborg D, Henriksen JF, Andersen M, Hagen C, Hangaard J, Rasmussen PE, Schousboe K, Hermann AP. Prevalence of endocrine diseases and abnormal glucose tolerance tests in caucasian premenopausal women with hirsutism as the referral diagnosis. *Fertil Steril* 2004; 82:1570-9

Glueck CJ, Wang P, Kobayashi S, Phillips H, Sieve-Smith L. Metformin therapy throughout pregnancy reduces the development of gestational Diabetes in women with polycystic ovary syndrome. *Fertility and Sterility* 2002; 77(3):520-525.

Glueck CJ, Wang P, Goldenberg N, Sieve L. Pregnancy loss, polycystic ovary syndrome, thrombophilia, hypofibrinolysis, enoxaparin, metformin. *Clin Appl Thromb Hemost* 2004; 10: 323-34

Glueck CJ, Awadalla SG, Phillips H, et al. Polycystic ovary syndrome, infertility, familial thrombophilia, familial hypofibrinolysis, recurrent loss of in vitro fertilized embryos, and miscarriage. *Metabolism* 1999; 48:1589-95.

Gordon CM. Menstrual disorders in adolescents. Excess androgens and the polycystic ovary syndrome. *Pediatr Clin North Am.* 46(3):519-43,1999.

Govind A, Obhrai MS, Clayton RN. Polycystic ovaries are inherited as an autosomal dominant trait: analysis of 29 polycystic ovary syndrome and 10 control families. *J Clin Endocrinology and Metabolism* 1999: 84:38-43.

Govoni, S. Estrogens as neuroprotectants: Hypotheses on the mechanism of action. Third International Symposium Women's Health and Menopause, June, 1998

Gracia CR, Sammel MD, Freeman EW, et al. Predictors of decreased libido in women during the late reproductive years. *Menopause* 2004;11:144-150.

Grady D, Herrington D, Bittner V, et al. for the HERS Research Group. Heart and estrogen/progestin replacement study follow-up (HERS II): Part 1: cardiovascular outcomes during 6.8 years of hormone therapy. *J Am Med Assoc* 288-49-57, 2002.

Grundy SM, Brewer HB Jr., Cleeman JI, et al. Definition of metabolic syndrome: report of the National Heart, Lung, and Blood Institute/American Heart Association conference on scientific issues related to definition. *Circulation* 2004; 109:433-438

Grundy SM, Cleeman JI, Bairey Merz N, et al. Implications of recent trials for the National Cholesterol Education Program Adult Treatment Panel III Guidelines. *Circulation.*

2004;110:227-239.

Grundy SM, Brewer B, Cleeman JI, et al. Definition of the metabolic syndrome. *Circulation.* 2004;109:433-438.

Gulekli B, Buckett WM, Chian RC, Child TJ, Abdul-Jalil AK, Tan SL. Randomized, controlled trial of priming with 10,000 IU versus 20,000 IU of human chorionic gonadotropin in women with polycystic ovary syndrome who are undergoing in vitro maturation. *Fertil Steril* 2004; 82: 1458-9

Guyatt G, Weaver B, Cronin L, Dooley JA, Azziz R. Health-related quality of life in women with polycystic ovary syndrome, self administered questionnaire, was validated. *J Clin Epidemiol* 2004, 57:1279-87

Haffner SM, Lehto S, Ronnemaa T, et al. Mortality for coronary heart disease in subjects with type 2 *Diabetes* and in nondiabetic subjects with and without prior myocardial infarction. *N Engl J Med.* 1998;339:229-234.

Hague WM, Adams J, Reeders ST, et al. Familial polycystic ovaries: a genetic disease? *Clinical Endocrinology* 1988;29:593-605.

Hart R, Hickey M, Franks S. Definitions, prevalence and symptoms of polycystic ovaries and polycystic ovary syndrome. *Best Pract Res Clin Obstet Gynaecol* 2004;18: 671-83

Hashemipour M, Faghihimani S, Zolfaghary B, Hovsepian S, Ahmadi F, Haghighi S. Prevalence of Polycystic Ovary Syndrome in Girls Aged 14-18 Years in Isfahan, Iran. *Horm Res* 2004; 62: 278-282

Heart Outcomes Prevention Evaluation Study Investigators. Effects of ramipril on cardiovascular and microvascular outcomes in people with *Diabetes* mellitus: results of the HOPE study and MICROHOPE substudy. *Lancet.* 2000;355:253-259.

Homburg R. Management of infertility and prevention of ovarian hyperstimulation in women with polycystic ovary syndrome. *Best Pract Res Clin Obstet Gynaecol* 2004; 18:773-88

Hu FB, Manson JE, Stampfer MJ, et al. Diet, lifestyle and the risk of type 2 *Diabetes* in women. *N Engl J Med.* 2001;345:790-797

Huang CW, Hsueh S, Chang MY. Angiogenic myeloid metaplasia in an ovarian steroid cell tumor with virilization: a case report. *J Reprod Med.* 2004; 49: 765-8

Hulley S, Grady D, Bush T, et al. Randomized trial of estrogen plus progestin (HERS) for secondary prevention of coronary heart disease in postmenopausal women. *J Am Med Assoc* 280:6-5-613, 1998.

Hurst RT, Lee RW. Increased incidence of coronary atherosclerosis in type 2 *Diabetes* mellitus: mechanisms and management. *Ann Intern Med.* 2003;139:824-834.

Ibanez L, deZegher P, Potau N. Anovulation after precocious pubarche: early markers and time course in adolescence. *J Clin Endocrinology* and *Metabolism* 1999; 84:2691-2695.

Jarrett JC, Ballejo G, Tsibris JDM, et al. Insulin binding to human ovaries. JCEM 1985; 60:460

Jarvela IY, Sladkevicius P, Kelly S, Ojha K, Campbell S, Nargund G. Comparison of follicular vascularization in normal versus polycystic ovaries during in vitro fertilization as measured using 3-dimensional power Doppler ultrasonography. *Fertil Steril* 2004; 82:1358-63

Jaussi R, Watson G, Paigen K. Modulation of androgen-responsive gene expression by estrogen, *Mol Cell Endocrinol.* 1992; 86:187.

Jones AE. Diagnosis and treatment of polycystic ovarian syndrome. *Nurs Times.* 2005 Jan 18-24;101(3):40-3

Judd HL, Lucas WE, Yen SS. Effect of oophrectomy on circulating testosterone and androstenedione levels in patients with endometrial *Cancer.* Am J. *Obstet Gynecol* 1974;118:793-8

Judd HL, Fournet N. Changes of ovarian hormonal function with aging. *Experiment Gerontol* 1994; 29:285-98

Kahsar-Miller M, Boots LR, Bartolucci A, Azziz R. Role of a CYP17 polymorphism in the regulation of circulating dehydroepiandrosterone sulfate levels in women with polycystic ovary syndrome. *Fertil Steril* 2004; 82: 973-5

Kamel N, Tonyukuk V, Emral R, et al. Role of ovary and adrenal glands in hyperandrogenemia in patients with polycystic ovary syndrome. *Exp Clin Endo Diabetes.* 2005 Kfeb; 113(2):115-121

Kashyap S, Claman P. Polycystic ovary disease and the risk of pregnancy-induced hypertension. *J Reprod Med* 2000; 45:991-4.

Katsambas AD, Stefanaki C, Cunliffe WJ. Guidelines for treating acne. *Clin Dermatol.* 2004; 22: 439-44

Kaye, S.A., Folsom, A.R., Soler, J.T., Prineas, R.J. and Potter, J.D. Association of body mass and fat distribution with sex hormone concentrations in postmenopausal women. *Int. J. Epidemiol.*, 20, 151-6

Keizer H, Janssen GME, Menheere P, and Kranenburg G. Changes in basal plasma testosterone, cortisol, and dehydroepiandrosterone in previously untrained males and females preparing for a marathon. *Int. J. Sports Med.* 10, S139, 1989.

Kelly CJ, Speirs A, Gould GW, et al. Altered vascular function in young women with polycystic ovary syndrome. *J Clin Endocrinol Metab* 2002;87:742-6

Khastgir G, Studd JWW. Hysterectomy, ovarian failure and depression. *Menopause* 5:113-122, 1998.

Kicman AT, Bassindale T, Cowan DA, et al. Effect of androstenedione ingestion on plasma testosterone in young women: a dietary supplement with potential health risks. *Clin Chem* 2003;49:167-9

Kilic-Okman T, Guldiken S, Kucuk M. Relationship between Homocysteine and Insulin Resistance in Women with Polycystic Ovary Syndrome. *Endocr J* 2004; 51: 505-8

Kip KE, Marroquin OC, Kelley DE, et al. Clinical importance of obesity versus the metabolic syndrome in cardiovascular risk in women. *Circulation.* 2004;109:806-713.

Kip KE, Marroquin OC, Kelley DE, et al. Clinical importance of obesity versus the metabolic syndrome in cardiovascular risk in women. *Circulation.* 2004;109:706-713.

Kistner RW. Peri-tubal and peri-ovarian adhesions subsequent to wedge resection of the ovaries. *Fertility and Sterility* 1969;20:35-42

Knowler WC, Barrett-Connor E, Fowler SE, et al. *Diabetes* Prevention Research Group. Reduction in the incidence of type 2 *Diabetes* with lifestyle intervention or metformin. *N Engl J Med.* 2002;346:393-403.

Krautheim A, Gollnick HP. Acne: Topical treatment. *Clin Dermatol.* 2004; 22: 398-407

La Marca A, Orvieto R, Giulini S, Jasonni VM, Volpe A, De Leo V. Mullerian-inhibiting substance in women with polycystic ovary syndrome: relationship with hormonal and metabolic characteristics. *Fertil Steril* 2004; 82: 970-2

Labrie F. Extragonadal synthesis of sex steroids: intracrinology. Ann Endocrinol 2003;64:95-107

Labrie F, Luu-The V, Lin SX, et al. Intracrinology: role of the family of 17B-hydroxysteroid dehydrogenases in human physiology and disease. *J Mol Endocrinol* 2000; 25:1-16

Labrie F, Luu-the V, Labrie C, et al. Endocrine and intracrine sources of androgens in women: inhibition of breast *Cancer* and other roles of androgens and their precursor dehydroepiandrosterone. *Endoc Rev* 2003; 24: 152-82

Lajic S, Nordenstrom A, Ritzen EM, Wedell A. Prenatal treatment of congenital adrenal hyperplasia. *Eur J Endocrinol.* 2004; 151 (Suppl 3): U63-9

Legro RS, Kunselman AR, Dodson WC and Dunaif A. Prevalence of impaired glucose tolerance and *Diabetes* in women with polycystic ovary syndrome: a prospective controlled study in 254 affected women. *J Clin Endocriology and Metabolism* 1999; 84: 165-169.

Legro RS, Driscoll D, Strauss II JF, et al. Evidence for a genetic basis for hyperandrogenemia in polycystic ovary syndrome, *Proc. Natl Acad Sci* (USA)1998; 95:14956-14960.

Legro RS, Finegood D, Dunaif A. A fasting glucose to insulin ratio is a useful measure of insulin sensitivity in women with polycystic ovary syndrome. *J Clin Endocrin and Metab* 1998;83:2694-2698

Liu FTY, Lin HS, Johnson DC. Serum FSH, LH and the ovarian response to exogenous gonadrtropins in alloxan diabetic immature female rats. *Endocrinology* 1972; 91:1172

Long DN, Wisniewski AB, Migeon CJ. Gender role across development in adult women with congenital adrenal hyperplasia due to 21-hydroxylase deficiency. J Pediatr *Endocrinol Metab.* 2004;17: 1367-73

Longcope C. Androgen Metabolism and the Menopause. Sem Reprod Endocrinol 1998; 16:111-5

Longcope C. Adrenal and gonadal androgen secretion in normal females. JCEM 1986; 15:213-28

Longcope C, Hunter R, Franz C. Steroid secretion by the postmenopausal ovary. Am J *Obstet*

Gynecol 1980; 1 38: 564-9

Longcope C, Franz C, Morello C, et al. Steroid and gonadotropin levels in women during the peri-menopausal years. *Maturitas* 1986;8:189-196

Lopez E, Gunby J, Daya S, Parrilla JD, Abad L, Balasch J . Ovulation induction in women with polycystic ovary syndrome: randomized trial of clomiphene citrate versus low-dose recombinant FSH as first line therapy. *Reprod Biomed Online* 2004 ;9: 382-90

Lord J, Wilkin T. Metformin in polycystic ovary syndrome. *Curr Opin Obstet Gynecol* 2004; 16: 481-6

Lowe P, Kovacs G, Howlett D. Inncidence of polycystic ovaries and polycystic ovary syndrome amongst women in Melbourne, Australia. *Aust NZ J Obstet Gynaecol.* 2005 Feb; 45(1):17-9

Ludwig DS. The glycemic index. Physiological mechanisms relating to obesity, *Diabetes* and cardiovascular disease. *JAMA.* 2002;287:2414-2423. Abstract

Maciel GA, Baracat EC, Benda JA, Markham SM, Hensinger K, Chang RJ, Erickson GF. Stockpiling of transitional and classic primary follicles in ovaries of women with polycystic ovary syndrome. *J Clin Endocrinol Metab* 2004; 89: 5321-7

Major outcomes in high-risk hypertensive patients randomized to angiotensin-converting enzyme inhibitor or calcium channel blocker vs diuretic: The Antihypertensive and Lipid Lowering Treatment to Prevent Heart Attack Trial (ALL HAT). *JAMA.* 2002;288:2981-2997.

Malkawi HY, Qublan HS. Laparoscopic ovarian drilling in the treatment of plycystic ovary syndrome: How many punctures per ovary are needed to improve the reproductive outcome? *J Obstet Gynaecol Res.* 2005 Apr; 31(2):115-9

Margolis E, Zhornitzki T, Kopernik G, et al. Polycytstic ovary sundrome in post-menopausal women-marker: the metabolic syndrome *Maturitas*, 2005 Apr 11; 50(4): 331-6

Marroquin OC, Kip KE, Kelly DE, et al. Metabolic syndrome modifies the cardiovascular risk associated with angiographic coronary artery disease in women: a report from the Women's Ischemia Syndrome Evaluation. *Circulation.* 2004;109:714-721.

Martin MB, White C, Kammerer C, Witchel SF. Mutational analysis of the melanocortin-4 receptor in children with premature pubarche and adolescent girls with hyperandrogenism. *Fertil Steril* 2004; 82: 1460-2

Mattison Dr, Plowchalk DR, Meadows MJ, et al. Reproductive Toxicity: male and female reproductive systems as targets for chemical injury. *Medical Clinics of North America* 1990; 74:391-411.

Mayer KC, Talbot M, Teede H. Effect of implanon on insulin resistance in women with Polysystic Ovary Syndrome. *Aust NZ J Obstet Gynaecol.* 2005 Apr;45(2):155-8

Mayer JA, Chuong CM, Widelitz R. Rooster feathering, androgen alopecia and hormone dependent tumor growth: What is in common? *Differentiation* 2004; 72: 474-88

Mazzone T. Strategies in ongoing clinical trials to reduce cardiovascular disease in patients with Diabetes mellitus and insulin resistance. *Am J Cardiol.* 2004;93S:27C-31C.

McCook JG, Reame NE, Thatcher SS. Health-related quality of life issues in women with poly-cystic ovary syndrome. *J. Obstet Gynecol Neonatal Nurs.* 2005 Jan-Feb;34(1):12-20

Miettinen H, Lehto S, Salomaa V et al. Impact of *Diabetes* on mortality after the first myo-cardial infarction. The FINMONICA myocardial infarction register study group. *Diabetes Care.* 1998;21:69-75.

Mitkov M, Pehlivanov B, Terzieva D. Combined use of metformin and ethinyl estradiol-cy-proterone acetatein polycystic ovary syndrome. *Eur J Obstet Gynecol Reprod Biol.* 2005 Feb 1;118(2):209-213

Mitwally MF, Kuscu NK, Yalcinkaya TM. High ovulatory rates with use of troglitazone in clomiphene-resistant women with polycystic ovary syndrome. *Hum Reprod* 1999 Nov; 14(11):2700-03

Moran L, Norman RJ. Understanding and managing disturbances in insulin *Metabolism* and body weight in women with polycystic ovary syndrome. *Best Pract Res Clin Obstet Gynaecol* 2004; 18: 719-36

Morin-Papunen LC, Kouuiven RM, Roukonene A, et al. Metformin treatment improves the menstrual pattern with minimal endocrine and metabolic effects in women with PCOS. *Fertil Steril* 1998;69:691-6

Mozzanega B, Mioni R, Granzotto M, et al. Obesity reduces the expression of GLUT4 in the endometrium of normoinsulinemic women affected by the polycystic ovary syndrome. *Ann NY Acad Sci* 2004 Dec; 1034:364-74

Must A, Jacques PF, Dallal GE, Bajema CJ, Dietz WH: Long-term morbidity and mortality of overweight adolescents: a follow-up of the Harvard Growth Study of 1922 to 1935. *N Engl J Med* 327:1350-1355, 1992

Muth S, Norman J, Sattar N, Fleming R. Women with polycystic ovary syndrome (PCOS) often undergo protracted treatment with metformin and are disinclined to stop: indications for a change in licensing arrangements? *Hum Reprod* 2004; 19: 2718-20

Myers LS, Dixen J, Morrissette D, et al. Effects of estrogen, androgen, and progestin on sexual psychophysiology and behavior in postmenopausal women. *J Clin Endocrinol Metab* 1990;70:1124-31

Nelson VL, Qin KN, Rosenfield RL, et al. The biochemical basis for increased testosterone production in theca cells propagated from patients with polycystic ovary syndrome. *J Clin Endocrinology and Metabolism* 2001; 86: 5925-5933.

Nestler JE, Jakubowicz DJ, Evans WS, et al. Effects of metformin on spontaneous and Clomiphene-induced ovulation in the PCOS. *NEJM* 1998;338-l876-80

Nestler JE, Jakubowica DJ. Decvreases in ovarian cytochrome P450c17a activity and serum free testosterone and reduction of insulin secretion in PCOS. *NEJM* 1996;335:617-23

Nesto R. C reactive protein, its role in inflammation, type 2 *Diabetes* and cardiovascular disease, and the effects of insulin-sensitizing treatment with thiazolidinediones. *Diabetes Med.* 2004;21:810-817.

Nieschlag E, Behre HM (Editors) Testosterone: Action, Deficiency, Substitution, 2nd Edition. *Springer-Verlag*, Berlin. 1998

Norman RJ. Editorial: Metformin--comparison with other therapies in ovulation induction in polycystic ovary syndrome. *J Clin Endocrinol Metab* 2004; 89: 4797-800

Norman RJ, Masters S, Hague W. Hyperinsulinemia is common in family members of women with polycystic ovary syndrome. *Fertility and Sterility* 1996; 66: 942-947.

Notelovitz M. Androgen effects on bone and muscle. *Fertil Steril* 2002;77:S34-S41

Orio F Jr, Palomba S, Cascella T, Tauchmanova L, Nardo LG, Di Biase S, Labella D, Russo T, Savastano S, Tolino A, Zullo F, Colao AM, Lombardi G. Is plasminogen activator inhibitor-1 a cardiovascular risk factor in young women with polycystic ovary syndrome? *Reprod Biomed Ondine* 2004; 9: 505-510

Orio F., Jr., Palomba S, Cascella T, De Biase S, Labella D, Russo T, Savastano S, Zullo F, Colao A, Vettor R, Lombardi G. Lack of an association between peroxisome proliferator-activated receptor-gamma gene Pro12Ala polymorphism and adiponectin levels in the polycystic ovary syndrome. *J Clin Endocrinol Metab* 2004; 89: 5110-5115

Palomba S, Orio F., Jr., Nardo LG, Falbo A, Russo T, Corea D, Doldo P, Lombardi G, Tolino A, Colao A, Zullo F. Metformin administration versus laparoscopic ovarian diathermy in clomiphene citrate-resistant women with polycystic ovary syndrome: a prospective parallel randomized double-blind placebo-controlled trial. *J Clin Endocrinol Metab* 2004; 89: 4801-9

Palomba S, Orio F., Jr., Falbo A, Russo T, Lombardi G, Zullo F. Are laparoscopic ovarian diathermy and gonadotropin administration the only therapeutic second-steps in clomiphene-citrate resistant women with polycystic ovary syndrome? *Hum Reprod* 2004; 19: 2682-3

Panidis D, Farmakiotis D, Rousso D, et al. Decrease in adiponectin levels in women with polycystic ovary syndrome after an oral glucose tolerance test. *Fertil Steril.* 2005 Jan; 83(1):232-4

Pasquali R, Patton L, Pagotto U, et al. Metabolic alterations and cardiovascular risk factors in the polycystic ovary syndrome. *Minerva Ginecole.* 2005 Feb;57(1):79-85

Perez-Bravo F, Echiburu B, Maliqueo M, et al. Trytophan 64-->arginine polymorphism of beta-3-andrehnergic receptor in Chilean women with polycystic ovary syndrome. *Clin Endocrinol* (Oxf). 2005 Feb;62(2):126-31

Peterson HB et al. The risk of menstrual abnormalties after tubal sterilization. *N Engl J Med* 2000 Dec. 7; 343:1681-7

Poretsky L, Grogorescu F, Sibel M, et al. Distribution and characterization of insulin and IGF receptors in normal human ovary. *JCEM* 1987; 61:728

Practice Committee of the American Society for Reproductive Medicine. The evaluation and treatment of androgen excess. *Fertil Steril*. 2004; 82 (Suppl 1): S173-80

Quinkler M, Sinha B, Tomlinson JW, Bujalska IJ, Stewart PM, Arlt W. Androgen generation in adipose tissue in women with simple obesity--a site-specific role for 17betahydroxysteroid dehydrogenase type 5. *J Endocrinol*. 2004;183: 331-42

Rautio K, Tapanainen JS, Ruokonen A, et al. Effects of metformin and ethinyl estradiol-cyproterone acetate on lipid levels in obese and non-obese women with polycystic ovary syndrome. *Eur J. Endo*. 2005 Feb;152(2):269-75

Redmond GP. *Androgenic Disorders*, Raven Press, New York, 1995.

Ridker PM, Buring JE, Cook NR, et al. C-reactive Protein,the metabolic syndrome, and risk of incident cardiovascular events: an 8 year follow-up of 14,719 initially healthy American women. *Circulation* 2003; 107:391-397

Ridker PM, Buring JE, Cook NR, Rifai N: C-reactive protein, the metabolic syndrome, and risk of incident cardiovascular events: an 8-year follow-up of 14,719 initially healthy American women. *Circulation* 107:391-397, 2003

Rossouw JE, Anderson GL, Prentice RL, et al. Risks and benefits of estrogen plus progestin in healthy postmenopausal women: principal results from the Women's Health Initiative randomized controlled trial. *JAMA* 2002;288:3231-333

Saleh HA, El-Nwaem MA, El-Bordiny MM, Maqlad HM, El-Mohandes AA, Eldaqaq EM. Serum leptin elevation in obese women with PCOS: a continuing controversy. *J Assist Reprod Genet* 2004; 21: 361-6

Scarabin P, Oger E, Plu-Bureau G (for the EStrogen and THromboEmbolism Risk [ESTHER] Study Group. Differential association of oral and transdermal oestrogen replacement therapy with venous thromboembolism risk. *Lancet* 2003; 362:428-432.

Scheen AJ. Thiazolidinediones and liver toxicity. *Diabetes Metab* 2001 Jun; 27(3):305-13

Scheinfeld N. Impact of phenytoin therapy on the skin and skin disease. *Expert Opin Drug Saf*. 2004; 3: 655-65

Schernthaner G, Matthews DR, Charbonnel B, et al. Efficacy and safety of pioglitazone versus metformin in patients with type 2 *Diabetes* mellitus: a double-blind, randomized trial. *J Clin Endocrinol Metab*. 2004;89:6068-6076.

Schmid J, Kirchengast S, Vytiska-Binstorfer E, Huber J. Infertility caused by PCOS–health-related quality of life among Austrian and Moslem immigrant women in Austria. *Hum Reprod* 2004; 19: 2251-7

Schneider, HPG. The view of the International *Menopause* Society on the women's health initiative (WHI). *Climacteric* 5:211-216, September, 2002.

Schneider, HPG. Guidelines for the hormone treatment of women in the menopausal transition and beyond. Position Statement by the Executive Committee of the International *Menopause* Society. *Climacteric* 2004;7:8-11.

Schroder AK, Tauchert S, Ortmann O, Driedrich K, Weiss JM. Insulin resistance in patients with polycystic ovary syndrome. *Ann Med* 2004; 36: 426-39

Shanti A, Murphy A. Surgical approaches to ovulation induction. *Sem Repro Endo* 1997; 15-2:183-191

Shen ZJ, Chen XP,Chen YG. Inhibin B, Activin A, and follistatin and the pathogenesis of polycystic ovary syndrome. *Int J. Bynaecol Obstet* 2005 Mar;88(3):336-7. E pub 2005

Shinozaki K, Kashiwagi A, Masada M, et al. Stress and vascular responses: oxidative stress and endothelial dysfunction in the insulin-resistant state. *J Pharmacol Sci* 2003;91:187-91

Simpson ER. Aromatization of androgens in women: current concepts and findings. *Fertil Steril* 2002; 77:S6-S10

Sir-Petermann T, Angel B, Maliqueo M, Santos JL, Riesco MV, Toloza H, Perez-Bravo F. Insulin secretion in women who have polycystic ovary syndrome and carry the Gly972Arg variant of insulin receptor substrate-1 in response to a high-glycemic or low-glycemic carbohydrate load. *Nutrition* 2004; 20: 905-10

Somboonporn W, Davis SR. Testosterone effects on the breast: implications for testosterone therapy for women. *Endocrine Reviews* 2004; 25(3):374-388.

Souter J, Sanchez LA, Perez M, Bartolucci AA, Azziz R. The prevalence of androgen excess among patients with minimal unwanted hair growth. *Am J Obstet Gynecol* 2004; 191: 1914-20

Speroff, L. Postmenopausal estrogen-progestin therapy and breast *Cancer*: a clinical response to epidemiological reports. *Climacteric: The Journal of the International Menopause Society* 2000:3:3-12

Spranger J, Mohlig M, Wegewitz U, Ristow M, Pfeiffer AF, Schill T, Schlosser HW, Brabant G, Schofl C. Adiponectin is independently associated with insulin sensitivity in women with polycystic ovary syndrome. *Clin Endocrinol* (Oxf) 2004; 61: 738-746

Spritzer PM, Comim FV, Capp E, et al. Influence of Leptin, Androgens and Insulin Sensitivity on increased GH response to Coonidine in lean patients with polysycstic ovary syndrome. *Horm Metab Res* 2005 Feb; 37(2):94-8

Stein, IF, Leventhal ML, Amenorrhea associated with bilateral polycystic ovaries. *Am J Obstet Gynecol*. 1935;29:181

Stein, IF. Wedge resection of the ovaries; the Stein-Leventhal syndrome. In Greenblat,RB(ed.) Ovulation: stimulation, suppresion, detection. Philadelphia: JB Lippincott, 1966, 150-157

Stern MP, Williams K, Gonzalez-Villalpando C, et al. Does the metabolic syndrome improve identification of individuals at risk of type 2 Diabetes and/or cardiovascular disease? *Diabetes Care*. 2004; 27:2676-2681.

Stickler RC. Women's health initiative results: a glass more empty than full. *Fertility and Sterility* 2003; 80:488-90.

Stikkelbroeck NM, Hermus AR, Schouten D, Suliman HM, Jager GJ, Braat DD, Otten BJ. Prevalence of ovarian adrenal rest tumours and polycystic ovaries in females with congenital adrenal hyperplasia: results of ultrasonography and MR imaging. *Eur Radiol*. 2004;14:1802-6

Stott CA. Steroid hormones: *Metabolism* and mechanism of action. In Yen SS, Jaffe RB, Barbieri RL (eds). Reproductive *Endocrinology*: Physiology, Pathophysiology, and Clinical Management. 4 ed. Philadelphia WB Saunders Co, 1999:124

Stout DL, Fugate SE. Thiazolidinediones for treatment of polycystic ovary syndrome. *Pharmacotherapy*.2005 Feb;25(2):244-52

Talbott EO, Guzick DS, Sutton-Tyrell K, et al. Evidence for association between polycystic ovary syndrome and premature carotid atherosclerosis in middle-aged women. *Arterioscler Thromb Vasc Biol* 2000;20:2414-21.

Talbott EO, Zborowki JV, Boudreaux MY, McHugh-Pemu KP, Sutton-Tyrrell K, Guzick DS. The relationship between C-reactive protein and carotid intima media wall thickness in middle-aged women with polycystic ovary sindrome. *J Clin Endocrinol Metab* 2004; 89:6061-7

Talbott EO, Zborowski JV, Rager JR, Boudreaux MY, Edmundowicz DA, Guzick DS. Evidence for an association between metabolic cardiovascular syndrome and coronary and aortic calcification among women with polycystic ovary syndrome. *J Clin Endocrinol Metab* 2004; 89: 5454-61

Tanaka YO, Tsumoda H, Kitagawa Y, Ueno T, Yoshikawa H, Saida Y. Functioning ovarian tumors: direct and indirect findings at MR imaging. *Radiographics* 2004; (Suppl.1): S147-166

Tarkun I, Canturk Z, Arslan BC, Turemen E, Tarkun P. The plasminogen activator system in young and lean women with polycystic ovary syndrome. *Endocr J* 2004; 51: 467-72

Tarkun I, Arslan BC, Canturk Z, et al. Endothelial dysfunction in young women with polycystic ovary syndrome: raltionship with insulin resistance and low-grade chronic inflammation. *Obstet Gynecol Surv*. 2005 (Mar;60(3): 180-1

Tarkun I, Arslan BC, Canturk Z, Turemen E, Sahin T, Duman C. Endothelial dysfunction in young women with polycystic ovary syndrome: relationship with insulin resistance and low-grade chronic inflammation. *J Clin Endocrinol Metab* 2004; 89: 5592-6

Tchernof A, et al. *Menopause*, central body fatness, and insulin resistance: effects of hormone-replacement therapy. *Coron Artery Dis*. 9(8):503-11, 1998.

The Rotterdam ESHRE/ASRM-Sponsored PCOS Consensus Workshop Group revised 2003 consensus on diagnostic criteria and long-term health risks related to polycystic ovary syndrome. *Fertility and Sterility* 2004; 81:19-25.

The Writing Group for the PEPI Trial. Effects of estrogen or estrogen/progestin regimens on heart disease risk factors in postmenopausal women: the postmenopausal estrogen/progestin intervention (PEPI) trial. JAMA 273:199-208, 1995.

The Writing Group for the Women's Health Initiative Investigators. Risks and benefits of estrogen plus progestin in healthy postmenopausal women. *JAMA* 2002;288:321-333.

Thiboutot D. Acne: Hormonal concepts and therapy. *Clin Dermatol.* 2004; 22: 419-28

Thijssen JHH, Nieuwenhuyse H (Editors). DHEA: A Comprehensive Review. The Parthenon Publishing Group, New York and London, 1999.

Toaff R, Toaff ME, Peyser MR. Infertility following wedge resection of the ovaries. *Am Jrnl Ob-Gyn* 1976; 124:92-96

Tominaga M, Eguchi H, Manaka H, et al. Impaired glucose tolerance is a risk factor for cardiovascular disease but not impaired fasting glucose. The Funagata Diabetes Study. *Diabetes Care.* 1999;22:920-924.

Trent M, Austin SB, Rich M, et al. Overweight status of adolescent girls with polycystic ovary syndrome: body mass index as mediator of quality of life. *Ambul Pediatr.* 2005 March-April; 5(2):107-111

Tuomilehto J, Lindstron J, Eriksson JG, et al. Prevention of type 2 *Diabetes* mellitus by changes in lifestyle among subjects with impaired glucose tolerance. *N Engl J Med.* 2001;344:1343-1350.

Unluhizarci K, Gokce C, Atmaca H, Bayram F, Kelestimur F. A detailed investigation of hirsutism in a Turkish population: idiopathic hyperandrogenemia as a perplexing issue. *Exp Clin Endocrinol Diabetes.* 2004;112: 504-9

Valimaki N, Harkonen M, and Ylikahri R. Acute effects of alcohol on female sex hormones. Alcohol Clin Exp Res 7: 289-293, 1983. Vermeulen A. Plasma androgens in women. *J Reprod Med* 1998; 43: 725-33

Van der Spuy ZM, Dyer SJ. The pathogenesis of infertility and early pregnancy loss in polycystic ovary syndrome. *Best Pract Res Clin Obstet Gynaecol* 2004; 18:755-71

Velasquez E, Mendoza SG, Hamer T, et al. Metformin therapy in PCOS reduces hyperinsulinism, insulin resistance, hyperandrogenemia and systolic blood pressure while facilitating normal menses and pregnancy. *Metabolism* 1994; 43:647-54

Vermeulen A, Verdonck L. Plasma androgen levels during the menstrual cycle. *Am J. Obstet Gynecol* 1976;125:491-4

Vintamaki T, Tuimala R. Can *Climacteric* women self-adjust therapeutic estrogen doses using symptoms as markers? *Maturitas,* 1998; 199-203.

Viser M, Bouter LM, McQuillan GM, et al. Low grade systemic inflammation in overweight children. *Pediatrics* 2001; 149:139-150.

Visser M, Bouter LM, McQuillan GM, Wener MH, Harris TB: Low-grade systemic inflammation in overweight children. *Pediatrics* 107:E13, 2001

Vliet, EL. *Savvy Woman's Guide to Testosterone.* HER Place Press, Tucson AZ, 2005

Vliet, EL. Hormone connections in urinary incontinence in women. *Top Ger Rehab;* 15(4):16-30, 2000.

Vliet, EL. *It's My Ovaries, Stupid!* Scribner, New York, 2003.

Vliet EL. Menopause and perimenopause: role of ovarian hormones in common neuroendocrine syndromes in primary care. *Primary Care Clinics in Office Practice,* 2002, 29:43-67.

Vliet EL, Davis VL New perspectives on the relationship of hormonal changes to affective disorders in the perimenopause. In Clinical Issues in Women's Health, Vol. 2, (4): *Midlife Women's Health,* Oct-Dec, JB Lippincott, Philadelphia, 1991, pp 453-472.

Vliet, EL. *Screaming to Be Heard: Hormone Connections Women Suspect and Doctors Still Ignore.* (Revised edition) M. Evans and Company, New York, 2001.

Vliet, EL. *Women, Weight and Hormones.* M. Evans and Company, New York, 2001.

Vrbikova J, Hill M, Starka L, et al. The effects of long-term metformin treatment on adrenal and ovarian steroidogenesis in women with polycystic ovary syndrome. *Eur J Endocrinol* 2001; 144 (6):619-28

Weiss R, Dziura J, Burgert TS, Tamborlane WV, Taksali SE, Yeckel CW, Allen K, Lopes M, Savoye M, Morrison J, Sherwin RS, Caprio S: Obesity and the metabolic syndrome in children and adolescents. *N Engl J Med* 350:2362-2374, 2004

Whitehead M. (Ed.) *The Prescriber's Guide to Hormone Replacement Therapy.* Parthenon Publishing Group, New York and London, 1998.

Whitehead, M. Oestrogens: relative potencies and hepatic effects after different routes of administration. J Obstet Gynecology 3(suppl) S11-16,1982.

Whitten PL, Lewis C, Russell E, Naftolin F. Potential adverse effects of phytoestrogens. Journal of Nutrition 125(Suppl):S 776, 1995.

Wild RA. Long-term health consequences of PCOS. Human Reproduction Update 2002; 8:231-241.

Willis D, Mason H, Gilling-Smith H, et al. Modulation by insulin of FSH and LH actions in human granulose cells of normal and PCO ovaries. J Clin Endocrin Metab 1996;81:302-9

Witkowski JA, Parish LC. The assessment of acne: An evaluation of grading and lesion counting in the measurement of acne. Clin Dermatol. 2004; 22: 394-7

Wren BG, McFarland K, Edwards P, et al. Effect of sequential transdermal progesterone cream on endometrium, bleeding pattern, and plasma progesterone and salivary progesterone levels in postmenopausal women. Climacteric 2000;3:155-160

Wu FC, von Eckardstein A. Androgens and coronary artery disease. Endocr Rev 2003;24:183-217.

Xita N, Georgiou I, Tsatsoulis A, Kourtis A, Kukuvitis A, Panidis D. A polymorphism in the resistin gene promoter is associated with body mass index in women with polycystic ovary syndrome. Fertil Steril 2004; 82:1466-7

Yen SS. Effects of lifestyle and body composition on the ovary (review). Endocrinol Metab Clin North Am.27(4):915-926,1998.

Yildiz BO, Woods KS, Stanczyk F, Bartolucci A, Azziz R. Stability of adrenocortical steroidogenesis over time in healthy women and women with polycystic ovary syndrome. J Clin Endocrinol Metab 2004; 89: 5558-62

Yildiz BO. Recent advances in the treatment of polycystic ovary syndrome. Expert Opin Investig Drugs 2004; 13: 1295-1305

Zawar V, Samkalecha C. Facial hirsutism following danazol therapy. Cutis 2004; 74: 301-

Zhou J, Ng S, Andesanya-Famuiya O, et al. Testosterone inhibits estrogen-induced mammary epithelial proliferation and suppresses estrogen receptor expression. FASEB J 2000;14:1725-30

Zoubulis CC, Degitz . Androgen action on human skin–from basic research to clinical significance. Exp Dermatol 2004; 13 (Suppl. 4): 5-10

Zumoff B, Strain GW, Miller LK, et al. Twenty-four hour mean plasma testosterone concentration declines with age in normal premenopausal women. J Clin Endocrinol Metab 1995;80:1329-30